# Live Advise
## Medical Terminology

W9-BAO-434

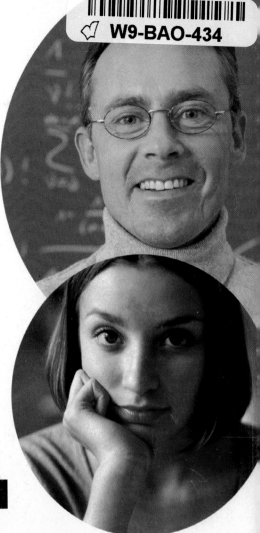

## Lippincott Williams & Wilkins
*offers online teaching advice and student tutoring with this textbook!*

### Instructors—have you ever wanted to:

…get help generating classroom activities or discussion ideas from an expert in your discipline?

…ask questions about the content of your adopted textbook or ancillary package, and have someone get back to you right away?

…have your lesson plans evaluated?

### Students— have you ever needed:

…help studying for a test at a time your instructor was not available?

…questions answered outside of class?

…feedback on assignments before turning them in?

**If so, LiveAdvise: Medical Terminology is the service you need!**

Our tutors are handpicked educators that we train to help you. They are very familiar with the textbook you are using in class and the text's ancillary package. You can connect live to a tutor during certain hours of the week, or send e-mail style messages to which the tutor will respond quickly – often within 24 hours.

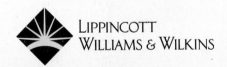

## LIPPINCOTT WILLIAMS & WILKINS

# And the best part—the service is free with the purchase of your textbook!

**Instructors**—to use this service, please visit **http://connection.LWW.com/LiveAdvise**

**Students**—see the codebook inside the front cover of this book for more details.
In it you'll find instructions for using this great service, along with your own personal code to log on and get started.

# A *Short* Course in
# Medical
# Terminology

# A *Short* Course in
# Medical
# Terminology

## C. Edward Collins

Adjunct Professor
Lambton College
Sarnia, Ontario

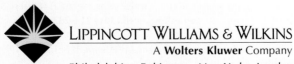

LIPPINCOTT WILLIAMS & WILKINS
A **Wolters Kluwer** Company

Philadelphia • Baltimore • New York • London
Buenos Aires • Hong Kong • Sydney • Tokyo

*Senior Acquisitions Editor: John Goucher*
*Managing Editor: Kevin C. Dietz*
*Development Editors: Rose Foltz, Nancy Peterson*
*Marketing Manager: Hilary Henderson*
*Production Editor: Kevin P. Johnson*
*Designer: Risa Clow*
*Compositor: Techbooks*
*Printer: R. R. Donnelley and Son's*

Copyright © 2006 Lippincott Williams & Wilkins

351 West Camden Street
Baltimore, MD 21201

530 Walnut Street
Philadelphia, PA 19106

All rights reserved. This book is protected by copyright. No part of this book may be reproduced in any form or by any means, including photocopying, or utilized by any information storage and retrieval system without written permission from the copyright owner.

The publisher is not responsible (as a matter of product liability, negligence, or otherwise) for any injury resulting from any material contained herein. This publication contains information relating to general principles of medical care that should not be construed as specific instructions for individual patients. Manufacturers' product information and package inserts should be reviewed for current information, including contraindications, dosages, and precautions.

*Printed in the United States of America*

**Library of Congress Cataloging-in-Publication Data**
Collins, C. Edward.
  A short course in medical terminology / C. Edward Collins.
    p. ; cm.
  Includes bibliographical references.
  ISBN 0-7817-4767-8 (case)
  1. Medicine—Terminology.   2. Medical sciences—Terminology.
  [DNLM:  1. Terminology—Problems and Exercises.  W 15 C1712s 2006]
I. Title. R123.C594 2006
610'.1'4—dc22

2005022886

*The publishers have made every effort to trace the copyright holders for borrowed material. If they have inadvertently overlooked any, they will be pleased to make the necessary arrangements at the first opportunity.*

To purchase additional copies of this book, call our customer service department at **(800) 638-3030** or fax orders to **(301) 824-7390.** International customers should call **(301) 714-2324.**

**Visit Lippincott Williams & Wilkins on the Internet: http://www.LWW.com.** Lippincott Williams & Wilkins customer service representatives are available from 8:30 am to 6:00 pm, EST.

05 06 07
1 2 3 4 5 6 7 8 9 10

# About the Author

C. Edward (Ed) Collins worked for more than a decade as a technical writer in the aviation and aerospace industry. During that period, he wrote and edited scores of technical documents on subjects ranging from the operation of carrier-based jet aircraft to the effects of protracted space missions on the human body. His college teaching career, during which he taught medical terminology and other subjects over the next 27 years, was overlapped by a third career: writing college textbooks, as well as articles for such publications as Flying, Kitplanes, and The Aviation Quarterly.

As an adjunct professor and curriculum consultant at Lambton College, Ed teaches the occasional course while continuing to write books and articles. A Short Course in Medical Terminology is his ninth textbook on language subjects and his second on medical terminology.

# Preface

## THE ACQUISITION OF MEDICAL LANGUAGE

Learning new words requires more than a simple association of sound and meaning. The process works best when the learner can associate the word with an experience. For example, a toddler remembers the word "hot" after touching a hot stove. But experiences can be dangerous or impractical for one reason or another, and in such cases we find it necessary to learn new words simply as words.

The history of words, called etymology, can help greatly in this kind of learning. Its usefulness becomes apparent to each medical terminology student with the discovery that most medical words have been adopted from either Greek or Latin and are thereby linked to each other. Indeed, memorizing a half-dozen or so word elements will enable a learner to define dozens of medical terms. To take full advantage of this phenomenon, the first three chapters of the book are devoted to medical word elements and their origins.

## COMMUNICATION MODES THAT HELP THE LEARNER

In its fundamental nature, language is linear, which simply means that language, both spoken and written, consists mostly of words following one another. But there are two other modes of written communication: graphic illustration and the parallel arrangement of words.

Graphic illustration is spatial by its very nature, and since a picture occupies space, we can look at it from left to right, top to bottom, center to edge, etc. In that way, every picture's spatial character provides a pattern that viewers subconsciously use in commiting information to memory. For that reason, this book contains more than 80 full-color illustrations. Words arranged in parallel make up another mode of communication that can be used to enhance the power of written words to convey information. Tables, which are the primary form of parallel communication, are used extensively throughout the book.

# Organization

Each chapter of A Short Course in Medical Terminology represents a major subdivision of medical language acquisition. After successfully completing the first four chapters, which make up Part I, users will be amazed to discover their ability to define many medical terms they have never seen before. In Part II, they will come to understand many more medical terms and enough human anatomy and physiology to continue building a medical vocabulary after completing the full study.

Chapter exercises and quizzes will help users retain the terms learned. Answers to all the exercises and quizzes are contained in an appendix.

The excerpts from medical documents in the "Deciphering Medical Documentation" feature appear in their original form. To retain an air of reality, the documentation excerpts remain unedited so that students may deal with them as they would appear in real work situations.

# Acknowledgments

This book would not have come into being without the talents of many people, first of whom are the members of the editorial staff of LWW, Inc. Very special thanks go to John Goucher for seeing the potential in the original idea, Kevin Dietz for directing the program, Development Editor Nancy Peterson, who is the real architect of the final product, Rose Foltz for her diligent work during the development phase, Renee Redding for a great job of editing and managing during the production process, and Sandy Bishop, who proofread the entire book.

Thanks also to Darla Riddell, R.N., for her contributions to the exercises and John C. McDonald for placing his artistic and editorial skills at my disposal many times during the project.

I wish also to offer special thanks to Bob Henry, Dean of International Education and former Dean of the School of Health Sciences at Lambton College, for his support and encouragement throughout all stages of the process.

# Reviewers

The publisher and author gratefully acknowledge the many professionals who shared their expertise and assisted in developing this textbook, appropriately targeting our marketing efforts, creating useful ancillary products, and setting the stage for subsequent editions. These individuals include:

## Proposal and Manuscript Reviewers:

Nancy Akery, MT, CMA-AC

North Harris Community College
Houston, TX

Lori Andreucci, MEd, CMT, CMA
Medical Assistant and Medical Transcription
Program Director
Gateway Technical College
Racine, WI

Denise G. Bender, JD, PT, GCS
Assistant Professor
University of Oklahoma Health Sciences Center
College of Allied Health
Department of Rehabilitation Sciences
Oklahoma City, OK

Dr. Pam Besser
Professor of Rhetoric
Jefferson Community College
Louisville, KY

Marie Bosscawen, RN, BSN
Raleigh, NC

Jean Fisher, RRT, MBA, MS
Director, Education and Distance Learning
West Virginia Hospital Association
Charleston, WV

Eva Hallis, MSRT(R)
University of Charleston
Charleston, WV

Chris Hollander, CMA, BS
Institute Director, Westwood College of
Health Careers
Denver, CO

Lynn M. Keenan, BA, LMT
Massage Therapy Instructor
Traviss Technical Center
Polk County Schools
Lakeland, FL

Diane M. Klieger, RN, MBA, CMA
Program Director - Medical Assisting
Pinellas Technical Education Centers
St. Petersburg, FL

Sandra. C. Speller, BA, RHIT
Instructor, Health and Public Safety Division
Cincinnati State Technical and
Community College
Cincinnati, OH

Sherry A. Welliver, Pharm.D
University of Minnesota
Minneapolis, MN

Brandy G. Ziesemer, RHIA, CCS
Lake-Sumter Community College
Leesburg, FL

## Marketing Reviewers:

Karen Ashby, RN, BN

Joyce L. Beaver, RN, BSN

Deborah J. Bedford, CMA

Patricia Bell, RVT, BSc

Julie E. Boles, MS, RHIA

Ada Boone Hoerl, COTA, BS

Joan Brown, RN, MSN, CNS

Jean M. Chenu, AAS, BS, MS

Linda Clarkson, BA, PTA

E. Roxann Clifton, MEd, MT

Candice Coffin, PhD

Connie Danko, OTR/L

Cecilia S. Democko, PT, DPT

Jewel Diller, RN, MSEd, MSN, FNP

Linda H. Donahue, RHIT, CCS-P, CPC

Susan S. Erue, RN, BSN, MS, PhDc

Karen M. Escolas, EdD, MT(ASCP)

Mary Fabick, MSN, MEd, RN, CEN

Karen B. Fanwick, MT(ASCP)SH

Pamela Fleming, RN, CMA, MPA

Michelle A. Green, MPS, RHIA

Susan L. Guinn

JoAnne Habenicht, MPA, RT (R)(T)(M)

Kay A. Hanna, BS, MT(ASCP)

Glenda Hatcher, BSN, RN, CMA

Rachel Hofstetter, RN, BSN, MSN

Geri Kale-Smith, MS, CMA

Christine J. Kasinskas, MSPT

Mari P. King, EdD, RT(R), CDT

Donna M. Kubesh, RN, PhD

Laura Logan, RN, BSN

Karen S. Long, MS, CLS(NCA), MT(ASCP)

Maryagnes Luczak, BS, AS, CMA, CPT, CHUC

Donna Lukich, RN, MSN, EdD

Donna L. Maher, MS, RD, CD

Lois Manning, RDH, MHE

Melissa J. Marchisotto, MPA, RPA-C

Patricia J. Martin, BS, COTA/L

Siri S. McElliott, MS

Jacqueline C. McNair, BA, RHIT

Ann Minks, MT

Dawn Couch Moore, MMSc, RT(R)

Karen L. Murphy, RN, BSN

Mary Olson, MEd, RHIT

A. William Paulsen, MMSc, PhD, CCE, AAC

Fred R. Pearson, PhD

Sally Pestana, CLS(NCA), MT(ASCP)

Fontaine C. Piper, PhD

Roberta L. Pohlman, PhD

Marsha Ray, RN, BSN, MSN

Pamela J. Reynolds, PT, EdD

Donna L. Robinson, BA, CDA, EFDA

Margie Roos, PT, MS, NCS

Marsha Rutland, PT, MEd, OCS, CSCS

Jody M. Seabright, RN, MSN

Luise Speakman, RN, PhD

Sandra C. Speller, BA, RHIT

Carol Vanlandingham, MS, RD

June Vermillion, RN, BSN

Jean Zorko, BS Bio, BSMT, MS Path

# Dedication

*For Con and Ada*

# Table of Contents

# PART 1

# INTRODUCTION TO MEDICAL TERMINOLOGY

# Analyzing Medical Terms

CHAPTER CONTENTS

Most medical terms have Latin or Greek roots, and for that reason, some people think that medical terminology is internationally recognized, like metric symbols. However, that notion is false. Medical terms are always part of the language that includes them, and they often vary when translated. For example, the word *artery* is English; in French, it is *artère,* but it is *arteria* in Spanish and *pulsader* in German. It follows, then, that in the English-speaking world, medical terms are English words.

Nevertheless, learning the Latin and Greek elements that make up medical terms is a useful way to study them. In fact, such knowledge will enable you to decipher some terms the first time you encounter them. Here are six examples of terms ending with the word element *-logy,* which means "study of." See how many of them you can you define.

1. psychology
2. pathology
3. hematology
4. cardiology
5. dermatology
6. gerontology

*Logy Always refers to the Study*

Most readers will probably know psychology and cardiology. *Psych* (from the Greek word for "mind") coupled with *-logy* tells us that psychology is the study of mental processes and behavior. *Card* (from the Greek word for "heart") indicates that cardiology is the medical specialty dealing with the heart. The roots *path, hem, derm,* and *ger* mean, respectively, disease, blood, skin, and old age. Given those meanings, write definitions in the spaces below for all the words in the above list:

1. psychology:      the study of      _mind_
2. pathology:       the study of      _Disease_
3. hematology:      the study of      _Blood_
4. cardiology:      the study of      _HEArt_
5. dermatology:     the study of      _Skin_
6. gerontology:     the study of      _Aging - Elderly_

Did you get all of them right?

1. psychology:      the study of mental processes and behavior
2. pathology:       the study of disease processes
3. hematology:      the study of blood and blood disorders
4. cardiology:      the study of the heart and its diseases
5. dermatology:     the study of the skin and its diseases
6. gerontology:     the study of the aging process and its accompanying diseases

The good news is that there are only about 300 Latin and Greek word elements, from which thousands of medical terms may be formed. Once you have learned those word elements, you can forget about Greek and Latin, since medical terms are, as already stated, English words. In learning medical terminology, you are not studying a foreign language. You are adding to your English vocabulary.

## COMBINING WORD ELEMENTS

In the previous exercise, you may have noted that one or more vowels, or a vowel-consonant combination, appears between each root and the word element *-logy*. Those letters are required to make medical terms pronounceable.

|   |   |   |   |
|---|---|---|---|
| 1. psych + *o* + logy | = | psychology |
| 2. path + *o* + logy | = | pathology |
| 3. hemat + *o* + logy | = | hematology |
| 4. cardi + *o* + logy | = | cardiology |
| 5. dermat + *o* + logy | = | dermatology |
| 6. ger + *onto* + logy | = | gerontology |

For this reason, each root hereafter introduced in this book will include its most common accompanying vowels or vowel-consonant combinations, separated by forward slant bars, as shown below:

1. psych/o
2. path/o
3. hem/o, hemat/o
4. card/i/o
5. derm/o, dermat/o
6. ger/o, geront/o

A suffix, which by definition comes last in a word, will be preceded by a hyphen. Thus, the suffix *-logy*, when it appears by itself in this book, will be written *-logy*, with the hyphen indicating that one or more word elements will always come before it.

When a prefix is present in a word, it comes first, and this book therefore presents it with a following hyphen to indicate that one or more word elements normally follow. For example, the *pre-* in prefix is itself a prefix meaning "before," a meaning that may help you remember the meaning of the word prefix: namely, a word element that comes before.

## PRONOUNCING MEDICAL WORDS

Beginning with Chapter 4, all the medical words introduced will include a phonetic spelling so you can begin learning how to pronounce them. Phonetic spelling indicates the sound of the word. For example, a phonetic spelling of psychology would be "sy-KOL-uh-jee." Capitalization indicates the syllable upon which the accent falls. As a further help in learning to pronounce medical terms, a CD-ROM with an audio pronunciation glossary is included with this book.

## SUPPLEMENTING THE WORD ELEMENTS METHOD OF LEARNING TERMS

Learning Latin and Greek word elements to decipher medical terms, such as *psychology*, does not provide a full understanding of all terms. Therefore, beginning with Chapter 5, terms are introduced in the context of anatomic systems.

## A FEW WORD ELEMENTS TO GET YOU STARTED

The roots and suffixes in Tables 1-1 and 1-2 include those you have already learned in the previous paragraphs, along with a few new ones. The roots refer to a variety of anatomic systems, which you will study in some depth later in the book. They are mentioned here so that you can practice what you have learned by completing the exercises at the end of this chapter.

| TABLE 1-1 | COMMON ROOTS OF MEDICAL TERMS |
|---|---|
| Root | Refers to |
| card/i/o | heart |
| derm/o, dermat/o | skin |
| ger/o, geront/o | aged |
| hem/o, hemat/o | blood |
| neur/o | a nerve cell, the nervous system |
| oste/o | bone |
| path/o | disease |
| psych/o | mind |

| TABLE 1-2 | COMMON SUFFIXES IN MEDICAL TERMS |
|---|---|
| Suffix | Meaning |
| -algia | pain |
| -derm | skin |
| -dynia | pain |
| -itis | inflammation |
| -logy | study of, specialty of |
| -path/y | disease |

 Exercises

### Exercise 1-1 Combining Roots and Suffixes

Combine the suffixes *-logy, -itis, -algia, -dynia, -path/y,* and *-derm* with as many of the roots on the next page as you can. Try to find at least one appropriate root for each suffix and write the resulting words in the "Word" column. Then write a brief definition in the "Meaning" column for each of your choices. You may use as many combinations as you think are appropriate.

| Root | Suffix | Word | Meaning |
|------|--------|------|---------|
| 1. psych/o | ____ | _____ | _____ |
| 2. path/o | ____ | _____ | _____ |
| 3. card/i/o | ____ | _____ | _____ |
| 4. hem/o, hemat/o | ____ | _____ | _____ |
| 5. derm/o, dermat/o | ____ | _____ | _____ |
| 6. ger/o/nt/o | ____ | _____ | _____ |
| 7. neur/o | ____ | _____ | _____ |
| 8. oste/o | ____ | _____ | _____ |

# Exercises

## Exercise 1-2 Matching Word Elements with Meanings

Match the numbers in Column 1 with the letters in Column 2 according to the corresponding terms and definitions they designate.

| | | |
|---|---|---|
| 1. _____ -itis | A. a suffix meaning "pain" |
| 2. _____ neur/o | B. another suffix meaning "pain" |
| 3. _____ -algia | C. a root meaning "skin" |
| 4. _____ -logy | D. a suffix meaning "the study of" |
| 5. _____ hemat/o | E. a root referring to the mind |
| 6. _____ -dynia | F. a suffix meaning "inflammation" |
| 7. _____ psych/o | G. a root referring to the nervous system |
| 8. _____ dermat/o | H. a root meaning "blood" |
| 9. _____ path/o | J. a root meaning "bone" |
| 10. _____ oste/o | K. a word root that can also be a suffix |

## ✓ Pre-Quiz Checklist

_____ Complete all exercises and check your answers in Appendix A.
_____ Review the word elements and definitions in the study table.
_____ Recognize and understand the similarities between the suffixes -algia and -dynia.
_____ Recognize and understand the dual function of the word elements derm and path.

## Chapter Quiz

Write the answers to the following questions using the spaces provided to the right of each question.

1. What two word roots discussed in this chapter also function as suffixes?

    1. _____

2. What special knowledge does a physician who practices gerontology need?

    2. _____

3. If a patient has neuralgia, what body system is involved?

    3. _____

4. The suffix -*algia* means "pain." What other suffix means "pain"?

    4. _____

5. What is dermatitis?

    5. _____

6. A cardiologist treats diseases of what body organ?

    6. _____

7. What science deals primarily with mental processes and behavior?

    7. _____

# Chapter 2

# Common Suffixes

The word *suffix* comes to us from the Latin word *suffixum,* which may be translated "to attach under or to the end of." By definition, then, the word element called a suffix must come at the end of the word. Although the suffix is last in a medical term, it most often comes first in its definition. For example, appendicitis means "inflammation *(-itis)* of the appendix." So the suffix, in this case *-itis,* provides us with the first word of the defining phrase. That fact also gives us a reason for learning suffixes before learning roots and prefixes. For convenience of study, however, this chapter introduces a few roots to combine with the suffixes you will learn.

Do not assume that a root must always be followed by a suffix. Roots are often combined with one another. Sometimes such a combination is followed by a suffix, and sometimes it stands alone.

## CATEGORIES OF SUFFIXES

Dividing suffixes into functional categories makes them easier to learn. Here are the four divisions:
- suffixes that signify medical conditions
- suffixes that signify diagnostic terms, test information, or surgical procedures.
- suffixes associated with a medical specialty or specialist
- suffixes that convert a noun to an adjective

### Suffixes That Signify Medical Conditions

Table 2-1 lists suffixes that signify medical conditions.

| TABLE 2-1 | SUFFIXES THAT SIGNIFY MEDICAL CONDITIONS |
|---|---|
| Suffix | Refers to |
| -algia | pain |
| -cele | protrusion, hernia |
| -dynia | pain |
| -ectasis, -ectasia | expansion or dilation |
| -emia | blood |
| -iasis | presence of; formation of |
| -itis | inflammation |
| -malacia | softening |
| -megaly | enlargement |
| -oma | tumor |
| -osis | condition |
| -penia | reduction of size or quantity |
| -plasia | abnormal formation |
| -plegia | paralysis |
| -ptosis | downward displacement |

| TABLE 2-1 | SUFFIXES THAT SIGNIFY MEDICAL CONDITIONS *(continued)* |
|---|---|
| Suffix | Refers to |
| -rrhage | flowing forth, as occurs in a hemorrhage: hem/a/t/o (blood) + -rrhage |
| -rrhea | discharge |
| -rrhexis | rupture |
| -spasm | muscular contraction |
| -pnea | breath, respiration |

In a few terms, the root *cardio* indicates the stomach rather than the heart. For example, *cardiospasm* refers to a stomach condition. *Cardia* is the name given to one of the upper parts of the stomach.

## Suffixes That Signify Diagnostic Terms, Test Information, or Surgical Procedures

Table 2-2 lists suffixes that indicate terms relating to diagnoses, test information, or surgical procedures.

| TABLE 2-2 | SUFFIXES THAT SIGNIFY DIAGNOSTIC TERMS, TEST INFORMATION, OR SURGICAL PROCEDURES |
|---|---|
| Suffix | Refers to |
| -centesis | surgical puncture |
| -desis | surgical binding |
| -ectomy | surgical removal |
| -gen, -genic, -genesis | origin, producing |
| -gram | written or pictorial record |
| -graph | device for graphic or pictorial recording |
| -graphy | act of graphic or pictorial recording |
| -meter | device for measuring |
| -metry | act of measuring |
| -pexy | surgical fixation |
| -plasty | surgical repair |
| -rrhaphy | suture |
| -scope | device for viewing |
| -scopy | act of viewing |
| -tomy | incision |
| -tripsy | crushing |

*[handwritten notes:]* Emesis- Vomiting    rrhea- discharge/Flow
Malacia- softning    gram- recording

Please note that *gen* can be a root or a suffix and that terms formed with the suffix *-genic* are adjectives, owing to the *-ic* ending. As you will see later in this chapter, *-ic* is also a suffix by itself.

## Suffixes Associated with a Medical Specialty or Specialist

Ordinary English speakers use the terms *technician* and *technologist* interchangeably, but engineers, noting the *-ian* and *-ist* suffixes, observe distinctions between them. Those working in the health sciences observe similar distinctions. However, since suffixes or other word elements are not always reliable guides, students must learn each one individually.

For example, consider the terms *psychologist* and *psychiatrist.* A psychologist is a person who has a Ph.D. in psychology, and a psychiatrist is a person who has an M.D. with a specialty in psychiatry. The two terms are, therefore, not interchangeable even though both begin with *psych* and end with *ist.* On the other hand, a *psychiatrist* and a *pediatrician* are both medical doctors in a medical specialty. The following suffixes occur in terms naming the study or practice of a medical specialty:

- -ist
- -ian
- -iatrist
- -logist

The following suffixes are associated with the study or practice of a medical specialty:

- -logy
- -ics
- -iatry
- -iatrics

> Please note that *-logy* sometimes signals the study of a field AND the specialty, e.g., *psychology* refers to both the field and the specialty. In other cases, however, the field and the specialty are differentiated, as in *gerontology,* which means "the study of the aging process," and *geriatrics,* which refers to the specialty of treating patients who suffer from the diseases brought on by aging.

## Suffixes That Denote Adjectives

Like suffixes that signify medical specialties and specialists, suffixes used to create adjective forms are not governed by a clear set of rules. Nevertheless, there are rules that come into play: i.e., the rules of English pronunciation. For example, we replace the final letter, *x,* in the word appendix with a *c* to form the adjective *appendicitis,* because *appendixitis* doesn't sound much like an English word.

In creating adjectives, you will also sometimes change noun terms that name specialties. For example, *psychiatry* and *pediatrics* are the names of specialties. Dropping the *y* from *psychiatry* and adding the adjective suffix *-ic* converts the specialty name to an adjective:

psychiatric medicine                    psychiatric hospital

With *pediatrics,* on the other hand, all one needs to do to form the adjective is drop the *s:*

pediatric medicine                       pediatric hospital

The following suffixes convert root nouns to adjectives:

- -ac
- -al
- -aneous
- -ar
- -ary
- -derm
- -eal
- -eous
- -iatric
- -ic
- -oid
- -otic
- -ous
- -tic
- -ular

## ADDITIONAL SUFFIXES

The suffixes given in Table 2-3 will come into play when you study the terminology concerned with individual body systems. For now, it will be sufficient for you to be exposed to their meanings without learning roots that are better left for introduction in those later chapters.

| **TABLE 2-3** | ADDITIONAL SUFFIXES |
|---|---|
| Suffix | Meaning |
| -cyte | cell |
| -edema | excessive fluid in intracellular tissues (edema is a word and, technically, not a suffix) |
| -emesis | vomiting |
| -globin | the protein of hemoglobin (globin is a word and, technically, not a suffix) |
| -iasis | a suffix used to convert a verb to a noun indicating a condition |
| -ism | a noun-forming suffix indicating a practice or a doctrine |
| -lith | a stone, calculus, calcification |
| -lysis | a suffix used to convert a verb to a noun indicating a condition |
| -mania | a morbid impulse toward a specific object or thought |
| -opsy | visual examination |
| -pathy | producing |
| -phobia | a word meaning fear, often appearing as a suffix |
| -poiesis | unchanging, level |

| TABLE 2-3 ADDITIONAL SUFFIXES *(continued)* | |
|---|---|
| Suffix | Meaning |
| -sclerosis | not really a suffix, but a root meaning "hard" that sometimes combines with other roots to indicate a condition of hardness |
| -sis | condition |
| -stasis | level: unchanging |
| -stenosis | narrowed, blocked |
| -stomy | permanent opening |
| -tome | instrument for cutting |

## STUDY TABLE SUFFIXES

| Suffix | Meaning |
|---|---|
| -ac, -al, -ar, -al, -iatric, -ic, -ous, -oid, -aneous, -eous, -otic, -ular, -ous | converts a root or a noun term to an adjective |
| -cele | protrusion, hernia |
| -centesis | surgical puncture |
| -cyte | cell |
| -desis | surgical binding |
| -dynia | pain |
| -ectasis, -ectasia | expansion or dilation |
| -ectomy | surgical removal |
| -edema | excessive fluid in intracellular tissues |
| -emesis | vomiting |
| -emia | blood |
| -gen, -genic, -genesis | origin, producing |
| -globin | the protein of hemoglobin |
| -gram | written or pictorial record |
| -graph | device for graphic or pictorial recording |
| -graphy | act of graphic or pictorial recording |
| -ian, -iatrist, -ist, -logist, -logy, -ics, -iatry, -iatrics | specialty of, study of, practice of |
| -iasis | a suffix used to convert a verb to a noun indicating a condition |
| -ism | a noun-forming suffix indicating a practice or a doctrine |
| -itis | inflammation |
| -lith | a stone, calculus, calcification |
| -lysis | disintegration |
| -malacia | softening |
| -mania | a morbid impulse toward a specific object or thought |
| -megaly | enlargement |
| -meter | device for measuring |

## STUDY TABLE SUFFIXES *(continued)*

| Suffix | Meaning |
|--------|---------|
| -metry | act of measuring |
| -oma | tumor |
| -opsy | visual examination |
| -osis | condition |
| -pathy | disease |
| -penia | reduction of size or quantity |
| -pexy | surgical fixation |
| -phobia | a word meaning fear, often appearing as a suffix |
| -plasia | abnormal formation |
| -plasty | surgical repair |
| -plegia | paralysis |
| -poiesis | producing |
| -ptosis | downward displacement |
| -rrhage | flowing forth |
| -rrhaphy | suture |
| -rrhea | discharge |
| -rrhexis | rupture |
| -sclerosis | not really a suffix, but a root meaning "hard" that sometimes combines with other roots to indicate a condition of hardness |
| -scope | device for viewing |
| -scopy | act of viewing |
| -sis | condition |
| -spasm | muscular contraction |
| -stasis | level: unchanging |
| -stenosis | narrowed, blocked |
| -stomy | permanent opening |
| -tome | instrument for cutting |
| -tomy | incision |
| -tripsy | crushing |

## 🖎 Exercises

### Exercise 2-1 Combining Roots and Suffixes That Signify Medical Conditions

NOTE: Since the object of this chapter is to introduce suffixes, not whole terms, these particular roots were selected for use only because they combine easily with more than one suffix. Additional roots will be introduced within the various anatomic system chapters. Build terms by combining the correct form of each of the roots below with the suffixes appearing next to it. Write a definition for each term in the space to the right.

| Root | Suffix | Word | Meaning |
|------|--------|------|---------|
| 1. card/i/o | -cele | _____ | _____ |
|  | -dynia | _____ | _____ |
|  | -ectasia | _____ | _____ |
|  | -itis | _____ | _____ |
|  | -malacia | _____ | _____ |
|  | -megaly | _____ | _____ |
|  | -ptosis | _____ | _____ |
|  | -plegia | _____ | _____ |
|  | -rrhexis | _____ | _____ |
|  | -spasm | _____ | _____ |
| 2. derm/o, | -itis | _____ | _____ |
|    dermat/o | -oma | _____ | _____ |
|  | -megaly | _____ | _____ |
|  | -osis | _____ | _____ |
| 3. ger/o | -derma | _____ | _____ |
| 4. hem/o, | -cele | _____ | _____ |
|    hemat/o | -genesis | _____ | _____ |
|  | -genic | _____ | _____ |
|  | -oma | _____ | _____ |
|  | -osis | _____ | _____ |
| 5. neur/o | -algia | _____ | _____ |
|  | -ectasis | _____ | _____ |
|  | -ectasia | _____ | _____ |
|  | -itis | _____ | _____ |
|  | -oma | _____ | _____ |
| 6. oste/o | -dynia | _____ | _____ |
|  | -ectasia | _____ | _____ |
|  | -oma | _____ | _____ |
|  | -malacia | _____ | _____ |
|  | -penia | _____ | _____ |
|  | -osis | _____ | _____ |
|  | -itis | _____ | _____ |
| 7. path/o | -osis | _____ | _____ |
| 8. psych/o | -osis | _____ | _____ |
|  | -algia | _____ | _____ |

# Exercises

### Exercise 2-2 Combining Roots and Suffixes That Signify Diagnostic Terms, Test Information, or Surgical Procedures

Build terms by combining the correct form of each of the roots below with the suffixes appearing next to it. Write a definition for each term in the space to the right.

| Root | Suffix | Word | Meaning |
|------|--------|------|---------|
| 1. card/i/o | -genic | _____ | _____ |
|  | -gram | _____ | _____ |
|  | -graph | _____ | _____ |
|  | -graphy | _____ | _____ |
|  | -pathy | _____ | _____ |
|  | -rrhaphy | _____ | _____ |
| 2. dermat/o | -plasty | _____ | _____ |
| 3. hemat/o | -genesis | _____ | _____ |
|  | -metry | _____ | _____ |
| 4. neur/o | -ectomy | _____ | _____ |
|  | -genic | _____ | _____ |
|  | -genesis | _____ | _____ |
| 5. oste/o | -rrhaphy | _____ | _____ |
|  | -plasty | _____ | _____ |
|  | -genesis | _____ | _____ |
|  | -ectomy | _____ | _____ |
|  | -tomy | _____ | _____ |
| 6. path/o | -gen | _____ | _____ |
|  | -genic | _____ | _____ |
|  | -genesis | _____ | _____ |
| 7. psych/o | -genic | _____ | _____ |
|  | -genesis | _____ | _____ |
|  | -metry | _____ | _____ |
|  | -path/o | _____ | _____ |

## Exercises

**Exercise 2-3** Combining Roots and Suffixes Associated with a Medical
Specialist or Specialty

Build terms by combining the correct form of each of the roots below with
the suffixes appearing next to it. Write a definition for each term in the space to
the right.

| Root | Suffix | Word | Meaning |
|------|--------|------|---------|
| 1. card/i/o | -logy | _____ | _____ |
|  | -logist | _____ | _____ |
| 2. derm/o, dermat/o | -logy | _____ | _____ |
|  | -logist | _____ | _____ |
| 3. ger/o/nt/o | -iatrics | _____ | _____ |
|  | -logy | _____ | _____ |
|  | -logist | _____ | _____ |
| 4. hem/o, hemat/o | -logy | _____ | _____ |
|  | -logist | _____ | _____ |
| 5. neur/o | -logy | _____ | _____ |
|  | -logist | _____ | _____ |
| 6. ocul/o | -ist | _____ | _____ |
| 7. oste/o | -logy | _____ | _____ |
|  | -logist | _____ | _____ |
| 8. path/o | -logy | _____ | _____ |
|  | -logist | _____ | _____ |
| 9. pediatr/o | -atrics | _____ | _____ |
|  | -ician | _____ | _____ |
| 10. psych/o | -logy | _____ | _____ |
|  | -iatry | _____ | _____ |
|  | -iatrist | _____ | _____ |
|  | -logist | _____ | _____ |
|  | -path | _____ | _____ |

# Exercises

## Exercise 2-4 Combining Roots and Suffixes That Denote Adjectives

Build terms by combining the correct form of each of the roots below with the suffixes appearing next to it. Write a definition for each term in the space to the right.

| Root | Suffix | Word | Meaning |
|---|---|---|---|
| 1. card/i/o | -ac | _____ | _____ |
|  | -al | _____ | _____ |
| 2. hem/o, hemat/o | -ic | _____ | _____ |
|  | -oid | _____ | _____ |
| 3. derm/o, dermat/o | -al | _____ | _____ |
|  | -ic | _____ | _____ |
| 4. ger/o/, geront/o | -iatric | _____ | _____ |
|  | -al | _____ | _____ |
| 5. neur/o | -al | _____ | _____ |
|  | -ic | _____ | _____ |
|  | -oid | _____ | _____ |
| 6. spin/o | -al | _____ | _____ |
|  | -ous | _____ | _____ |
| 7. oste/o | -al | _____ | _____ |
|  | -oid | _____ | _____ |

# Exercises

## Exercise 2-5 Matching Suffixes with Meanings

Choose the letter next to the Column 2 definition corresponding to each suffix in Column 1 and write it in the space provided.

| Column 1 | Column 2 |
|---|---|
| 1. _____ -cyte | A. a morbid impulse toward a specific object or thought |
| 2. _____ -edema | B. a noun-forming suffix indicating a practice or a doctrine |
| 3. _____ -emesis | C. a stone, calculus, calcification |
| 4. _____ -globin | D. a suffix used to convert a verb to a noun indicating a condition |
| 5. _____ -iasis | E. disease |
| 6. _____ -ism | F. a word meaning fear, often appearing as a suffix |

| | | |
|---|---|---|
| 7. _____ -lith | | G. cell |
| 8. _____ -mania | | H. condition |
| 9. _____ -opsy | | J. excessive fluid in intracellular tissues |
| 10. _____ -pathy | | K. instrument for cutting |
| 11. _____ -phobia | | L. level: unchanging |
| 12. _____ -poiesis | | M. narrowed; blocked |
| 13. _____ -sis | | N. not really a suffix, but a root meaning hard that sometimes combines with other roots or prefixes to indicate a condition of hardness |
| 14. _____ -stasis | | O. permanent opening |
| 15. _____ -stenosis | | P. producing |
| 16. _____ -stomy | | Q. the protein of hemoglobin |
| 17. _____ -tome | | R. unchanging; level |
| 18. _____ -lysis | | S. visual examination |
| 19. _____ -sclerosis | | T. vomiting |

## ✓ Pre-Quiz Checklist

_____  Complete all exercises and check your answers in Appendix A.

_____  Review the suffixes and definitions in the study table.

_____  Note and understand that *gen* can be either a root or a suffix, and understand that terms formed with the suffix *-genic* are adjectives, owing to the *-ic* ending.

## Chapter Quiz

For each of the following questions or statements, write the answers in the spaces to the right.

1. What two suffixes mean "pain"?

    1. _____

2. *Angi* is a root meaning "blood vessel." What term means "dilation of a blood vessel"?

    2. _____

3. Angioid means "resembling blood vessels." What part of speech is "angioid"?

    3. _____

4. Define *angiorrhaphy.*

    4. _____
    _____

5. What suffix would you add to the root *ang/i/o* to form a term meaning "the act of making a pictorial record of blood vessels"?

    5. _____

6. What is an angioma?

    6. _____

7. What does *-plasty* mean?

    7. _____
    _____
    _____
    _____

8. What term denotes a skin specialist?

    8. _____

9. A gerontologist treats patients in what age group?

    9. _____

10. What is the difference between *gerontology* and *geriatrics*?

    10. _____
    _____
    _____
    _____

Chapter **3**

# Common Prefixes

Aprefix is a word element that comes at the beginning of a word. You may have noticed that the word *prefix* itself contains a prefix, namely, "pre-." The second part of the word *prefix* is "fix," and that additional fact gives us a perfect definition of *prefix*: something attached (fixed) in front of or before (pre-) something else.

Most of the prefixes occurring in medical terms are also found in everyday English. That is, you probably already use most of the prefixes contained in this chapter. Even so, you may not be aware of their exact meanings or even that they are prefixes, since most English speakers have no reason to analyze the words they use. For example, when we are admitted to an anteroom, we may not stop to think that the prefix *ante-* means "before" and that an anteroom is so called because it is a room we enter *before* entering another room. Likewise, when we say, "My workday starts at 8 AM," most of us don't realize that AM is an abbreviation for ante meridiem. In that word, *ante-* means "before" and *meridiem* means "noon."

More often than not, medical terms do not include a prefix. But when one is present, it always comes at the very beginning of the word and is critical to its meaning. For example, *hyper*glycemia ("high blood sugar") and *hypo*glycemia ("low blood sugar") name conditions that are exact opposites. In this chapter, you will concentrate on learning prefixes by identifying them in common English words. Learning prefix meanings as parts of common words has two distinct advantages over learning them as parts of medical terms. The first is that you will learn the meaning of each prefix as part of a word you already know or have probably at least heard. The second, even more important advantage is that you will not be prematurely exposed to medical term roots that are best learned in connection with anatomic systems, all of which are subjects of subsequent chapters.

Pay attention to similar-sounding prefix pairs, such as *hyper-* and *hypo-*. *Hyper-* means "above" or "beyond normal"; *hypo-* means "below" or "below normal." Also watch out for the pair *ante-* and *anti-*, which are pronounced alike but have different meanings. *Ante-* means before, and *anti-* means against.

## CATEGORIES OF PREFIXES

Dividing prefixes into functional categories, just as we did with suffixes, makes them easier to learn. There are four logical divisions:

- prefixes of time or speed
- prefixes of direction
- prefixes of position
- prefixes of size or number

### Prefixes of Time or Speed

Table 3-1 lists prefixes that indicate a time or speed.

| **TABLE 3-1** | PREFIXES OF TIME OR SPEED |
|---|---|
| Prefix | Refers to |
| ante-, pre- | before |
| brady- | abnormally slow rate of speed |
| neo- | new |
| post- | after |
| tachy- | rapid, abnormally high rate of speed |

## Prefixes of Direction

Table 3-2 lists prefixes that indicate direction.

| **TABLE 3-2** | PREFIXES OF DIRECTION |
|---|---|
| Prefix | Refers to |
| ab- | away from, outside of, beyond |
| ad- | toward, near to |
| con-, sym-, syn- | with |
| contra- | against |
| dia- | across, through |

## Prefixes of Position

Table 3-3 lists prefixes that indicate position.

| **TABLE 3-3** | PREFIXES OF POSITION |
|---|---|
| Prefix | Refers to |
| ec- | outside |
| ecto- | outside |
| en- | inside |
| endo- | within |
| epi- | upon, subsequent to |
| ex- | outside |
| exo- | within |
| extra- | beyond |
| hyper- | above, beyond normal |
| hypo- | below, below normal |
| infra- | inside or below |
| inter- | between |

| TABLE 3-3   PREFIXES OF POSITION *(continued)* | |
| --- | --- |
| Prefix | Refers to |
| intra- | inside |
| meso- | middle |
| meta- | beyond |
| pan- | all or everywhere |
| para- | alongside, like |
| retro- | backwards, behind |

### Prefixes of Size or Number

Table 3-4 lists prefixes that indicate size or number.

| TABLE 3-4   PREFIXES OF SIZE OR NUMBER | |
| --- | --- |
| Prefix | Refers to |
| bi- | two |
| hemi-, semi- | half |
| macro- | big |
| micro- | small |
| mono- | one |
| olig-, oligo- | a few |
| pan- | all or everywhere |
| quadri- | four |
| tri- | three |
| uni- | one |

| STUDY TABLE COMMON PREFIXES | |
| --- | --- |
| Prefix | Meaning |
| ab- | away from, outside of, beyond |
| ad- | toward, near to |
| ante-, pre- | before |
| anti- | against, opposed |
| bi- | two |
| brady- | abnormally slow rate of speed |
| con-, sym-, syn- | with |
| contra- | against |
| dia- | across, through |
| dys- | bad, difficult |
| ec-, ecto- | outside |

📖 **STUDY TABLE** COMMON PREFIXES *(continued)*

| Prefix | Meaning |
|---|---|
| en-, endo- | inside |
| epi- | upon, subsequent to |
| ex-, exo- | outside |
| extra- | beyond |
| hemi-, semi- | half |
| hyper- | above, beyond normal |
| hypo- | below, below normal |
| infra- | inside or below |
| inter- | between |
| intra- | inside |
| macro- | big |
| meso- | middle |
| meta- | beyond |
| micro- | small |
| mono-, uni- | one |
| neo- | new |
| oligo- | a few |
| pan- | everywhere |
| para- | alongside, like |
| post- | after |
| quadri- | four |
| retro- | backward, behind |
| tachy- | abnormally high rate of speed |
| tri- | three |

📝 Exercises

### Exercise 3-1 Adding Prefixes of Time or Speed

Add each prefix in the list below to the word appearing next to it and write the definition of the word thus formed in the space to the right, referring to a standard English dictionary if you need to.

| Prefix | Word | Word Formed | Meaning |
|---|---|---|---|
| 1. ante- | room | _____ | _____ |
| 2. brady- | seismic | _____ | _____ |
| 3. neo- | classic | _____ | _____ |
| 4. post- | glacial | _____ | _____ |
| 5. pre- | dominant | _____ | _____ |
| 6. tachy- | meter | _____ | _____ |

## Exercises

### Exercise 3-2 Adding Prefixes of Direction

Add each prefix in the list below to the word appearing next to it and write the definition of the word thus formed in the space to the right, referring to a standard English dictionary if you need to.

| Prefix | Word | Word Formed | Meaning |
|---|---|---|---|
| 1. ab- | normal | | |
| 2. ad- | joining | | |
| 3. con- | centric | | |
| 4. contra- | lateral | | |
| 5. dia- | gram | | |
| 6. sym- | pathetic | | |
| 7. syn- | thesis | | |

## Exercises

### Exercise 3-3 Adding Prefixes of Position

Add each prefix in the list below to the word or word part appearing next to it and write the definition of the word thus formed in the space to the right, referring to a standard English dictionary if you need to.

| Prefix | Word | Word Formed | Meaning |
|---|---|---|---|
| 1. ec- | centric | | |
| 2. ecto- | morph | | |
| 3. en- | slave | | |
| 4. endo- | cardial | | |
| 5. epi- | demic | | |
| 6. ex- | change | | |
| 7. exo- | sphere | | |
| 8. extra- | terrestrial | | |
| 9. hyper- | sensitive | | |
| 10. hypo- | thesis | | |
| 11. infra- | structure | | |
| 12. inter- | collegiate | | |
| 13. intra- | mural | | |
| 14. meso- | sphere | | |
| 15. meta- | physics | | |
| 16. pan- | orama | | |
| 17. para- | legal | | |
| 18. retro- | rocket | | |

# Exercises

## Exercise 3-4 Adding Prefixes of Size or Number

Add each prefix in the list below to the word appearing next to it and write the definition of the word thus formed in the space to the right, referring to a standard English dictionary if you need to.

| Prefix | Word | Word Formed | Meaning |
|--------|------|-------------|---------|
| 1. bi- | annual | _____ | _____ |
| 2. hemi- | sphere | _____ | _____ |
| 3. macro- | cosm | _____ | _____ |
| 4. micro- | scope | _____ | _____ |
| 5. mono- | rail | _____ | _____ |
| 6. olig- | archy | _____ | _____ |
| 7. quadri- | lateral | _____ | _____ |
| 8. semi- | annual | _____ | _____ |
| 9. tri- | angle | _____ | _____ |
| 10. uni- | cycle | _____ | _____ |

### ✓ Pre-Quiz Checklist

_____  Review the four categories of prefixes: time or speed, direction, position, size or number.

_____  Review the study table.

_____  Check your answers to the exercises with those given in the Appendix and correct any errors before attempting the quiz.

## Chapter Quiz

For each of the following questions or statements, write the answers in the spaces to the right.

1. The prefixes *ab-* and *ad-* are opposites; which one means "toward"?

   1._____

2. The prefix *pre-* means "before"; what other prefix means the same thing?

   2._____

3. Write a brief definition of bradycardia.

   3._____
   _____
   _____

4. What does the prefix *extra-* mean in the word extrasensory?

   4._____

5. What prefix would you use in a term that means "high blood pressure"?

   5._____

6. Given the meaning of *anti-*, what would be the purpose of anticollision radar?

   6._____
   _____

7. Given the meaning of the prefix *tri-*, how many engines does a trijet have?

   7._____

8. Does the prefix *micro-* refer to the physical size of a microscope? If not, what does its presence in the word tell us?

   8._____
   _____
   _____
   _____

9. Write a medical term by combining the prefix *endo-* with the root *card/i/o*, meaning "heart," and the suffix that means "inflammation." Using only your knowledge of these three word elements, write the best definition you can for the term.

   9._____
   _____
   _____
   _____
   _____

10. The suffix *-pnea*, meaning "breathing" or "respiration," can follow both *tachy-* and *dys-*. Define the terms *tachypnea* and *dyspnea*.

    10._____
    _____
    _____
    _____
    _____
    _____
    _____

# Chapter 4

# The Body's Organization

To begin building medical terms, we must first come to understand how the human body is constructed and how it works. The first distinction to be made is between the terms *anatomy* and *physiology.* Briefly, anatomy is the study of the body, and physiology is the study of the body's functions. Insofar as construction is concerned, the body is like all other material objects. It is made up of atoms that can combine to become chemical molecules.

The human body has a chemical basis, and the chemicals act together to form cells and to power the biologic "machinery" contained within them. This machinery processes the food we eat and the air we breathe. It carries away unwanted substances and enables cells to reproduce themselves, each cell according to the DNA code it contains. The wonder of all this activity becomes even more mind-boggling when one discovers that the average adult human body contains about 70 trillion cells.

Those cells combine to form tissues that compose the various organs, both internal and external, about which you will learn in the chapters that follow. In this chapter, you will learn the terms associated with the general make-up of the body and the ways of discussing locations within it.

## THE MAJOR BODY CAVITIES

The two major body cavities, one in the front of the body and one in the back, are divisible into subcavities. The front body cavity is called the *ventral cavity.* The Latin word *venter* means "belly," and the English adjective *ventral* consists of a shortened version of that Latin word combined with the suffix *-al,* which you learned in Chapter 2. The cavity in the back of the body is called the *dorsal cavity,* from the shortened Latin word *dorsum,* which means "back," and the suffix *-al.* The ventral cavity is subdivided into the *thoracic* and *abdominopelvic* cavities. The *dorsal cavity* is subdivided into the *cranial* and *spinal* cavities, as shown in Table 4-1 and Figure 4-1.

| TABLE 4-1 THE TWO MAJOR BODY CAVITIES AND THEIR SUBDIVISIONS | |
|---|---|
| Ventral Cavity | Dorsal Cavity |
| **Subcavities** | **Subcavities** |
| 1. thoracic – Chest | 1. cranial |
| 2. abdominopelvic | 2. spinal |

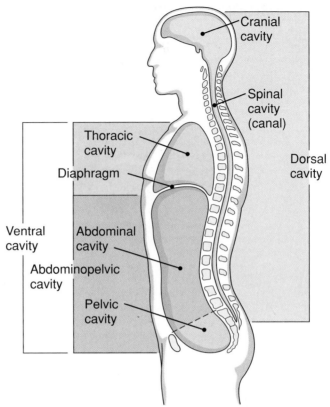

FIGURE **4-1** The major body cavities. *Reprinted with permission from:*
*Cohen, B. Memmler′s The Human Body in Health and Disease.*
*10th ed. Philadelphia: Lippincott Williams & Wilkins; 2005.*

The new word roots used to form the adjectives referring to the subcavities of the body are listed in Table 4-2.

| TABLE 4-2 | NEW ROOTS RELATED TO BODY CAVITIES | |
|---|---|---|
| Root | Origin | Meaning |
| abdomin/o | abdomen (French for "abdomen") | abdomen |
| crani/o | cranium (from Greek *kranion*) | skull |
| thorac/o | thorax (Greek for breastplate) | chest |

The dorsal cavity contains the brain and spinal cord, which make up the central nervous system, about which you will learn in Chapter 16. The ventral cavity contains all the other internal organs, sometimes referred to as *viscera* (singular *viscus*). When we add the *-al* suffix, we get the adjective *visceral*. The root used in building all the related terms is *viscer/o.* Many of the suffixes you learned in Chapter 2 can be combined with these roots (see Exercise 4-1).

## THE ANATOMIC POSITION AND DIRECTIONAL TERMS

In the *anatomic position,* the body is erect and facing forward with the palms of the hands also facing forward (Figure 4-2 and Table 4-3).

Referring to Figure 4-2, you can see that the ear is lateral to the nose, the elbow is proximal to the wrist, the ankle is distal to the knee, the nose is superior to the chest and medial to the ear, etc.

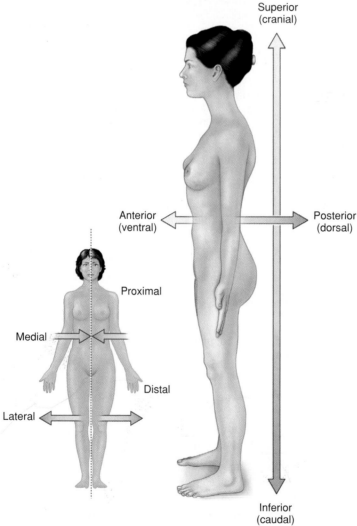

FIGURE **4-2** The anatomic position with directional terms. *Adapted from:* Cohen, B. *Memmler's The Human Body in Health and Disease.* 10th ed. Philadelphia: Lippincott Williams & Wilkins; 2005.

| TABLE 4-3 | DIRECTIONAL ADJECTIVES |
|---|---|
| Anatomic Position | Direction |
| anterior or ventral | toward the front and away from the back of the body |
| distal | away from the attachment point of a limb (arm or leg) |
| inferior | away from the head |
| lateral | away from the middle of and toward the side of the body |
| medial | toward the middle of the body |
| posterior or dorsal | toward the back and away from the front of the body |
| proximal | toward the attachment point of a limb (arm or leg) |
| superior or cranial | toward the head |

## BODY SYSTEMS

Apart from their locations in body cavities, each of the organs, tissues, bones, and so on, belongs to one or more specific body system, in which they work together to carry out physiologic functions. The body systems are listed below.

- Integumentary System - *Skin - Dermatology*
- Skeletal System   - *Ortho*
- Muscular System
- Heart
- Blood and Blood Vessels  - *Internal Medicine*
- Respiratory System - *Cardiologist / Pulmonologist*
- Digestive System
- Endocrine System - *Internal Medicine*
- Immune System
- Urinary System  - *Urologist*
- Reproductive System -
- Nervous System - *Neurologist*
- Eye   } *ENT*
- Ear

The first unfamiliar word you encountered in the list above was probably *integumentary*. The Latin word *integumentum* means "covering." Thus, the *integumentary system* includes the skin, fingernails, toenails, and hair. To remember that definition, all you have to do is ask yourself what makes up the outer layer of our bodies. And you will think of skin, nails, and hair.

The eye and the ear are not body systems by themselves but belong to several other systems, namely, the integumentary, nervous, blood and blood vessel, and muscular systems. They are discussed separately, however, because of their complexity and importance. As a matter of fact, no system works independently. Each is a part of the living body and relies on the others for life and good health. In the chapters to come, you will learn about the organs and tissues that make up all of these systems.

Table 4-4 lists a few new roots that are related to the systems listed above and are in addition to those you have already learned.

| TABLE 4-4 | NEW ROOTS RELATED TO BODY SYSTEMS | |
|---|---|---|
| Root | System | Meaning |
| angi/o | blood and immune | vessel |
| my/o | muscular | muscle |
| pneum/o, pneumon/o, pneumat/o | respiratory | lung |

## STUDY TABLE  TERMS RELATED TO BODY ORGANIZATION

| Term and Pronunciation | Meaning |
|---|---|
| abdominopelvic (ab-DOM-ih-no-PELV-ihk) | adjective meaning abdomen and pelvis; used to describe one of the body subcavities contained in the ventral cavity |
| angiography (an-jee-OG-ruh-fee) | x-ray of vessels |
| angioid (AN-jee-oyd) | resembling blood vessels |
| angioplasty (AN-jee-oh-plass-tee) | surgical repair effected by opening a clogged blood vessel by means of balloon dilation |
| anterior (an-TEER-ee-uhr) | toward the front of the body; can be a noun or an adjective |
| ventral (VEHN-trahl) | adjective meaning toward the front and away from the back of the body |
| cranial (CRAY-nee-ahl) | adjectival form of cranium or skull |
| craniopathy (cray-nee-OP-ah-thee) | abnormal condition of any of the cranial bones |
| craniotomy (cray-nee-OT-oh-mee) | incision into the cranium |
| distal (DISS-tahl) | away from the attachment point to the body; can be a noun or an adjective |
| dorsal (DOR-sahl) | adjective meaning the back |
| inferior (ihn-FEER-ee-ohr) | below or in the direction away from the cranium; can be a noun or an adjective |
| integumentary (in-tehg-yu-MEN-tah-ree) | adjectival form of integument, meaning the covering of the body |
| lateral (LAT-eh-rahl) | adjective meaning away from the middle of and toward the side of the body |
| medial (MEE-dee-ahl) | toward the midline of the body |
| myalgia (my-AL-jee-ah) | muscle pain |
| myocele (MY-oh-seel) | protrusion of muscle tissue through surrounding tissue |
| pneumatocele (nu-MAT-oh-seel) | protrusion of lung tissue through the chest wall |
| pneumonopexy (NOO-moh-noh-pex-ee) | fixation of two layers of the lung |
| posterior (poss-TEE-ree-ohr) | toward the back of the body |
| proximal (PROX-ih-mahl) | toward the point of fixation to the body |
| superior (soo-PEER-ee-ohr) | above; toward the cranium |
| thoracic (tho-RASS-ik) | adjective for chest area |
| ventral (VEHN-trahl) | toward the front of the body |
| visceromegaly (VISS-her-oh-MEG-ah-lee) | abnormal enlargement of an organ |

OSIS- Condition OR disorder
Emesis- Vomiting

# Exercises

## Exercise 4-1 Defining Terms Constructed of New Roots and Old Suffixes

Recalling the meanings of the suffixes you learned in Chapter 2, write definitions for the following terms.

| Term | Definition |
|---|---|
| 1. visceromegaly | |
| 2. craniotomy | |
| 3. craniopathy | |

# Exercises

## Exercise 4-2 Defining Terms Constructed of New Roots and Old Suffixes

Recalling the meanings of the suffixes you learned in Chapter 2, write definitions for the following terms.

| Term | Definition |
|---|---|
| 1. angioplasty | |
| 2. angiography | |
| 3. angioid | |
| 4. myalgia | |
| 5. myocele | |
| 6. pneumatocele | |
| 7. pneumonopexy | |

## Pre-Quiz Checklist

_____  Review the names and locations of the major body cavities, as shown in Figure 4-1 and Table 4-1, along with the roots in Table 4-2.

_____  Review the anatomic position, shown in Figure 4-2, and its associated directional terms, listed in Table 4-3.

_____  Review the body systems.

_____  Check your answers to the exercises with the Appendix and correct any errors before attempting the quiz.

## Chapter Quiz

Write the answers to the following ten questions using the spaces provided to the right of each question.

1. What is the difference between *anatomy* and *physiology*?

1. _____
   _____

2. What are the names of the two main body cavities?

2. _____
   _____

3. Which of the two main body cavities is located in the front of the body?

3. _____
   _____

4. What word describes the position of the ear in relation to the nose?

4. _____
   _____

5. What does *posterior* mean?

5. _____
   _____

6. What word describes the position of the elbow in relation to the wrist?

6. _____
   _____

7. When the body is in the anatomic position, which direction are the palms of the hands facing?

7. _____
   _____

8. What does *myalgia* refer to?

8. _____
   _____

9. What does *visceromegaly* mean?

9. _____
   _____

10. What does "superior to" mean in the context of body location?

10. _____
    _____

# PART 2

## BODY SYSTEM TERMINOLOGY

## Chapter 5

# The Integumentary System

## CHAPTER CONTENTS

*I*ntegumentum is Latin for "covering" or "shelter," and thus the skin, nails, and hair covering our bodies is called, collectively, the *integumentary system*. There are only two layers of skin, the *epidermis* and the *dermis*. The epidermis is divisible into five sublayers and the dermis into two sublayers, the names of which will be given later. Table 5-1 lists word elements that are used in forming terms related to the integumentary system.

| **TABLE 5-1**  WORD ELEMENTS RELATED TO THE INTEGUMENTARY SYSTEM | | |
|---|---|---|
| Word or Element | Type | Refers to |
| corium (KO-ree-uhm) | Latin word for "skin" | synonym for dermis |
| cutis | Latin word meaning "skin"; sometimes used to form a medical phrase, such as *cutis anserina*, the technical name for "goose flesh"; *cutis* is also the origin of the adjective *cutaneous*, which refers to the skin. | skin |
| cyan/o | root | blue |
| -cyte | suffix | cell |
| derm/o; dermat/o | root | skin |
| epi- | prefix | upon |
| follicul/o | root | follicle |
| kerat/o | root | horn-like |
| leuk/o | root | white |
| melan/o | root | black |
| onych/o | root | nail |
| -phyte | suffix | plant |
| pil/o | root | hair |
| sub- | prefix | below |
| sudor/i | root | sweat |
| xer/o | root | dry |

## THE PRACTICE AND THE PRACTITIONERS

As shown in the preceding table, *dermat/o* means "skin," and as you have already learned, *-logy* means "study of." Coupling the root *dermat/o* with the suffix *-logy* gives us the term *dermatology,* which names the specialty dealing with the skin. Dropping the *-y* and adding *-ist* gives us *dermatologist,* the word for a physician who specializes in dermatology and who diagnoses and treats skin abnormalities.

## THE SKIN

The skin is said to be the body's largest organ, and since the skin covers the entire body—more than 20 square feet on average—and weighs about 24 pounds, the claim would seem to be true. As already noted earlier, the skin is composed of two parts: the *epidermis* is the outer layer, and the *dermis* is the inner layer.

### The Epidermis

The epidermis protects the body from the outside world, a pretty big job for something only three one-thousandths of an inch thick. The epidermis on the palms of our hands and the soles of our feet is somewhat thicker than that, but even there, it is only about two one-hundredths of an inch thick. The epidermis is divisible into five sublayers, which are listed with brief descriptions in Table 5-2.

| TABLE 5-2   SUBLAYERS OF THE EPIDERMIS | |
|---|---|
| Epidermal Skin Layer | Brief Description |
| stratum corneum | the tough, waterproof outer sublayer of the skin |
| stratum lucidum | the transparent, barely discernible sublayer just below the stratum corneum |
| stratum granulosum | the grainy sublayer between the stratum lucidum and stratum spinosum |
| stratum spinosum | the spiny sublayer just below the stratum ganulosum; contains cells that create an immune response to protect the body against foreign bodies that get through the first three outer sublayers of skin |
| stratum germinativum | the innermost sublayer of skin, which butts against the loose connective tissue of the dermis; forms epidermal ridges that connect with the dermis and also gives the stratum corneum its distinctive pattern, as in a fingerprint |

The epidermis is also sometimes referred to as *epithelial tissue* because it is *avascular*, which means "without blood vessels." However, epithelial tissue is found elsewhere in the body, and for that reason, you should remember that the phrase *epithelial tissue* is NOT synonymous with the term *epidermis*.

### The Dermis

The dermis, which may also be called the *corium,* has two sublayers: the *papillary sublayer* and the *reticular sublayer,* the latter being the deeper of the two. Unlike the epidermis, the dermis contains blood vessels and nerves. So if you get a scratch that hurts and/or bleeds, you will know that the scratch extends through the epidermis and into the dermis. The dermis also contains both *sebaceous* (oil-producing) glands and *sudoriferous* (sweat-producing) glands.

 Note the difference between *corium,* a synonym for the dermis, and *corneum,* as in "stratum corneum," the outermost layer of the epidermis.

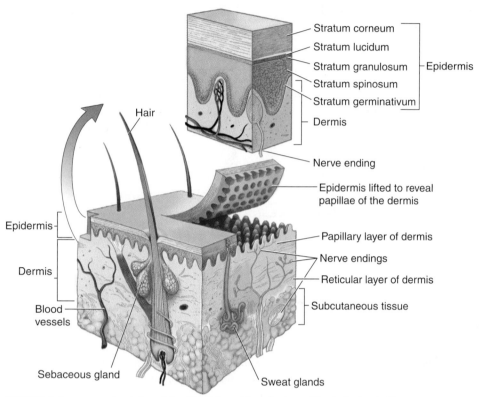

FIGURE 5-1 A cross-sectional view of the skin. *Adapted from:* Stedman, TE, ed. *Stedman's Medical Dictionary.* 27th ed. Baltimore: Lippincott Williams & Wilkins; 2000.

## Subcutaneous Tissue

A layer of subcutaneous tissue, located just beneath the dermis, is composed of connective tissue. Synonyms for subcutaneous tissue include *hypodermis, subfascia,* and *the fat layer* because subcutaneous tissue stores lipids. The Latin word *cutis,* which means "skin," gives us the English adjectives *cutaneous* and *subcutaneous.* Although the subcutaneous tissue is, categorically speaking, separate from the skin, its proximity and physiology dictate that it be considered in discussions of the skin and its abnormalities (Figure 5-1).

## Keratin and Melanin

Composed of *keratinocytes, keratin* is a protein that toughens the outer layer of skin and is a key component in the formation of hair and nails. *Melanin,* a pigment composed of *melanocytes* present in the dermis, gives the skin its color and provides protection against the sun's ultraviolet (UV) rays. Hair and nails are both composed of epithelial cells filled with keratin. Keratinocytes and melanocytes are simply the cells that make up keratin and melanin (recall that the suffix *-cyte* means "cell").

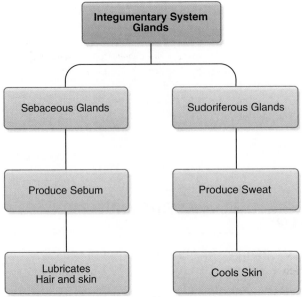

FIGURE 5-2 Glands, secretions, and functions of the integumentary system.

 Be careful to distinguish *keratinocytes*, which are cells that form keratin, from *keratocytes*, which are cells in the cornea of the eye.

## GLANDS WITHIN THE SKIN

The sebaceous and sudoriferous glands provide the skin, hair, and nails with the secretions needed to keep the integumentary system in good health (Figure 5-2).

## THE STRUCTURE OF HAIR AND NAILS

A hair *follicle* is a mass of cells that forms a cavity, out of which a hair grows. The word *follicle* is derived from a Latin word meaning "small sac." Most sebaceous glands are located close to, but are not part of, hair follicles. Although they are distinct from hair follicles, sebaceous glands share hair follicle ductwork to transmit their oily secretions to each hair and its adjacent skin. Certain hairless areas of skin, mostly on the face, chest, or back, contain sebaceous glands that have their own follicles and ductwork.

Nails are composed of layers of hardened cells of the stratum corneum (the outermost sublayer of the epidermis).

## DECIPHERING MEDICAL DOCUMENTS

**Read the following excerpt from a hospital discharge statement and answer the questions:**

*On day two under spinal anesthesia, the left hip was pinned percutaneously with three cannulated screws. Postoperatively she did well and was quite stable. Hematocrit was 32.0, hemoglobin 10.9.*

1. Identify and analyze the word that means "through the skin."
2. To what time period does "postoperatively" refer?
3. What kind of tests are hematocrit and hemoglobin?
   A. biopsies
   B. common blood tests
   C. urinalysis

## COMMON INTEGUMENTARY SYSTEM DISORDERS AND PROCEDURES

Table 5-3 lists common integumentary system disorders and some of the procedures used in their diagnosis and treatment.

| TABLE 5-3 | COMMON DISORDERS AND PROCEDURES ASSOCIATED WITH THE INTEGUMENTARY SYSTEM |
|---|---|
| **Term** | **Definition** |
| dermatitis | inflammation of the skin |
| dermatoma | skin tumor |
| dermatomegaly | excessive skin, often hanging in folds |
| dermatomycosis | fungal infection of the skin |
| dermatopathy | any disease of the skin |
| dermatoplasty | plastic surgery performed on the skin |
| epidermatitis | inflammation of the epidermis |
| melanoma | tumor of the melanocytes |
| onychectomy | surgical removal of a nail |
| onychomalacia | softening of the nails |
| onychomycosis | fungal infection of a nail |
| onychopathy | any disease of the nails |
| onychoplasty | surgical repair of a nail |
| onychotomy | incision into a nail |
| paronychia | infection around a nail |

## 📖 STUDY TABLE  THE INTEGUMENTARY SYSTEM

| Term and Pronunciation | Analysis | Meaning |
|---|---|---|
| **STRUCTURE & FUNCTION** | | |
| avascular (ah-VASS-cue-luhr) | *a-* ("without"); vascular (adjectival form of the nouns *vessel* or *vein*) | absence of vessels or veins |
| corium (KO-ree-uhm) | from the Latin ("skin") | synonym for dermis |
| cutaneous (cue-TAYN-ee-uhs) | from the Latin word *cutis* ("skin") | adjective referring to the skin |
| dermis (DUR-muss) | from the Greek word *derma* ("skin") | inner layer of skin |
| epidermal (epp-ih-DUR-muhl) | *epi-* ("upon"); *dermis* ("skin"); *-al* (adjectival suffix) | adjectival form of epidermis |
| epidermis (epp-ih-DUR-muss) | *epi-* ("upon"); *dermis* ("skin") | outer layer of the skin |
| follicle (FAWL-ik-uhl) | from the Latin word *folliculus* ("a small sac") | small sac in the skin from which a hair grows |
| keratin (KERR-uh-tin) | from the Greek word *kera* ("horn") | protein that forms hair, nails, and the tough outer layer of skin |
| keratinocyte (keh-RAT-ih-no-site) | from the Greek word *kera* ("horn"); *-cyte* (cell) | cell that produces keratin |
| melanin (MELL-uh-nihn) | from the Greek word *melas* ("black") | dark pigment present in skin and other parts of the body |
| melanocyte (MEL-uh-no-site) | from the Greek word *melas* ("black"); *-cyte* (cell) | cell that produces melanin |
| sebaceous (she-BAY-shus) | from the Latin word *sebum* ("tallow" and by extension, grease, oil, fat) | adjective describing an oil-producing gland |
| stratum corneum (STRAT-uhm COR-nee-uhm) | Latin phrase meaning "tough layer of skin" | outermost sublayer of the epidermis |
| sudoriferous (soo-doe-RIFF-uh-russ) | from two Latin words: *sudor* ("sweat") and *fero* ("to carry") | adjective describing sweat-producing glands |
| **COMMON DISORDERS** | | |
| dermatitis (dur-muh-TY-tiss) | *derm/a/t/o* ("skin"); *-itis* ("inflammation") | inflammation of the skin |
| dermatoma (dur-muh-TOH-muh) | *dermat/o* ("skin"); *-oma* ("tumor") | tumor of the skin |
| dermatomegaly (DUR-mah-toh-MEG-ah-lee) | *dermat/o* ("skin"); *-megaly* ("enlarged") | excessive skin, often hanging in folds |
| dermatomycosis (DUR-matt-oh-MI-ko-sis) | *dermat/o* ("skin"); *myc/o* ("fungus"); *-osis* ("abnormal condition") | fungal infection of the skin |
| dermatopathy (DUR-mah-TOP-ah-thee) | *derm/a/t/o* ("skin"); *-pathy* ("disease") | any disease of the skin |
| epidermitis (epp-ih-dur-MY-tiss) | *epi-* ("upon"); *-dermis* ("skin"); *-itis* ("inflammation") | inflammation of the epidermis |
| melanoma (mel-uh-NO-muh) | *melan/o* ("black"); *-oma* ("tumor") | tumor of the melanocytes |
| onychomalacia (ON-ih-ko-muh-LAY-shee-uh) | *onych/o* ("nail"); *-malacia* ("softening") | softening of the nails |

## STUDY TABLE   THE INTEGUMENTARY SYSTEM *(continued)*

| Term and Pronunciation | Analysis | Meaning |
|---|---|---|
| **COMMON DISORDERS** | | |
| onychomycosis (ON-ih-ko-my-KO-sis) | *onych/o* ("nail"); *mycosis* ("fungal infection") | fungal infection of a nail |
| onychopathy (on-ih-KOP-uh-thee) | *onych/o* ("nail"); *-pathy* ("disease") | any disease of the nails |
| paronychia (pahr-oh-NIK-ee-ah) | *para-* ("adjacent"); *onych/o* ("nail"); *-ia* ("condition") | infection around a nail |
| **PRACTICE & PRACTITIONERS** | | |
| dermatologist (dur-muh-TAHL-uh-jist) | *dermat/o* ("skin"); *-logist* ("practitioner") | a specialist who diagnoses and treats skin diseases |
| dermatology (dur-muh-TAHL-uh-jee) | *dermat/o* ("skin"); *-logy* ("study") | study of the integumentary system |
| **SURGICAL PROCEDURES** | | |
| dermatoplasty (dur-MAT-oh-plass-tee) | *derm/a/t/o* ("skin"); *-plasty* ("surgical repair") | plastic surgery performed on the skin |
| onychectomy (ON-ihk-EHK-toh-mee) | *onych/o* ("nail"); *-ectomy* ("incision") | surgical removal of a nail |
| onychoplasty (on-ihk-oh-PLASS-tee) | *onych/o* ("nail"); *plasty* ("repair") | surgical repair of a nail |
| onychotomy (on-ih-KOT-oh-mee) | *onych/o* ("nail"); *-tomy* ("incision") | incision into a nail |
| **ENHANCEMENT TERMS** | | |
| cuticle (CUE-tih-kuhl) | from the Latin word *cutis* ("skin") | the common word used as a synonym for the eponychium |
| cyanosis (SY-uh-no-siss) | *cyan-* ("blue"); *-osis* ("abnormal condition") | abnormal condition signaled by bluish discoloration of tissue |
| epidermoid (epp-ih-DURM-oyd) | *epi-* ("upon"); *dermis* ("skin"); *-oid* ("resemblance") | resembling the epidermis |
| eponychium (ep-oh-NIK-ee-uhm) | *epi-* ("upon"); *onych/o* ("nail") | thin, transparent layer of skin located at the nail root |
| follicular (fah-LIK-u-luhr) | from the Latin word *folliculus* ("a small sac") | adjective form of the noun follicle |
| lunula (LOON-yu-luh) | from the Latin word *luna* ("moon") | white, crescent-shaped area of a nail |
| onychia (oh-NIK-ih-ya) | *onych/o* ("nail"); *-ia* ("condition") | infection of a nail bed |
| onychoid (ON-ik-oyd) | *onych/o* ("nail"); *-oid* ("resemblance") | adjective meaning nail-like in structure or form |
| piloid (PY-loyd) | *pil* ("hair"); *-oid* ("resemblance") | hair-like |
| pilosebaceous (PY-lo-she-BAY-shus) | *pil/o* ("hair"); *sebaceous* ("oil-producing") | adjective referring to the hair and sebaceous glands |
| vellus (VELL-uhs) | from the Latin ("fleece") | fine hair that covers much of the body |

## ABBREVIATION TABLE

### COMMON ABBREVIATIONS:
### The Integumentary System

| Abbreviation | Meaning |
| --- | --- |
| BSA | body surface area (used in describing skin damage assessment caused by burns) |
| derm | dermis |
| SPF | sun protection factor |
| UV | ultraviolet |

# Exercises

## Exercise 5-1 Choosing the Correct Term

Fill in the blanks.

The outer and inner layers of the skin are called, respectively, the 1) _Epidermis_ and the 2) _Dermis_. The dermis is sometimes called the 3) _Corium_ and contains 4) _Sudoriferous_ ~~Sebaceous~~ _Sebaceous_, or oil-producing glands, along with 5) _Sudoriferous_, or sweat-producing glands. Hair and nails are both composed of 6) ~~Keratinized~~ _Epithelial_ cells filled with 7) _Keratin_, but nails are made even tougher by hardened cells of the 8) _Stratum Corneum_, which is the outermost sublayer of the epidermis.

## Exercises

## Exercise 5-2 Converting Nouns to Adjectives

Convert each of the following nouns to its adjective form using one of the following suffixes: -al, -aneous, -eous, -otic, -ular, -oid, -ous.

| Noun | Adjective Form |
| --- | --- |
| 1. vessel | Vessalular |
| 2. epidermis | Epidermal |
| 3. sebum | Sebaceous |
| 4. cutis | Cutical |
| 5. cyanosis | Cyanotic |
| 6. follicle | Folliculus |
| 7. keratin | Kera |

# Exercises

## Exercise 5-3 Matching Terms with Definitions

Match the numbers in Column 1 with the letters in Column 2 according to the corresponding terms and definitions they designate.

| Term | Definition |
|------|------------|
| 1. _D_ melanin | A. oil-producing glands |
| 2. _E_ epidermis | B. protein that toughens the outer layer of the skin |
| 3. _F_ lunula | C. physician who specializes in dermatology and diagnoses and treats skin abnormalities |
| 4. _A_ sebaceous | D. responsible for pigment or color of skin |
| 5. _C_ dermatologist | E. the outer layer of the skin |
| 6. _I_ stratum corneum | F. the white, crescent-shaped area of the nail |
| 7. _H_ avascular | G. BSA |
| 8. _B_ keratin | H. without vessels or veins |
| 9. _J_ sudoriferous glands | I. the outermost sublayer of the epidermis |
| 10. _G_ body surface area | J. sweat-producing glands |

# Exercises

## Exercise 5-4 Identifying Skin Layers

Label the following skin layers on Figure 5-3.
* epidermis  1
* dermis  2
* nerve endings  5
* stratum germinativum  4
* subcutaneous tissue  3

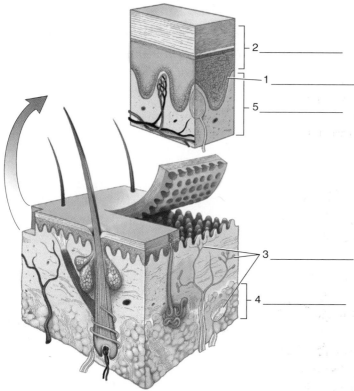

FIGURE **5-3** A cross-sectional view of the skin (Exercise 5-4).

## Exercises

### Exercise 5-5 True, False, and Correction

Read each statement, then indicate whether you think it is true or false. If false, fill in the correct answer in the "Correction, if False" box at the right.

| Statement | True | False | Correction, if False |
|---|---|---|---|
| 1. Eponychium is a thick white layer of skin located around the knuckles. | | ✓ | thin transpour located at Nail Root |
| 2. Stratum corneum is the inner lens aperture of the eye. | | ✓ | outer most Sub layer of the epidermis |
| 3. Piloid is a capsule-shaped cell found in the epidermis. | | ✓ | Hair like |
| 4. Dermatitis is an inflammation of the skin. | ✓ | | |
| 5. Dermis refers to the life cycle of the cuticle. | | ✓ | inner layer of skin |
| 6. Sebaceous describes an area consisting of several follicles. | | ✓ | oil Producing glands |

T      F

7. A sudoriferous gland produces sweat.      ✓   ___

8. Avascular is a crowded mass of veins.      ___   ✓   *absence*

9. Dermatoma is a fungus infection of the skin.   ___   ✓   *tumor*

10. Onychoplasty is the study of skin.      ___   ✓   *Dermatology*

11. Onychectomy is the surgical removal      ✓   ✓   ___
of a nail.

12. Onychomalacia is hardening of the skin.      ___   ✓   *Softning*

## Exercises

### Exercise 5-6 Complete the Sentences

Fill in the missing terms to complete the sentences.

1. Hairs grow from small sacs in the epidermis called *Follicles*

2. A tumor of the melanocytes is referred to as *Melanoma*

3. The white crescent-shaped moon-like area of the fingernail is called the *Lunula*

4. The protein *Keratin* forms hair, nails, and the tough outer layer of skin.

5. The outer layer of skin is the *epidermis*

6. The adjective *Avascular* signifies an absence of veins.

7. *Epidermal* is an adjective suffix pertaining to the epidermis.

8. Dermatomycosis is a fungal infection of the *Skin* .

9. Any disease of the nails may be referred to as an *onychopathy*

10. The study of the integumentary system is called *dermatology*

11. *Melanin* is the dark pigment found in skin and other body parts.

12. Epidermitis is an inflammation of the *epidermis*

☑ **Pre-Quiz Checklist**

_____ Study the word elements specific to the integumentary system.

_____ Review the definitions and etymologies listed in the study table.

_____ Check the exercises with the answers in the Appendix; consult the study table
again to correct any errors.

## Chapter Quiz

Write the answers to the following questions, using the spaces provided to the right of each question.

1. What are the two major layers of the skin called?

1. epidermis
   dermis

2. What is the function of the epidermis?

2. Protect body from Outside world

3. Which part of the skin do you know you have injured if you have a scratch that hurts and/or bleeds?

3. epidermus
   dermis

4. What is the layer of tissue just beneath the dermis, and what is it composed of?

4. Subcutaneous tissue

5. What protein is the key component in the formation of hair and nails?

5. Keratin

6. What term names the types of cells that make up the nails?

6. Epithelial

7. What is the purpose of melanin?

7. Curves Skin its color, Protects against Sun Ultraviolt ray

8. How many sublayers do the epidermis and dermis have?

8. Five

9. What do sudoriferous glands secrete?

9. Sweat

10. What is a lunula?

10. white crescent Shapped area of the nucy

Chapter **6**

# The Skeletal System

The human skeleton begins to form about 6 weeks after fertilization and continues to grow and develop until the person is 25 years old. The human skeleton, which includes approximately 206 bones, performs many duties. It serves as a rigid but *articulating* (which means "allowing for movement") framework for all our muscles and other tissues. It also protects our vital organs by forming a shield to ward off blows. Its less obvious jobs are to produce and store essential minerals and to make blood cells.

In this chapter, you will learn that the skeleton may be divided into two parts: the *axial* and *appendicular* skeletons. The axial skeleton consists of the skull and the chest bones, along with those of the spinal column, and the appendicular skeleton includes all the bones found in the shoulders, limbs, and pelvic area.

The appendicular skeleton has nothing whatever to do with the body's appendix. But the two do have a common classical word origin. *Appendix* is a Latin word referring to something that is attached to something else. Thus, the adjective *appendicular* indicates that the arms and legs, along with the shoulder and pelvic girdles, are attached to the axial skeleton, which forms the central core of the entire skeletal system.

## WORD ROOTS SPECIFIC TO THE SKELETAL SYSTEM

The roots shown in Table 6-1 are often found in terms related to the skeletal system. You will recognize them in many of the terms you will learn in this chapter.

| TABLE 6-1 | COMMON ROOTS RELATED TO THE SKELETAL SYSTEM |
|---|---|
| Root | Refers to |
| arthr/o | joint |
| brachi/o | arm |
| carp/o | wrist |
| chondr/o | cartilage |
| cost/o | rib |
| crani/o | cranium |
| dactyl/o | finger, toe |
| oste/o | bone |
| orth/o | correct |
| spondyl/o | vertebrae |
| vertebr/o | vertebrae |

## THE PRACTICE AND THE PRACTITIONERS

Skeletal or bone specialists include *osteologists, orthopedic surgeons, osteopaths,* and *rheumatologists.* The adjective *orthopedic* derives from the Greek word *orthos,* meaning "correct." A rheumatologist is a specialist in *rheumatology,* the specialty that involves the study, diagnosis, and treatment of rheumatic illnesses.

## THE BONES THAT MAKE UP THE HUMAN SKELETON

All human bones are part of one of the two divisions of the human skeleton mentioned at the beginning of this chapter—that is to say, axial or appendicular (Figure 6-1).

### The Axial Skeleton

The bones of the axial skeleton are the *cranial, facial,* and *thoracic* bones, along with the spinal column.

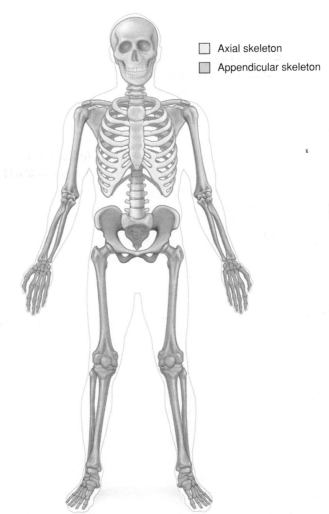

☐ Axial skeleton

☐ Appendicular skeleton

FIGURE **6-1** The axial and appendicular skeletons differentiated. The axial skeleton is shown in yellow; the appendicular is in blue.

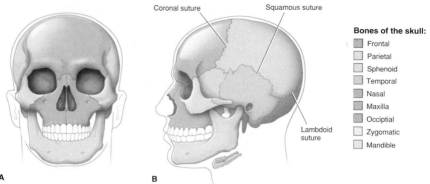

FIGURE **6-2** The skull, with the cranial and facial bones shown.

## Cranial Bones

The six main cranial bones are the *frontal bone,* two *parietal bones* (one on each side), two *temporal bones* (one on each side), and the *occipital bone* (Figure 6-2). These cranial bones are joined by *sutures,* which are fibrous membranes that occur between the bones.

## Facial Bones

The main facial bones are the *nasal bone, zygomatic bones* (two), *maxilla,* and *mandible.* The nasal bone forms the bridge of the nose, and the two zygomatic bones form the cheeks. The maxilla is the upper jawbone and the mandible is the lower jawbone.

> Although the mandible is regarded as "the jawbone," *maxilla* is the Latin word for jawbone. The Latin word *mandere,* from which "mandible" is derived, means "to chew or devour."

## Thoracic Bones

The adjective *thoracic* is formed from the word *thorax,* which is Latin for "breastplate" (chest armor), and thus *thoracic* refers to the chest area. The thoracic bones, which include the sternum, the ribs, and associated cartilage, are known collectively as the *thoracic cage* (Figure 6-3). It is a cage not in the sense of an enclosure to keep an animal from escaping, but is rather more akin to a roll cage on a car, in that it has the purpose of protecting that which is inside.

At the back (posterior), each of the 12 pairs of ribs is attached to its correspondingly numbered vertebra. (The spinal vertebrae are discussed below as part of the spinal column.) The anterior (front) rib attachments are to the sternum, but rib pairs 11 and 12 "float," which means that they do not attach to the sternum, but only to the vertebrae.

The medical term for floating ribs is *costae fluctuantes.* Also, as you can see in Figure 6-3, rib pairs 7 through 10 share some of the same cartilage en route to their anterior attachments. For these reasons, rib pairs 8, 9, and 10, together with 11 and

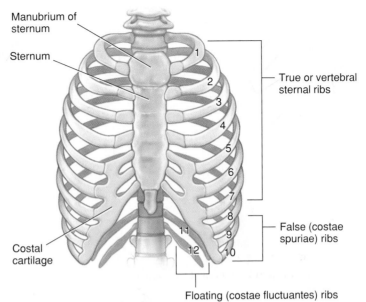

Manubrium of sternum

Sternum

True or vertebral sternal ribs

1
2
3
4
5
6
7
8
9
10
11
12

False (costae spuriae) ribs

Costal cartilage

Floating (costae fluctuantes) ribs

FIGURE 6-3 The thoracic bones.

12, are sometimes collectively called *false ribs* or *costae spuriae.* It follows, then, that the first seven pairs of ribs are *costae verae* ("true ribs").

If you know the English words *fluctuate, spurious,* and *verify,* you can associate them with the three terms above as a help in remembering them. If you don't know those English words, you might want to look them up in a good dictionary and make them part of your general vocabulary.

### The Spinal Column

The spinal column includes 33 *vertebrae* (singular: *vertebra*). The first 24 are numbered consecutively according to their positions along the first three sections of the body axis, each one having a prefix letter (*C* for *cervix; T* for *thorax;* and *L* for *lumbar*). The seven beginning with the letter C are the *cervical* vertebrae, so named because they are part of the neck (*cervix* is Latin for "neck"). *Lumbus* is Latin for "loin," and thus the lumbar region is part of the lower back.

The words *cervix* and *cervical* also refer to the "neck" of the uterus, part of the female reproductive system (see Chapter 15).

The numbering and distribution of the 24 vertebrae of the cervical, thoracic, and lumbar regions are as shown in Figure 6-4. As the illustration also shows, the remaining nine vertebrae are fused together to form only two bones, the *sacrum* and *coccyx.*

The sacrum is joined to the hip bones and, therefore, is part of the pelvic girdle, which is in turn part of the appendicular skeleton. Although the sacrum is not part of the axial skeleton, it is mentioned here because it is associated with the spinal column.

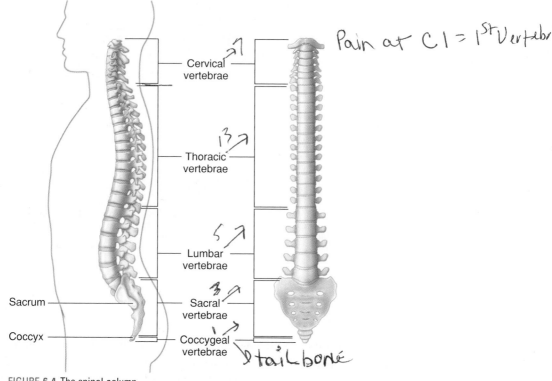

*Pain at C 1 = 1st Vertebr*

*↳ tail bone*

FIGURE 6-4 The spinal column.

## A Word about Joints

A *joint* (from the Latin *junctio,* meaning "junction") is simply a "meeting place" between bones. Some joints are highly movable (articulating), e.g., the knee and elbow joints, and some are capable of little or no movement. A joint with no movement is called a *synarthrosis,* and one with little movement is called an *amphiarthrosis.* Any of the suture joints in the cranium would be a good example of a synarthrosis, and the vertebral bodies within the spinal column are examples of amphiarthroses.

A joint that has free movement is called a *diarthrosis* or a *synovial joint.* The spaces within each synovial joint are filled with a viscous (thick) liquid called *synovial fluid.* Although the spaces in even a large joint are so tiny that less than $1/100^{th}$ of an ounce of synovial fluid is needed to fill each one, the fluid is needed to lubricate the joint as it moves and to cushion it against shock. Synovial fluid also carries nutrients and removes waste products.

*Bursae,* found wherever tendons or ligaments impinge on other tissues, consist of spaces within connective tissue that are filled with synovial fluid. *Bursitis* is a common English word that means "inflammation of a bursa," which may be, but is not always, connected to a joint cavity.

*Cartilage* is classified as connective tissue, but the term is included here because cartilage enables movement (articulation) in the synovial joints.

Joints are often named for the bones they join together; for example, the *humeroulnar* joint (the conjoining bones are the humerus and ulna) and the *humeroradial* joint (the conjoining bones are the humerus and radius) together make up the elbow.

One other term that you should know in connection with joints is *patella,* a Latin word meaning "small dish." The common name for the patella is kneecap.

### The Appendicular Skeleton

#### Shoulder Girdle

Shoulder bones, although they are associated with the chest, are part of the appendicular skeleton. The main bones of the shoulder girdle are the *clavicle* (collarbone) and the *scapula* (shoulder blade). The shoulder girdle is also sometimes called the *shoulder complex* or the *pectoral girdle* (*pectus* is Latin for "breast" (Figure 6-5).

#### Bones of the Arms and Hands

The long bone extending from the shoulder and ending at the elbow is called the *humerus,* not because it is the "funny bone" but because *humerus* is the Latin word for "shoulder." There is a connection with the word *humorous,* however. The phrase *funny bone* was coined as a joke because the ulnar nerve, which causes the pins-and-needles sensation when it is struck, is located where the humerus joins the elbow.

The *ulna* and *radius* extend from the elbow down to the wrist (Figure 6-6). The wrist includes eight bones called *carpals,* from the Latin word *carpus,* meaning

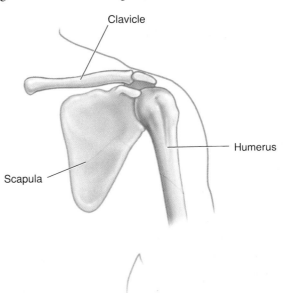

FIGURE **6-5** Bones of the shoulder girdle.

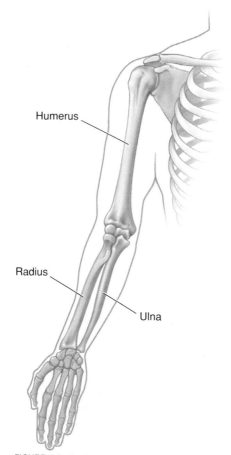

FIGURE 6-6 The bones of the arm.

"wrist." Figure 6-7 shows the location of the carpals, and their specific names are given in the following list:

1. capitate bone
2. hamate bone
3. lunate bone
4. pisiform bone
5. scaphoid bone
6. trapezium
7. trapezoid bone
8. triquetrum

As you learned in Chapter 3, *meta-* is a prefix meaning "beyond," and there-fore, the *metacarpals* lie "beyond" the carpals, connecting the wrist to the fingers. The *phalanges* make up the fingers. Phalanges is the plural form of *phalanx,* which is Greek for "line of soldiers." The bones of the wrist and hand are shown in Figure 6-7.

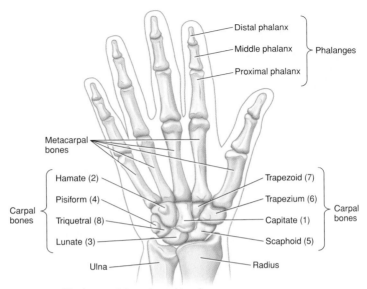

FIGURE **6-7** The bones of the wrist and hand.

### The Pelvic Girdle

The *pelvic girdle,* so named because it surrounds and protects the pelvic organs, consists of the two *hip bones,* right and left, along with the *sacrum,* noted earlier in connection with the spinal column. The hip bone, also called the *os coxae,* is a fusion of three bones: the *ilium,* the *ischium,* and the *pubis* (Figure 6-8).

### Bones of the Legs

The *femur,* Latin for "thigh," extends from the hip to the knee, and the *tibia* and *fibula* carry on from the knee to the ankle (Figure 6-8). The tibia, Latin for "shin," is the shin bone or heavy bone of the lower leg; the fibula, from the Latin word *figibula,* meaning "fastener," does not bear the body's weight, but together with the tibia, it is connected to the *talus* (ankle bone).

### Bones of the Ankles and Feet

*Tarsus* (from the Greek *tarsos,* "a flat surface") is sometimes used as a technical name for the ankle. Whatever one chooses to call it, the ankle is a complex mechanism, as any reader who has suffered a broken ankle already knows. The ankle includes seven bones:

- talus
- calcaneus (heel bone)
- cuboid
- navicular
- cuneiform bones (the name of three bones, respectively, preceded by the adjectives *lateral, intermediate,* and *medial*)

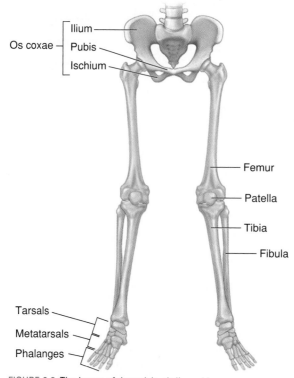

FIGURE **6-8** The bones of the pelvic girdle and legs.

The *tarsals* and *metatarsals* of the ankle and foot correspond with the carpal and metacarpal bones of the wrist and hand. The bones making up the fingers and toes are both called *phalanges*. Figure 6-9 shows the bones of the ankle and foot.

## ABBREVIATION TABLE

### COMMON ABBREVIATIONS
**The Skeletal System**

| Abbreviation | Meaning |
| --- | --- |
| C | cervical |
| CT | computed tomography |
| Fx | fracture |
| L | lumbar |
| MSS | musculoskeletal system |
| RA | rheumatoid arthritis |
| ROM | range of motion |
| S | sacral |
| T | thoracic |

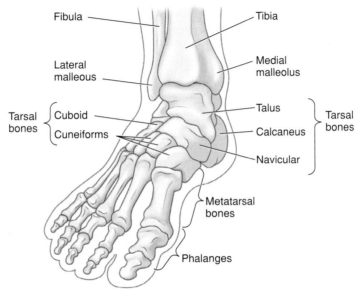

FIGURE **6-9** The bones of the ankles and feet. *From:* Moore, K.L., Dalley, A.F. II. *Clinical Oriented Anatomy.* 4th ed. Baltimore: Lippincott Williams & Wilkins; 1999.

 **DECIPHERING MEDICAL DOCUMENTS**

**Read the following excerpt from an orthopedic consultation report and answer the questions that follow:**

*I have reviewed the x-rays and the CT reconstructions of her lumbar spine. She has severe degenerative changes with osteopenia, vertebral body compression fractures of L1 and L2, age indeterminate.*

1. What does CT mean?
2. How do "degenerative changes" fit in with "osteopenia"?
3. To what do L1 and L2 refer?

## SKELETAL SYSTEM DISORDERS AND PROCEDURES

Table 6-2 lists skeletal system disorders and some of the procedures used to diagnose and correct them.

| TABLE 6-2 | COMMON DISORDERS AND PROCEDURES ASSOCIATED WITH THE SKELETAL SYSTEM |
|---|---|
| Term | Definition |
| arthralgia | pain in a joint |
| arthrectomy | excision of a joint |
| arthritis | inflammation of a joint |
| arthrocele | swelling of a joint |

| TABLE 6-2 | COMMON DISORDERS AND PROCEDURES ASSOCIATED WITH THE SKELETAL SYSTEM *(continued)* |
|---|---|
| Term | Definition |
| arthrocentesis | removal of fluid from a joint |
| arthrochondritis | inflammation of cartilage in a joint |
| arthrodynia | pain in a joint |
| arthrogram | radiograph of a joint |
| arthrometry | measurement of the amount of movement in a joint |
| arthropathy | any disorder of a joint |
| arthroplasty | surgical repair of a joint |
| arthroscopy | examination of the interior of a joint |
| arthroscope | device used in arthroscopy |
| arthrosis | disintegration of a joint |
| arthrotomy | surgical incision into a joint |
| brachialgia | pain in the arm |
| carpal tunnel syndrome | condition characterized by wrist pain, often occurring during sleep |
| carpectomy | excision of part of the wrist |
| chondrodynia | pain originating in cartilage |
| chondrogenesis | formation of cartilage |
| chondroid | resembling cartilage |
| chondromalacia | softening of cartilage |
| chondropathy | disease of cartilage |
| chondroplasty | surgical repair of cartilage |
| costalgia | pain in a rib(s) |
| costectomy | excision of a rib |
| costochondritis | inflammation of rib cartilage |
| dactylalgia | pain in a finger (or toe) |
| dactylodynia | pain in a finger (or toe) |
| dactylomegaly; more often: "megadactyly" (probably because "mega" has so many common uses as an English prefix) | enlargement of one or more fingers or toes |
| ostealgia | pain in a bone |
| ostectomy | surgical removal of bone |
| osteitis | inflammation of bone |
| osteochondritis | inflammation of bone and associated cartilage |
| osteodynia | pain in a bone |
| osteogenesis | formation of bone |
| osteology | study of bone(s) |
| osteomalacia | softening of bone |
| osteopenia | abnormally low bone density |
| osteoplasty | surgical repair of bone |
| osteoporosis | atrophy of bone tissue |
| osteorrhaphy | suturing together the parts of a broken bone |
| osteotomy | surgical cutting of bone |

## STUDY TABLE THE SKELETAL SYSTEM

| Term and Pronunciation | Analysis | Meaning |
|---|---|---|
| **STRUCTURE & FUNCTION** | | |
| appendicular (APP-ehn-DIHK-u-lahr) | adjective formed from the Latin word *appendicula* ("a small addition") | having to do with something attached |
| axial (AX-ee-uhl) | adjective formed from the Latin word *axis* ("axle") | straight line through a physical body |
| brachial (BRAY-kee-uhl) | adjective formed from the Latin word *brachium* ("radial") | having to do with an arm |
| calcaneus (kal-KAY-nee-uhs) | from the Latin word *calcaneum* ("heel") | the heel bone |
| capitate bone (KAP-ih-tayt) | adjective formed from the Latin word *caput* ("head") | one of the eight carpals |
| carpal (KAR-pahl) | from the Greek word *karpos* ("wrist") | a wrist bone |
| cervical (SUR-vih-kuhl) | adjective formed from the Latin word *cervix* ("neck") | adjective describing the vertebrae (C1–C7) in the neck region; also used in connection with the uterus, which is part of the female reproductive system |
| cervix | from the Latin ("neck") | neck (also the neck of the uterus) |
| chondrogenesis (konn-droh-JENN-uh-sihs) | chondr/o (cartilage); -genesis (origin) | formation of cartilage |
| chondroid (KONN-droyd) | chondr (cartilage); -oid (similar) | resembling cartilage |
| clavicle (KLAV-ih-cuhl); the adjectival form is clavicular (kla-VIK-yu-luhr) | from the Latin word *clavicula* ("a small key"), the connection probably being that the clavicle turns in key-like fashion to effect movements of the shoulder | the collarbone |
| coccyx (KOK-six); the adjectival form is coccygeal (kok-SIH-jee-uhl) | from the Greek ("cuckoo"), the etymological connection being that this bone resembles the beak of a bird | the tailbone, made up of the four fused vertebrae at the base of the spinal column |
| costae fluctuantes (KOS-tay fluk-chu-AN-tays) | plural form of the Latin noun *costa* ("rib") and from the Latin verb *fluctuare* ("to toss") | rib pairs 11 and 12 |
| costae spuriae (KOS-tay SPYUR-ee-ay) | plural form of the Latin words *costa* ("rib") and *spurius* ("illegitimate") | rib pairs 8 through 12 |
| costae verae (KOS-tay VER-ay) | plural form of the Latin words *costa* ("rib") and *veritas* ("truth") | rib pairs 1 through 7 |
| cranial bones (KRAY-nee-uhl) | adjective formed from cranium (the skull) | collectively, and along with other minor bones, the frontal bone, two parietal bones, two temporal bones, and the occipital bone |
| cuboid (CUBE-oyd) | from the Greek word *kybos* ("cube") and the suffix -*oid* ("like") | a bone of the ankle |
| cuneiform bones (KYU-nee-ih-form) | from the Latin word *cuneus* ("wedge") | three ankle bones, respectively preceded by the adjectives lateral, intermediate, and medial |
| diarthrosis (dy-ar-THRO-sihs) | from the Greek ("articulation") | synonym for synovial joint |

## STUDY TABLE THE SKELETAL SYSTEM (continued)

| Term and Pronunciation | Analysis | Meaning |
|---|---|---|
| femur (FEE-muhr) | from the Latin ("thigh") | thighbone |
| fibula (FIHB-yu-lah) | from the Latin ("clasp") | the lateral leg bone |
| frontal bone (FRUN-tihl) | adjective formed from the English word *front* | one of the six main cranial bones |
| hamate bone (HAM-ayt) | from the Latin word *hamus* ("hook") | one of the eight carpals |
| humerus (HUE-muh-ruhs) | from the Latin ("shoulder") | the long bone extending from the shoulder to the elbow |
| ilium (IL-ee-uhm) | from the Latin ("flank") | one of the three bones fused together to form the hip bone |
| ischium (IS-kee-uhm) | from the Greek word *ischion* ("hip") | one of the three bones fused together to form the hip bone |
| lumbar (LUM-bar) | adjective formed from the Latin word *lumbus* ("loin") | adjective describing the vertebrae (L1–L5) in the lower spinal column |
| lunate bone (LOON-ayt) | from the Latin word *luna* ("moon") | one of the eight carpals |
| mandible (MAN-dih-buhl); the adjectival form is mandibular (man-DIB-yu-luhr) | noun derived from the Latin verb *mandere* ("to chew," "to devour") | the jawbone |
| maxilla (MAX-ih-luh); the adjectival form is maxillary (MAX-ih-lahr-ee) | from the Latin ("jawbone") | the bone above the upper teeth |
| metacarpal (MEHT-uh-KAR-puhl) | from the Greek word *karpos* ("wrist") and the prefix *meta-* ("beyond") | one of the five bones extending from the wrist to the first knuckle in each hand |
| metatarsals (MEH-tah-TAHR-sahlz) | From the prefix *meta-* ("beyond") and the Greek word *tarsos* ("a flat surface") | the bones between the tarsals and the phalanges (toes) of the foot |
| nasal bone (NAY-zuhl) | adjective formed from the Latin word *nasus* ("nose") | a facial bone (nose) |
| navicular (na-VIK-yu-lahr) | from the Latin word *navicula* ("boat") | the central ankle bone |
| occipital bone (ox-SIP-it-uhl) | adjective formed from the Latin word *occipitium* ("the back of the head") | one of the six main cranial bones |
| os coxae (OSS COX-ay) | *oste/o* ("bone"); *coxae* ("hip") | hip bone |
| osteogenesis (oss-tee-oh-JENN-uh-suhs) | *oste/o* ("bone"); *-genesis* ("origin") | formation of bone |
| parietal bones (puh-RY-uh-tuhl) | adjective formed from the Latin ("wall") | two of the six main cranial bones |
| patella (pah-TELL-ah) | from the Latin ("a small dish") | kneecap |
| pectoral girdle (pek-TOR-uhl) | adjective formed from the Latin word *pectus* ("breast") | the shoulder girdle |
| phalanges (FAY-lanj-es) | from the Greek word *phalanx* ("a line of soldiers") | fingers |
| pisiform bone (PIHS-ih-form) | from the Latin word *pisum* ("pea") | one of the eight carpals |
| pubis (PYU-bihs) | from the Latin word for that particular bone | one of the three bones fused together to form the hip bone |

📖 **STUDY TABLE** THE SKELETAL SYSTEM *(continued)*

| Term and Pronunciation | Analysis | Meaning |
|---|---|---|
| radius (RAY-dee-uhs); the adjectival form is radial (RAY-dee-uhl) | from the Latin word ("stick") | one of the two bones (the other is the ulna) extending from the elbow to the wrist |
| sacrum (SAK-rum); the adjectival form is sacral (SAK-ruhl) | from the Latin ("a sacred thing") | bone formed from five vertebrae fused together near the base of the spinal column |
| scaphoid bone (SKAF oyd) | from the Greek word *scaphe* ("boat") and the suffix *-oid* ("like") | one of the eight carpals |
| scapula (SKAP-yu-luh); plural scapulae (SKAP-yu-lay); the adjectival form is scapular (SKAP-yu-luhr) | from the Latin ("shoulder") | the shoulder blade |
| sternum (STUR-nuhm) | from the Greek word *sternon* ("chest") | the breastbone |
| suture (SOO-chur) | from the Latin word *sutura* ("seam") | in the skeletal system, a fibrous membrane joining bones, especially the cranial bones |
| synovial (sy-NOH-vee-ahl) | *syn-* ("together"); *ovi-* ("ovum"); and the adjective suffix *-al* | adjective form of synovia, a synonym for synovial fluid |
| talus (TAY-luhs) | from the Latin ("ankle") | the bone in the ankle that articulates with the tibia and fibula |
| tarsals (TAR-sahlz) | from the Greek word *tarsos* ("a flat surface") | the bones of the sole of the foot |
| tarsus (TAR-suhs) | from the Greek word *tarsos* ("a flat surface") | instep or sole of the foot; collectively, the seven bones making up the bottom of the foot |
| temporal bones (TEMP-uh-ruhl) | adjective formed from the Latin word *tempora* ("the fatal spot") | two of the six main cranial bones |
| thoracic (tho-RASS-ik) | adjective formed from the Latin word *thorax* ("chest armor") | adjective form of thorax |
| thorax (THOR-ax) | from the Latin word *thorax* ("chest armor") | chest |
| tibia (TIH-bee-ah) | from the Latin ("shin bone") | shin bone |
| trapezium (tra-PEEZ-ee-uhm) | from the Greek word *trapizion* ("table") | one of the eight carpals |
| trapezoid bone (TRAP-eh-zoyd) | from the Greek word *trapizion* ("table") and the suffix *-oid* ("like") | one of the eight carpals |
| triquetrum (try-KWEET-rum) | from the Latin word *triquetras* ("three-cornered") | one of the eight carpals |
| ulna (ULL-nah); the adjectival form is ulnar (ULL-nahr) | from the Latin word for both "elbow" and "arm" | one of the two bones (the other is the radius) extending from the elbow to the wrist |
| vertebra (VUR-tuh-bruh); plural: vertebrae (VUR-tuh-bray) | from the Latin ("joint") | one of the 33 segments making up the spinal column |
| zygomatic bones (ZI-go-MAT-ik) | adjective formed from the Greek word *zygon* ("yoke") | a facial bone (cheek, one of two) |

📖 **STUDY TABLE** THE SKELETAL SYSTEM *(continued)*

| Term and Pronunciation | Analysis | Meaning |
|---|---|---|
| **COMMON DISORDERS** | | |
| arthralgia (ar-THRAL-jee-uh) | *arthr/o* ("joint"); *-algia* ("pain") | pain in a joint |
| arthritis (ar-THRY-tuhs) | *arthr/o* ("joint"); *-itis* ("inflammation") | inflammation of a joint |
| arthrocele (ARTH-roh-seel) | *arthr/o* ("joint"); *-cele* ("tumor") | swelling of a joint |
| arthrochondritis (ARTH-roh-konn-DRY-tihs) | *arthr/o* ("joint"); *chondr/o* ("cartilage"); *-itis* ("inflammation") | inflammation of cartilage in a joint |
| arthrodynia (arth-roh-DINN-ee-uh) | *arthr/o* ("joint"); *-dynia* ("pain") | pain in a joint |
| arthropathy (ARTH-roh-path-ee) | *arthr/o* ("joint"); *-pathy* ("disease") | any disorder of a joint |
| arthrosis (ar-THROW-sihs) | *arthr/o* ("joint"); *-osis* ("abnormal condition") | disintegration of a joint |
| brachialgia (BRAY-kee-AL-jee-uh) | *brachi/o* ("arm"); *-algia* ("pain") | pain in the arm |
| bursitis (burr-SY-tihs) | *bursa* (Latin for "purse"); *-itis* ("inflammation") | inflammation of a bursa |
| carpal tunnel syndrome (KAR-puhl TUN-uhl SINN-druhm) | carpal (adjective form of *carp/o,* "wrist"); tunnel (needs no explanation); *syn-* ("together"); *drome* (from the Greek word *dromos,* "running") | condition characterized by wrist pain, often occurring during sleep |
| chondrodynia (konn-droh-DINN-ee-uh) | *chondr/o* ("cartilage"); *-dynia* ("pain") | pain originating in cartilage |
| chondromalacia (konn-droh-muh-LAY-she-uh) | *chondr/o* ("cartilage"); *-malacia* ("softening") | softening of cartilage |
| chondropathy (KONN-droh-path-ee) | *chondr/o* ("cartilage"); *-pathy* ("disease) | disease of cartilage |
| costalgia (koss-TAL-jee-uh) | *cost/o* ("rib"); *-algia* ("pain") | pain in a rib(s) |
| costochondritis (KOSS-toh-kon-DRY-tihs) | *cost/o* ("rib"); *chondr* ("cartilage"); *-itis* ("inflammation") | inflammation of rib cartilage |
| dactylalgia (DAKK-tihl-AL-jee-uh) | *dactyl/o* ("digit"); *-algia* ("pain") | pain in a finger (or toe) |
| dactylodynia (DAKK-tihl-oh-DINN-ee-uh) | *dactyl/o* ("digit"); *-dynia* ("pain") | pain in a finger (or toe) |
| dactylomegaly (DAKK-tih-lo-MEG-uh-lee); more often "megadactyly" (meg-uh-DAKK-tuh-lee), probably because "mega" has so many common uses as an English prefix | *dactyl/o* ("digit"); *-megaly* ("enlargement") | enlargement of one or more fingers or toes |
| ostealgia (oss-tee-AL-jee-uh) | *oste/o* ("bone"); *-algia* ("pain") | pain in a bone |
| osteitis (oss-tee-EYE-tihs) | *oste/o* ("bone"); *-itis* ("inflammation") | inflammation of bone |

## STUDY TABLE THE SKELETAL SYSTEM (continued)

| Term and Pronunciation | Analysis | Meaning |
|---|---|---|
| osteochondritis (OSS-tee-oh-konn-DRY-tihs) | *oste/o* ("bone"); *chondr* ("cartilage"); *-itis* ("inflammation") | inflammation of bone and associated cartilage |
| osteodynia (oss-tee-oh-DINN-ee-uh) | *oste/o* ("bone"); *-dynia* ("pain") | pain in a bone |
| osteomalacia (OSS-tee-oh-muh-LAY-she-uh) | *oste/o* ("bone"); *-malacia* ("softening") | softening of bone |
| osteomyelitis (OSS-tee-oh-my-eh-LY-tihs) | *oste/o* ("bone"); *myel/o* ("marrow"); *-itis* ("inflammation") | inflammation of bone marrow |
| osteopenia (oss-tee-oh-PEEN-ee-uh) | *oste/o* ("bone"); *-penia* ("deficiency") | abnormally low bone density |
| osteoporosis (OSS-tee-oh-puh-RO-sihs) | *oste/o* ("bone"); *porosis* ("porous") | atrophy of bone tissue |
| syndrome (SIN-drum) | *syn-* ("together"); *drome* ("running") | collection of signs and symptoms occurring together and characterizing a medical condition |

**PRACTICE & PRACTITIONERS**

| Term and Pronunciation | Analysis | Meaning |
|---|---|---|
| osteology (oss-tee-AWL-uh-jee) | *oste/o* ("bone"); *-logy* ("study") | study, diagnosis, and treatment of skeletal disorders |
| osteologist (oss-tee-AWL-uh-jist) | *oste/o* ("bone"); *-logist* ("practitioner") | specialist in osteology |

**DIAGNOSIS & TREATMENT**

| Term and Pronunciation | Analysis | Meaning |
|---|---|---|
| arthrocentesis (arth-roh-senn-TEE-suhs) | *arthr/o* ("joint"); *-centesis* ("puncture") | removing fluid from a joint |
| arthrogram (ARTH-roh-gram) | *arthr/o* ("joint"); *-gram* ("recording; picture") | radiograph of a joint |
| arthrometry (arth-ROM-uh-tree) | *arthr/o* ("joint"); *-metry* ("measure") | measurement of the amount of movement in a joint |
| arthroscope (ARTH-roh-skope) | *arthr/o* ("joint"); *-scope* ("instrument for viewing") | device used in arthroscopy |
| arthroscopy (ahr-THRAH-skoh-pee) | *arthr/o* ("joint"); *-scope* ("instrument for viewing") | examination of the interior of a joint |

**SURGICAL PROCEDURES**

| Term and Pronunciation | Analysis | Meaning |
|---|---|---|
| arthrectomy (ar-THREK-tuh-mee) | *arthr/o* ("joint"); *-ectomy* (excision) | excision of a joint |
| arthroplasty (ARTH-roh-plass-tee) | *arthr/o* ("joint"); *-plasty* (repair") | surgical repair of a joint |
| arthrotomy (ar-THRAWT-uh-mee) | *arthr/o* ("joint"); *-tomy* ("incision") | surgical incision into a joint |
| carpectomy (kar-PEK-tuh-me) | *carp/o* ("wrist"); *-ectomy* ("excision") | excision of part of the wrist |
| chondroplasty (KONN-droh-plass-tee) | *chondr/o* ("cartilage"); *-plasty* ("repair") | surgical repair of cartilage |
| costectomy (koss-TEK-tuh-mee) | *cost/o* ("rib"); *-ectomy* ("excision") | excision of a rib |

## STUDY TABLE  THE SKELETAL SYSTEM  (continued)

| Term and Pronunciation | Analysis | Meaning |
|---|---|---|
| ostectomy (oss-TECK-tuh-mee) | oste/o ("bone"); -ectomy ("excision") | surgical removal of bone |
| osteoplasty (OSS-tee-oh-plass-tee) | oste/o ("bone"); -plasty ("repair") | surgical repair of bone |
| osteorrhaphy (OSS-tee-oh-raff-ee) | oste/o ("bone"); rrhaphy ("suturing") | suturing together the parts of a broken bone |
| osteotomy (oss-tee-AW-tuh-mee) | oste/o ("bone"); -tomy ("incision," "cutting") | surgical cutting of bone |
| vertebrectomy (ver-tuh-BREKK-tuh-mee) | vertebr/o ("vertebra"); -ectomy ("excision") | excision (resectioning) of a vertebra |

# Exercises

## Exercise 6-1 Choosing the Correct Term
Fill in the blanks.

The skeleton can be divided into two parts, the _____ skeleton, and the _____ skeleton. The bones covering the head are, collectively, called the _____, of which there are six. The main facial bones are the _____ bone, _____ bones, and the _____. The thoracic cage consists of the _____, the _____, and associated _____. In the spinal cord, 24 vertebrae are numbered, and each one is also labeled with a prefix letter. The prefix C refers to the _____ vertebrae, the prefix T refers to the _____ vertebrae, and L designates the _____ vertebrae.

The main bones of the pectoral girdle are the _____, or collarbone, and the _____, or the shoulder blade. The bones of the upper forearm include the _____, _____ , and _____. The wrist contains eight bones collectively called _____ . Extending from the hip to the knee is the _____ , which joins the _____ and _____ , which extend to the ankle. The tarsals and _____ of the ankle correspond with the carpal and _____ of the wrist and hand.

# Exercises

## Exercise 6-2 Converting Nouns to Adjectives
Convert each of the following nouns to its adjective form using one of the following suffixes: al, ar, ic, ary, ular.

| Noun | Adjective |
|---|---|
| 1. vertebra | _____ |
| 2. thorax | _____ |
| 3. maxilla | _____ |
| 4. mandible | _____ |

| Noun | Adjective |
|------|-----------|
| 5. sternum | _____ |
| 6. cervix | _____ |
| 7. lumbus | _____ |
| 8. sacrum | _____ |
| 9. appendix | _____ |
| 10. pectus | _____ |
| 11. ulna | _____ |
| 12. femur | _____ |
| 13. pelvis | _____ |
| 14. tibia | _____ |
| 15. clavicle | _____ |
| 16. humerus | _____ |
| 17. ischium | _____ |
| 18. scapula | _____ |

# Exercises

## Exercise 6-3 Matching Terms with Definitions

Match the numbers in Column 1 with the letters in Column 2 according to the corresponding terms and definitions they designate.

| Term | Definition |
|------|-----------|
| 1. _____ sutures | A. rib pairs one through seven |
| 2. _____ costae fluctuantes | B. inflammation of a joint |
| 3. _____ diarthrosis/synovial joint | C. the lower jawbone |
| 4. _____ zygomatic bones | D. the breastbone |
| 5. _____ arthritis | E. fibrous membranes that occur between cranial bones |
| 6. _____ sternum | F. the bone formed from five fused vertebrae near the base of the spinal column |
| 7. _____ costae verae | G. a joint that has free movement or articulation |
| 8. _____ cartilage | H. the "cheek" bones |
| 9. _____ sacrum | I. connective tissue |
| 10. _____ mandible | J. "floating ribs" (they are not attached at the sacrum) |
| 11. _____ phalanges | K. the heel bone |
| 12. _____ calcaneus | L. the wrist bones |

| Term | Definition |
|------|-----------|
| 13. _____ clavicle | M. the bones making up the fingers and the toes |
| 14. _____ tibia | N. the collarbone |
| 15. _____ carpals | O. the shin bone |

# Exercises

## Exercise 6-4 Identifying the Cranial Bones

Label the following parts on Figure 6-10.

* frontal
* mandible
* maxilla
* nasal
* occipital
* parietal
* sphenoid
* temporal
* zygomatic

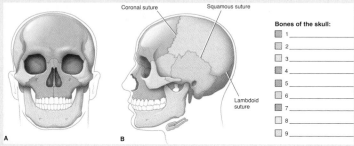

FIGURE **6-10**  The cranial bones (Exercise 6-4).

# Exercises

## Exercise 6-5 Identifying the Sections of the Spinal Column

Label the following parts on Figure 6-11.

* cervical vertebrae
* coccygeal vertebrae
* coccyx
* lumbar vertebrae
* sacral vertebrae
* sacrum
* thoracic vertebrae

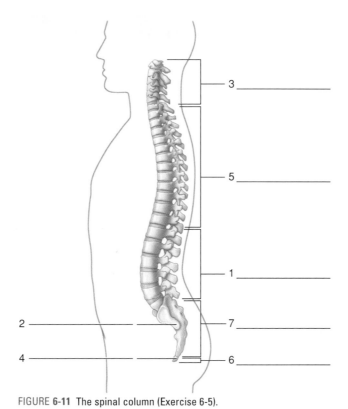

3 _____

5 _____

2 _____

4 _____

1 _____

7 _____

6 _____

FIGURE **6-11** The spinal column (Exercise 6-5).

## Pre-Quiz Checklist

_____ Study the word roots specific to the skeletal system.
_____ Using the study table, practice pronouncing the terms learned.
_____ Review the definitions and etymologies listed in the study table.
_____ Check the exercises with the answers in the Appendix to correct your errors before attempting the quiz.

## Chapter Quiz

Write the answers to the following questions in the spaces provided to the right of each question.

1. What are the three main jobs of the human skeleton ?         1. _____
   _____

2. What bones compose the axial skeleton ?         2. _____
   _____

☑ **Chapter Quiz** *(continued)*

3. What are the six main cranial bones ?                             3. _____

                                                                    _____

4. There are nine lower vertebrae fused together                    4. _____
   to form two bones. What are they ?
                                                                    _____

5. What would *C4* refer to in the spinal column?                   5. _____

                                                                    _____

6. Which bones form the upper and lower jaw ?                       6. _____

                                                                    _____

7. What is the main purpose of the thoracic cage ?                  7. _____

                                                                    _____

8. Which joint does *humeroradial* refer to ?                       8. _____

                                                                    _____

9. To what does the adjective *synovial* refer ?                    9. _____

                                                                    _____

10. How many vertebrae does the spinal column                       10. _____
    contain, and how many are numbered ?
                                                                    _____

11. The *os coxae* is a fusion of which three bones ?               11. _____

                                                                    _____

12. What condition, characterized by wrist pain, often              12. _____
    occurs during sleep ?
                                                                    _____

13. What bone in the ankle articulates with the tibia and fibula ?  13. _____

                                                                    _____

14. What are the two main bones of the pectoral girdle ?            14. _____

                                                                    _____

15. How did the phrase "funny bone" come about and                  15. _____
    where it is located ?
                                                                    _____

16. Which bone of the lower leg acts as a fastener, but does not    16. _____
    bear the body's weight ?
                                                                    _____

17. What bones make up the pelvic girdle ?                          17. _____

                                                                    _____

Chapter 7

# The Muscular System

CHAPTER CONTENTS

Y ou may recall having read in Chapter 6 that there are approximately 206 bones in the human body. The total number of muscles is harder to calculate because of the various ways to distinguish them. But it is safe to say that there are many more muscles than bones. In fact, muscles make up about half of the average person's total body weight.

Muscles are necessary for all the obvious activities, such as lifting objects, running, jumping, throwing a ball, and swinging a bat. However, muscles are also needed for seeing, talking, eating, digesting, breathing, smiling, frowning, blinking, and so on. And then, of course, there is the heart muscle, which is discussed in Chapter 8.

## WORD ROOTS SPECIFIC TO THE MUSCULAR SYSTEM

The roots shown in Table 7-1 are often found in terms related to the muscular system. You will recognize them in many of the terms you will learn in this chapter.

| **TABLE 7-1** COMMON ROOTS RELATED TO THE MUSCULAR SYSTEM | |
| --- | --- |
| Word Roots | Refers to |
| kine; kinesi/o | movement |
| ligament/o | ligament |
| muscul/o | muscle |
| my/o | muscle |
| tend/o; tendin/o | tendon |

## MUSCLE TYPES

There are three kinds of muscles: *skeletal, cardiac,* and *smooth.* Skeletal muscles are distinguished not only by the jobs they do, but also by their large size in comparison with the cardiac and smooth muscles. Skeletal muscles are sometimes referred to as *striated* (from the Latin verb *striare,* which means "to groove") because their fibers run parallel to each other. The cardiac muscle contains striated fibers, too, but they are much shorter and not as obvious. Chapter 8 deals with the heart.

The third type, smooth muscles that (like the heart) work involuntarily, include the *sphincter* muscles and others that surround internal organs such as the esophagus, which you will learn about in Chapter 11.

Since muscles serve in so many different ways, they occur in many different sizes, shapes, and forms, and include the *ligaments* and *tendons.* Ligaments, from the Latin noun *ligament,* meaning "string," connect muscles to bones, cartilage, or other tissue structures. They contain a protein called *elastin,* which makes them regain their shape after being stretched, much in the same way an elastic band does. Tendons are similar to ligaments and are located with the muscles of the appendicular skeleton. The Achilles tendon is an example with which nearly everyone is familiar. The name tendon comes from the Latin verb *tendo*, which means "stretch."

In this chapter, we will look at some of the skeletal muscles within the axial skeleton, along with the main ones associated with the appendicular skeleton.

> Muscle cells are elongated and are commonly called *muscle fibers* rather than *muscle cells*. However, you may wish to note that each muscle fiber has the same constituents as any other body cell.

## MUSCLES ASSOCIATED WITH THE AXIAL SKELETON

### Facial Muscles

A muscle called the *orbicularis oris* enables us to move our lips and to open and close our mouths. Another called the *corrugator supercilii* allows us to move our eyebrows. *Supercilium* means "eyebrow" in Latin. Another muscle, called the *orbicularis oculi*, makes it possible for us to close our eyes.

Muscles beginning with the word *orbicularis* are to be found "around" something. The orbicularis oris is around the mouth, and an orbicularis oculi is to be found around each eye (Figure 7-1).

### Muscles of the Tongue

The tongue has four muscles ending with the word element *glossus*, which comes from a Greek word *glossa*, meaning "language." The word root *gloss/o* also

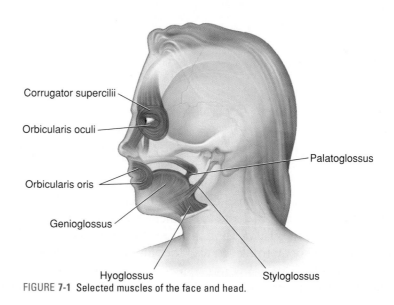

FIGURE 7-1 Selected muscles of the face and head.

means "tongue," and can be combined with many of the suffixes you already know, e.g., *glossodynia*. The names of the four tongue muscles are as follows:

- ◆ genioglossus
- ◆ hyoglossus
- ◆ palatoglossus
- ◆ styloglossus

## Muscles Surrounding the Spinal Column

The spinal column includes spinal extensors, also called the *erector spinae,* which enable one to move the head and neck and to extend and flex the spine. In addition, the *trapezius* and *latissimus dorsi* cover the back and facilitate movement of the trunk of the body (Figure 7-2).

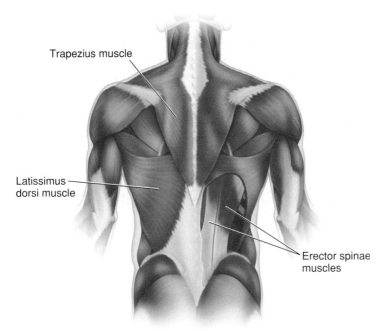

Trapezius muscle

Latissimus dorsi muscle

Erector spinae muscles

FIGURE **7-2** Spinal and back muscles.

## MUSCLES ASSOCIATED WITH THE APPENDICULAR SKELETON

### Shoulder Muscles

The *trapezius* muscles, mentioned earlier in connection with the axial skeleton, are actually part of both the axial and appendicular skeletons, in that they start at the neck and extend to the clavicles and the scapulae. Thus, they can help to move not only the neck and body trunk but also the shoulder girdle, depending on the action of associated muscles.

The other muscles that move the shoulder are shown in Table 7-2 and Figure 7-3.

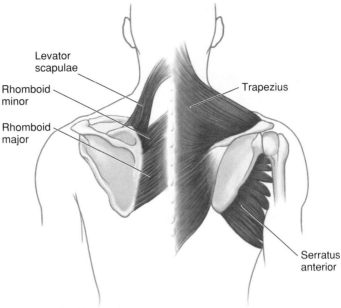

Levator
scapulae

Rhomboid
minor

Rhomboid
major

Trapezius

Serratus
anterior

FIGURE **7-3** Shoulder muscles.

| **TABLE 7-2** | **SHOULDER MUSCLES** |
|---|---|
| Muscles | Movement |
| serratus anterior | upward or upward rotation |
| levator scapulae | upward or upward rotation |
| pectoralis minor | downward or downward rotation |
| rhomboideus (both major and minor) | downward or downward rotation |
| subclavius | downward or downward rotation |

## Arm and Hand Muscles

The main muscles of the arm start with the *deltoid,* where the arm joins the shoulder. The *biceps brachii* and *triceps brachii,* located as shown in Figure 7-4, work in conjunction with the *brachialis.* In common speech, the words *biceps* and *triceps* are used indiscriminately to refer to the biceps and triceps in the arm. However, the leg also contains biceps and triceps.

The muscles associated with the ulna are the *flexor carpi ulnaris* and *extensor carpi ulnaris.* A similar pair, the *flexor carpi radialis* and the *extensor carpi radialis longus,* are associated with the radius. All these names contain "carpi," which means "wrist" or "hand," because they flex or extend the hand, depending on whether the name begins with "flexor" or "extensor."

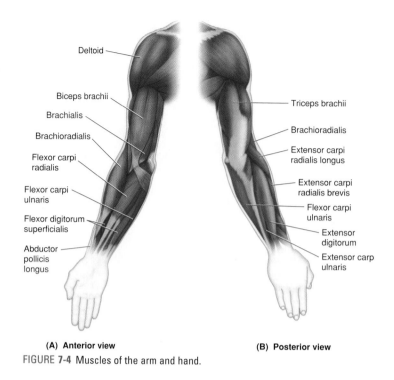

Deltoid

Biceps brachii

Brachialis

Brachioradialis

Flexor carpi
radialis

Flexor carpi
ulnaris

Flexor digitorum
superficialis

Abductor
pollicis
longus

Triceps brachii

Brachioradialis

Extensor carpi
radialis longus

Extensor carpi
radialis brevis

Flexor carpi
ulnaris

Extensor
digitorum

Extensor carp
ulnaris

**(A) Anterior view**   **(B) Posterior view**

FIGURE **7-4** Muscles of the arm and hand.

Similarly, any muscle that contains the word element *digiti* or *digitorum* will affect finger movement of some kind, and any muscle with *pollicis* (*pollex* is the Latin word for "thumb") in its name has to do with the thumb. Prominent terms include the *extensor digitorum* and the *abductor pollicis longus.* Table 7-3 indicates the functions of all the muscles just mentioned.

| TABLE 7-3 | MUSCLE ACTION IN THE ARMS AND HANDS |
|---|---|
| Muscle Name | Action |
| biceps brachii | flexes the upper arm and forearm |
| brachialis | flexes the forearm |
| deltoid* | rotates the arm sideways |
| triceps brachii | extends the forearm |
| flexor carpi ulnaris | flexes and curls the hand inward |
| flexor carpi radialis | flexes and curls the hand outward |
| extensor carpi radialis longus | extends and curls the hand outward |
| extensor carpi ulnaris | extends and curls the hand inward |

*Other authorities may refer to the deltoid as a shoulder muscle. Actually, it is located at the top of the humerus and is attached to the shoulder at the clavicle. It is listed here as an arm muscle because of its function in moving the arm.*

## Muscles of the Lower Extremities

The *gluteus maximus,* the muscle located within each buttock, helps to rotate the thigh. Beneath the gluteus maximus lies the *gluteus medius* and beneath that, the *gluteus minimus,* both of which facilitate walking by supporting the pelvis.

The major muscles in the front (anterior) of the thigh, known collectively as the *quadriceps femoris,* comprise the *vastus lateralis, vastus medialis, vastus intermedias,* and *rectus femoris,* all of which serve to extend the leg. The longest muscle in the leg (and in the whole body, by the way) is the *sartorius,* which flexes and rotates the thigh. This motion is the one we use to cross our legs when we are sitting down (Figure 7-5, A).

The posterior of the thigh contains a muscle group commonly called the hamstring. The hamstring is made up of three muscles: the *biceps femoris,* the *semitendinosus,* and the *semimembranosus.* Together, they flex the leg and extend the thigh (Figure 7-5, A).

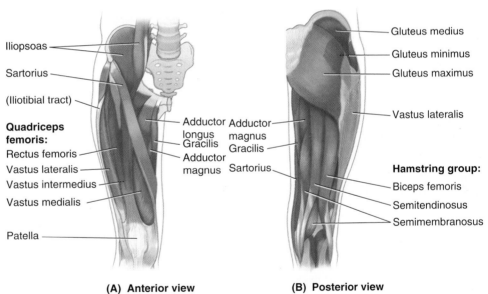

**(A) Anterior view**    **(B) Posterior view**

FIGURE 7-5 The muscles of the thigh and leg. A. Anterior view. B. Posterior view.

The main muscles we use to move our feet and toes are shown in Figure 7-6. The anterior muscles controlling the feet are the *tibialis anterior,* the *peroneus tertius,* and the *peroneus longus.* The posterior muscle group controlling the foot is called the *triceps surae.*

The anterior muscles controlling the toes are the *extensor hallucis longus* and the *extensor digitorum longus.* The posterior muscles controlling toe movement are the *flexor hallucis longus* and the *flexor digitorum longus.* Just as "pollicis" is derived from *pollex* ("thumb"), "hallucis" is derived from *hallux* ("great toe").

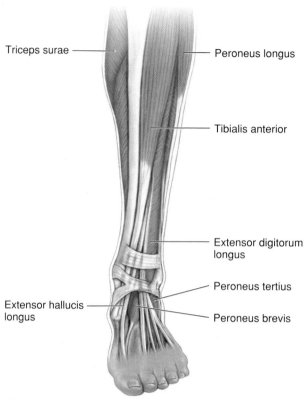

Triceps surae

Peroneus longus

Tibialis anterior

Extensor digitorum longus

Peroneus tertius

Extensor hallucis longus

Peroneus brevis

FIGURE 7-6 Muscles that move the feet and toes.

 **DECIPHERING MEDICAL DOCUMENTS**

**Read the following excerpt from a physical therapy note and answer the questions:**

*The patient should perform this exercise without discomfort or unstable feeling. This exercise was chosen to improve motor control strategies through manipulation of the serratus anterior and levator scapulae.*

1. What two terms denote muscles?
2. Where are these two muscles located?
3. What motions are involved?

## MUSCULAR SYSTEM DISORDERS AND PROCEDURES

Table 7-2 lists abnormal conditions, along with some of the procedures to diagnose and correct them.

| TABLE 7-2 | COMMON DISORDERS AND PROCEDURES ASSOCIATED WITH THE MUSCULAR SYSTEM |
|---|---|
| **Term** | **Definition** |
| kinesalgia; kinesialgia | pain caused by muscle movement |
| kinesiology | study of movement |
| myasthenia | muscular weakness |
| myectomy | excision of part or all of a muscle |
| myelitis | inflammation of a muscle |
| myocele | protrusion of muscle tissue through a tear in its outer sheath |
| myodynia | muscle pain |
| myogenesis | formation of muscle cells |
| myoid | adjective meaning "resembling a muscle" |
| myology | study of muscles |
| myoma | benign neoplasm of muscle tissue |
| myomalacia | softening of muscle tissue |
| myositis | inflammation of a muscle |
| myospasm | muscle contraction |
| tenodynia, tenontodynia | pain in a tendon |
| tendonitis | inflammation of a tendon |
| tenontoplasty | reparative or plastic surgery of the tendons |
| tenorrhaphy | suturing of a tendon |
| tenotomy, tendotomy | surgical division of a tendon |

## STUDY TABLE   THE MUSCULAR SYSTEM

| Term and Pronunciation | Analysis | Meaning |
|---|---|---|
| **STRUCTURE & FUNCTION** | | |
| abductor pollicis longus (ab-DUK-tor POL-ih-siss LONG-guss) | *abductor* ("outward"); *pollicis* ("thumb"); *longus* ("long") | extends and curls the thumb outward |
| biceps brachii (BY-sepps BRAY-kee-eye) | *bi-* ("two"); *caput* (Latin for "head"); *brachium* (Latin for "arm") | a "two-headed" muscle located in the upper arm |
| biceps femoris (BY-sepps FEE-mohr-uhs) | *bi-* ("two"); *caput* ("head"); *femoris* ("thigh") | posterior thigh muscle; in conjunction with the semitendinosus and semimembra-nosus, makes up the hamstring |
| brachialis (bray-kee-AL-iss) | *brachium* ("arm") | the third major muscle of the upper arm; flexes the forearm |
| corrugator supercilii (KOR-uh-gay-tuhr soop-ehr-SIL-ee-eye) | from a Latin verb *corrugo* ("to wrinkle"); *super* ("above"); *cilii* ("eyelash") | muscle above the eyelid |
| deltoid (DEL-toyd) | from *delta*, a Greek letter shaped like a triangle; *-oid* ("similar") | triangular-shaped arm muscle that joins with the shoulder |
| digiti (DIHJ-ih-ty), digitorum (dihj-ih-TOR-uhm) | Latin for "fingers" or "toes" | words denoting a muscle that facilitates movement in either the fingers or toes |
| elastin (eh-LASS-tihn) | from the Latin word *elasticus* | the major connective tissue pro-tein of tendons and ligaments, as well as large blood vessels |
| erector spinae (ee-REK-tohr SPY-nay) | *erector* ("to extend or make erect"); *spinae* ("relating to the spine") | name given to the spinal exten-sors that make it possible to extend and flex the spine |
| extensor carpi radialis longus (ex-TENSE-ohr kar-pee ray-dee-AL-iss LONG-guss) | from the Latin words *extendo* ("stretch"), *carpus* ("wrist"), *radialis* ("angle"), and *longus* ("long") | extends and curls the hand out-ward |
| extensor carpi ulnaris (ex-TENSE-ohr kar-pee uhl-NAHR-iss) | from the Latin words *extendo* ("stretch"), *carpus* ("wrist"), and *ulna* ("elbow") | extends and curls the hand inward |
| extensor digitorum (ex-TEN-sohr dij-ih-TOR-uhm) | from the Latin words *extendo* ("stretch") and *digitorum* ("fingers") | extends the fingers |
| extensor digitorum longus (ex-TENSE-ohr dij-ih-TOR-uhm LONG-guss) | *extensor* ("extend"); *digitorum* ("toes"); *longus* ("long") | anterior muscle controlling the toes |
| extensor hallucis longus (ex-TENSE-ohr hah-LUCE-ihs LONG-guss) | *extensor* ("extend"); *hallux* ("great toe"); *longus* ("long") | anterior muscle controlling the great toe |
| flexor carpi radialis (FLEX-ohr kar-pee-ray dee-AL-iss) | from the Latin words *flecto* ("bend"), *carpus* ("wrist"), and *radialis* ("angle") | flexes and curls the hand out-ward |
| flexor carpi ulnaris (FLEX-ohr kar-pee uhl-NAHR-iss) | from the Latin words *flecto* ("to bend"), *carpus* ("wrist"), and *ulna* ("elbow") | flexes and curls the hand inward |
| flexor digitorum longus (FLEX-ohr dij-ih-TOR-uhm LONG-guss) | *flexor* ("extend"); *digitorum* ("toes"); *longus* ("long") | posterior muscle controlling the toes |

## STUDY TABLE THE MUSCULAR SYSTEM (continued)

| Term and Pronunciation | Analysis | Meaning |
|---|---|---|
| flexor hallucis longus (FLEX-ohr hah-LUCE-ihs LONG-guss) | *flexor* ("flex"); *hallux* ("great toe"); *longus* ("long") | posterior muscle controlling the great toe |
| genioglossus (jeen-ee-oh-GLOSS-uhs) | *gen/i/o* ("origin"); *-glossus* ("tongue") | one of the four tongue muscles |
| gluteus maximus (GLU-tee-uhs MAX-ih-muss) | from the Greek *boutos* ("buttock"); *maximus* ("outer") | the outer muscle of the buttock |
| gluteus medius (GLU-tee-uhs MEED-ee-uss) | from the Greek *boutos* ("buttock"); *medius* ("middle") | the middle muscle of the buttock |
| gluteus minimus (GLU-tee-uhs MIN-ih-muss) | from the Greek *boutos* ("buttock"); *minimus* ("inner") | the inner muscle of the buttock |
| hyoglossus (HY-oh-gloss-uhs) | *hy/o* ("relating to a U-shaped bone"); *-glossus* ("tongue") | one of the four tongue muscles |
| latissimus dorsi (la-TISS-ih-muhs DOR-see) | latissiumus is related to *lateralis*, a Latin adjective for "side," and *dorsi* is the plural form of *dorsum,* which is Latin for "back" | muscles that wrap around the side and back |
| levator scapulae (leh-VAY-tor SKAP-yu-lay) | from the Latin verb *levo* ("to lift") and the Latin word *scapula* ("shoulder blade") | a shoulder muscle that facilitates upward movement |
| ligament (LIG-ah-ment) | from the Latin noun *ligamen* ("string") | a type of muscle tissue connecting bones, cartilage, or other tissue structures |
| myogenesis (my-oh-JENN-ih-sihs) | *my/o* ("muscle"); *-genesis* ("origin") | formation of muscle cells |
| myoid (MY-oyd) | *my/o* ("muscle"); *-oid* ("similar") | resembling muscle |
| orbicularis oculi (or-BIK-yah-lahr-iss AWK-yu-ly) | formed from two Latin words: *orbiculus* ("small disc") and *oculi* ("plural form of eye") | muscle around the eye |
| orbicularis oris (or-BIK-yah-lahr-iss OR-iss) | formed from two Latin words: *orbiculus* ("small disc") and *ora* (plural form of mouth") | muscle around the mouth |
| palatoglossus (PAL-ah-toe-gloss-uhs) | *palat/o* (relating to the palate); *-glossus* ("tongue") | one of the four tongue muscles |
| pectoralis minor (pek-toh-RAL-iss MY-nohr) | from the Latin word *pectus* ("chest"); *minor* ("small") | a shoulder muscle that facilitates downward movement |
| peroneus longus (peh-ROH-nee-uhs LONG-guss) | *peroneus* ("clasp"); *longus* ("long") | anterior muscle of the lower leg |
| peroneus tertius (peh-ROH-nee-uhs TERSH-ee-uhs) | *peroneus* ("clasp"); *tertius* ("third") | anterior muscle of the lower leg |
| pollicis (POL-ih-sis) | possessive case of the Latin word *pollex* ("thumb") | refers to thumb movement when used in the name of a muscle |
| quadriceps femoris (KWA-drih-sepps FEE-mohr-uss) | *quadri-* ("four"); *caput* ("head"); *femoris* ("thigh") | the collective name of the anterior thigh muscles |
| rectus femoris (REK-tuss FEE-morh-uss) | *rectus* ("straight"); *femoris* ("thigh") | An interior thigh muscle (part of the quadriceps femoris) |

📖 **STUDY TABLE** THE MUSCULAR SYSTEM *(continued)*

| Term and Pronunciation | Analysis | Meaning |
|---|---|---|
| rhomboideus major and minor (rohm-BOY-dee-uhs MAY-juhr); (rohm-BOY-dee-uhs MY-nuhr) | *rhomboid* (an English noun meaning "equilateral parallelogram"; *major* ("large"); *minor* ("small") | shoulder muscles that facilitate downward movement |
| sartorius (sar-TOR-ee-uhs") | from the Latin word *sartor* ("tailor") | the longest muscle in the leg (and the body) |
| semimembranosus (SEM-ee-mehm-brah-NO-suhs) | *semi-* ("half"); *membranosus* ("membrane") | posterior thigh muscle; in conjunction with the semitendinosus and biceps femoris, makes up the hamstring |
| semitendinosus (SEM-ee-tend-ih-NO-suhs) | *semi-* ("half"); *tendinosus* ("tendon") | posterior thigh muscle; in conjunction with the biceps femoris and semimembranosus, makes up the hamstring |
| serratus anterior (serr-RAT-uhs an-TEER-ee-ohr) | possibly from the Latin word *serra* ("saw"); *anterior* ("front") | a shoulder muscle that facilitates upward movement |
| sphincter (SFINK-tehr) | from the Greek word *sphinkter* ("band") | a muscle that surrounds a duct, tube, or orifice |
| striated (STRY-ayted) | from the Latin verb *striare* ("to groove") | adjective describing skeletal muscles |
| styloglossus (STYL-oh-gloss-uhs) | from the Greek word *stylos* ("post"); *-glossus* ("tongue") | one of the four tongue muscles |
| subclavius (sub-KLAY-vee-uhs) | *sub-* ("beneath"); *clavius* ("collar bone") | a shoulder muscle that facilitates downward movement |
| tendon (TEN-dun) | from the Latin verb *tendo* ("stretch") | a type of muscle structure, such as the Achilles tendon, associated with appendicular muscles |
| tibialis anterior (tihb-ee-AL-ihs an-TEE-ree-ohr) | *tibialis* ("shin"); *anterior* ("front") | one of the muscles that move the feet |
| trapezius (trah-PEEZ-ee-uhs) | from the Greek word *trapezion* ("table"): relevance to the trapezius muscle is obscure | a muscle surrounding the spinal column |
| triceps brachii (TRY-sepps BRAY-kee-eye) | *tri-* ("three"); *caput* (Latin for head"); *brachium* (Latin for arm") | a "three-headed" muscle located in the upper arm |
| triceps surae (TRY-sepps SHUR-ay) | *tri-* ("three"); *caput* ("head"); *surae* ("calf of the leg") | the posterior muscle group controlling the foot |
| vastus intermedius (VASS-tuhs ihn-tehr-MEE-dee-ihs) | *vastus* ("great"); *intermedius* ("inside") | An interior thigh muscle (part of the quadriceps femoris) |
| vastus lateralis (VASS-tuhs lat-uhr-AL-ihs) | *vastus* ("great"); *lateralis* ("side") | An interior thigh muscle (part of the quadriceps femoris) |
| vastus medialis (VASS-tuhs mee-dee-AL-ihs) | *vastus* ("great"); *medialis* ("middle") | An interior thigh muscle (part of the quadriceps femoris) |
| **COMMON DISORDERS** | | |
| glossodynia (gloss-oh DINN-ee-yuh) | *glosso-* ("tongue"); *-dynia* ("pain") | pain in the tongue |
| kinesalgia (kin-ee-SAL-jee-uh); kinesialgia (kih-nee-see-AL-jee-uh) | *kines/io* ("motion"); *-algia* ("pain") | pain resulting from movement |

## STUDY TABLE  THE MUSCULAR SYSTEM *(continued)*

| Term and Pronunciation | Analysis | Meaning |
|---|---|---|
| myelitis (my-uh-LY-tuhs) | *myel/o* ("muscle"); *-itis* ("inflammation") | inflammation of a muscle |
| myocele (MY-oh-seel) | *my/o* ("muscle"); *-cele* ("protrusion," "hernia") | hernia of a muscle |
| myodynia (my-oh-DINN-ee-yuh) | *my/o* ("muscle"); *-dynia* ("pain") | pain in a muscle |
| myoma (my-OH-muh) | *my/o* ("muscle"); *-oma* ("tumor") | benign neoplasm of muscle tissue |
| myomalacia (MY-oh-mah-LASH-ee-yuh) | *my/o* ("muscle"); *-malacia* ("softening") | softening of muscle |
| myositis (my-oh-SY-tihs) | *my/os* ("muscle"); *-itis* ("inflammation") | inflammation of muscle |
| myospasm (MY-oh-spaz-uhm) | *my/o* ("muscle"); *-spasm* ("contraction") | involuntary contraction of a muscle |
| tenalgia (tehn-AL-jee-uh), tenodynia (ten-oh-DINN-ee-uh) | from the Latin verb *tendo* ("extend"); *-algia* ("pain"); *-dynia* ("pain") | pain in a tendon |
| tendonitis (ten-doe-NY-tiss); also sometimes spelled tendinitis (TEN-dih-NY-tiss) | from the Latin verb *tendo* ("extend"); *-itis* ("inflammation") | inflammation of a tendon |
| **PRACTICE & PRACTITIONERS** | | |
| kinesiology (kih-nee-see-AWL-uh-jee) | from the Greek word *kinesis* ("motion"); *-logy* ("study of") | study of muscle motion |
| myology (my-AWL-uh-jee) | *my/o* ("muscle"); *-logy* ("study of") | study of muscles |
| **SURGICAL PROCEDURES** | | |
| myectomy (my-EKK-tuh-mee) | *my/o* ("muscle"); *-ectomy* ("excision") | excision of part of a muscle |
| tenontoplasty (teh-NON-toe-plass-tee); tendinoplasty (TEN-dih-no-plass-tee); tendoplasty (TEN-doe-plass-tee); tenoplasty (TEN-oh-plass-tee) | from the Latin verb *tendo* ("extend"); *-plasty* ("surgery") | surgical repair of a tendon |
| tenorrhaphy (TEN-oh-raff-ee) | from the Latin verb *tendo* ("extend"); *-rrhaphy* ("suturing") | suturing of a tendon |
| tenotomy (ten-AW-tuh-mee); also sometimes tendotomy (ten-DAW-tuh-mee) | from the Latin verb *tendo* ("extend"); *-tomy* ("incision into") | incision into a tendon |

## ABBREVIATION TABLE

**COMMON ABBREVIATIONS:**
**The Muscular System**

| Abbreviation | Meaning |
|---|---|
| ACMU | accessory muscles |
| APF | ankle plantar flexor muscles |
| EDL | extensor digitorum longus |
| EMG | electromyography |
| ESSM | electrostimulation of large skeletal muscles |
| IM | intramuscular |
| JCM | jaw-closing muscles |
| JOM | jaw-opening muscles |
| RICE | rest, ice, compression, elevation |

# Exercises

## Exercise 7-1 Completing Sentences

Fill in the missing terms to complete the following sentences.

1. Two muscles, the trapezius and the _____, cover the back and facilitate movement of the trunk and body.
2. The muscles associated with the ulna are the _____ and the _____.
3. Similarly, the muscles of the radius are called the _____ and the _____.
4. The major muscles in the anterior thigh are known collectively as the _____.
5. All of the muscles mentioned above are _____ muscles, the ones we move voluntarily. They are called _____ because they have a "grooved" appearance.
6. The abductor pollicis _____ extends and curls the thumb outward.
7. The extensor hallucis longus is the anterior muscle that controls the great _____.
8. The muscle that facilitates downward movement of the shoulder is the _____.
9. The four tongue muscles are called the _____, _____, _____, and _____.

# Exercises

## Exercise 7-2 Converting Nouns to Adjectives

Convert each of the following nouns to its adjective form using one of the following suffixes: *al, ar, or, ular.*

| Noun | Adjective |
|------|-----------|
| 1. muscle | _____ |
| 2. digit | _____ |
| 3. extension | _____ |
| 4. flexion | _____ |
| 5. abduction | _____ |
| 6. adduction | _____ |
| 7. gluteus | _____ |
| 8. erection | _____ |
| 9. hyoglossus | _____ |
| 10. digit | _____ |

# Exercises

## Exercise 7-3 Matching Terms with Definitions

Place the letter of the definition in the right column in the space next to the matching term in the left column.

| | Term | Definition |
|---|------|------------|
| 1. _____ | latissimus dorsi | A. the middle muscle of the buttock |
| 2. _____ | gluteus medius | B. the study of movement |
| 3. _____ | deltoid | C. a "three-headed" muscle located in the upper arm |
| 4. _____ | extensor | D. moving inward |
| 5. _____ | tendonitis | E. a muscle that extends the fingers |
| 6. _____ | myodynia | F. a muscle around the mouth |
| 7. _____ | adduction | G. the triangular-shaped arm muscle that joins with the shoulder |
| 8. _____ | triceps brachii | H. muscles that wrap around the side and back |
| 9. _____ | kinesiology | J. pain in a muscle |
| 10. _____ | orbicularis oris | K. inflammation of a tendon |

## Exercises

### Exercise 7-4 True, False, and Correction

Read each statement, and then indicate whether you think it is true or false. If false, fill in the correct answer in the "Correction, if False" box at the right.

| Statement | True | False | Correction, if False |
|---|---|---|---|
| 1. The orbicularis oculi is the muscle above the eyelid. | ___ | ___ | _____ |
| 2. The outer muscle of the buttock is the gluteus maximus. | ___ | ___ | _____ |
| 3. The biceps femoris is the "two-headed" muscle in the upper arm. | ___ | ___ | _____ |
| 4. The deltoid is a triangular-shaped muscle located in the chest. | ___ | ___ | _____ |
| 5. The rectus femoris is the inner muscle of the buttock. | ___ | ___ | _____ |
| 6. The semitendinosus is a posterior thigh muscle that, with the biceps femoris and semimembranosus, makes up the hamstring. | ___ | ___ | _____ |
| 7. The muscle surrounding the spinal column is called the trapezius. | ___ | ___ | _____ |
| 8. The formation of cartilage cells is called myogenesis. | ___ | ___ | _____ |
| 9. One of the muscles that moves the feet is the tibialis anterior. | ___ | ___ | _____ |
| 10. Rhomboideus is a consistent pain in the shoulder. | ___ | ___ | _____ |

## Exercises

### Exercise 7-5 Choosing from Options

Choose the term in the right column that correctly completes each sentence.

1. Inflammation of a tendon is _____.    tenalgia; tendonitis; tibialis

2. Pain in a tendon is _____.    tenalgia; tendonitis; tibialis

3. Inflammation of a muscle is referred to as _____.    myelitis; myocele; myoma

4. A hernia of a muscle is called a _____.    myelitis; myocele; myoma

5. Flexor digitorum longus is an anterior muscle that controls the _____.    fingers; legs; toes

6. The extensor digitorum extends the _____.    fingers; legs; toes

7. Surgical repair of a tendon is called a _____.    tenontoplasty; tenorrhaphy; tenotomy

8. Suturing of a tendon is a _____.    tenontoplasty; tenorrhaphy; tenotomy

9. Movement of the toes and fingers is facilitated by _____.    kinesiology; kinesalgia; digiti

10. The study of the motion of muscles is called _____.    kinesiology; kinesalgia; digiti

# Exercises

## Exercise 7-6 Misspelled Terms

Check the terms below and correct all misspellings that you find.

| Term | Correction |
|---|---|
| 1. biceps brachili | _____ |
| 2. deltoid | _____ |
| 3. erecter spinae | _____ |
| 4. extenser digitorum | _____ |
| 5. extenser hallucis longis | _____ |
| 6. genioglossis | _____ |
| 7. hyoglossus | _____ |
| 8. orbicularis oculi | _____ |
| 9. orbicularis oress | _____ |
| 10. palatoglossus | _____ |
| 11. peroneus longus | _____ |
| 12. peroneus tercias | _____ |
| 13. pollicus | _____ |
| 14. myospasm | _____ |
| 15. myomalaysia | _____ |
| 16. myoseal | _____ |
| 17. miology | _____ |
| 18. myectomy | _____ |
| 19. tenentoplasty | _____ |
| 20. tenorrhafy | _____ |

# Exercises

## Exercise 7-7 Identifying Selected Facial Muscles

Label the following muscles on Figure 7-7.

+ corrugator supercilii
+ genioglossus
+ hyoglossus
+ orbicularis oris
+ orbicularis oculi
+ palatoglossus
+ styloglossus

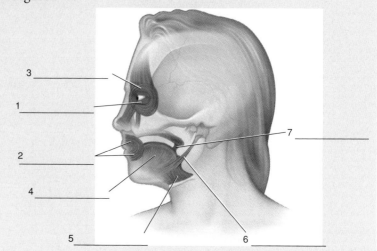

FIGURE 7-7 Selected facial muscles
(Exercise 7-7).

# Exercises

## Exercise 7-8 Identifying the Muscles of the Arms and Hands

Label the following muscles on Figure 7-8.

+ biceps brachii
+ extensor carpi ulnaris
+ flexor carpi ulnaris
+ flexor carpi radialis
+ triceps brachii

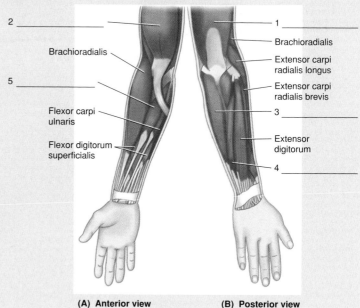

FIGURE 7-8 Muscles of the arms and hands
(Exercise 7-8).

## Pre-Quiz Checklist

_____ Study the word roots specific to the muscular system in Table 7-1.
_____ Review the definitions and etymologies listed in the study table.
_____ Check your answers to the exercises with the answers in the Appendix and consult the study table again to correct any errors.

## Chapter Quiz

Write the answers to the following ten items using the spaces provided to the right.

1. Name the four muscles containing the word element "glossus." On what part of the body do they effect movement?

1. _____
   _____
   _____
   _____

2. The trapezius muscles facilitate movement of which parts of the body?

2. _____
   _____

3. List the four main muscles of the arm.

3. _____
   _____
   _____
   _____

4. On what area of the body would a muscle containing the word element *digiti* or *digitorum* effect movement?

4. _____

5. What is the job of the gluteus maximus?

5. _____
   _____

6. Which four muscles serve to extend the leg?

6. _____
   _____
   _____
   _____

7. What is the longest muscle of the body, and what is its function?

7. _____
   _____
   _____
   _____

8. The hamstring is composed of which three muscles, and what is their job?

8. _____
   _____
   _____
   _____

9. Describe the difference in texture between the voluntary and involuntary muscles.

9. _____
   _____
   _____
   _____

10. Which two leg muscles facilitate walking by supporting the pelvis?

10. _____
    _____

Chapter 8

# The Heart

CHAPTER CONTENTS

The heart, which is part of the cardiovascular system, pumps blood to every cell in the body. That job is critical, because without the oxygen and nutrients that the blood delivers, body cells quickly die. This chapter introduces terms relating to the structure, function, and disorders of the heart, along with those that name some of the procedures and treatments that keep it working when it malfunctions. Chapter 9 deals with the rest of the cardiovascular system, i.e., the blood and blood vessels.

## WORD ELEMENTS SPECIFIC TO THE HEART

The word elements in Table 8-1 are often found in terms related to the heart. You will recognize them in many of the terms you will learn in this chapter.

| **TABLE 8-1** | COMMON WORD ELEMENTS RELATED TO THE HEART | |
|---|---|---|
| Word or Word Element | Type | Refers to |
| aort/o | root | aorta |
| atri/o | root | atrium |
| brady- | prefix | slow |
| card/i/o | root | heart |
| corona | from the Latin word for "crown" | the adjective form "coronary" is sometimes used to describe anatomic structures, such as nerves, ligaments, and blood vessels, especially the arteries of the heart |
| echo | English word from Greek mythology; Echo was a nymph who helped Zeus deceive his wife by distracting her with chatter | a reverberation of sound; not properly called a root (and therefore written without the slash before its final letter), *echo* has been adopted for use in forming some medical terms, such as *echogram* and *echocardiography*) |
| electr/o | root | electrical |
| endo- | prefix | inner, inside |
| -gram | suffix | written record |
| my/o | root | muscle |
| peri- | prefix | around, surrounding |
| -stenosis | suffix | a narrowing |
| tachy- | prefix | fast |
| valv/o, valvul/o | root | valve |
| ventricul/o | root | ventricle |

## THE LOCATION OF THE HEART

The heart is encased in and separated from the walls of the pericardial cavity by three linings: the *epicardium,* which forms the outer part of the heart; the *pericardial sac;* and the *pericardium.* The heart fits tightly inside the *pericardial cavity,* a sub-cavity of the thoracic cavity. The pericardial cavity is lined with a serous (thin) membrane called the *pericardium,* and the heart is within yet a second lining called the *pericardial sac.* This sac contains about half an ounce of fluid, which lies between it and the heart's outer lining (Figure 8-1).

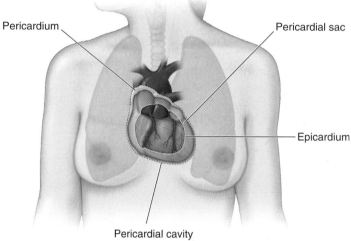

FIGURE **8-1** The location of the heart.

## THE STRUCTURE OF THE HEART

The membrane forming the outer lining of the heart is called the *epicardium.* Immediately beneath the epicardium is the *myocardium,* comprising the muscles, blood vessels, and nerve tissue that make up the bulk of the heart. The heart's inner surface is called the *endocardium.*

The heart has four chambers: the *right atrium,* the *right ventricle,* the *left atrium,* and the *left ventricle.* They are separated by *septa* (singular, *septum*). The names and locations of the septa are easy to remember because they include the names of the parts they separate. They are the *interventricular septum* (separates the two ventricles) and the *interatrial septum* (separates the two *atria*). Also, each atrium is divided from each ventricle by an *atrioventricular septum,* which contains various valves.

The *right atrioventricular valve,* also sometimes called the *tricuspid valve,* leads from the right atrium into the right ventricle. The *pulmonary semilunar valve* connects the right ventricle to the lungs, which also connect to the left ventricle through the left atrium by way of the *left atrioventricular valve,* also sometimes called the *bicuspid* or *mitral valve.* The *aortic semilunar valve* leads out of the left ventricle (Figure 8-2).

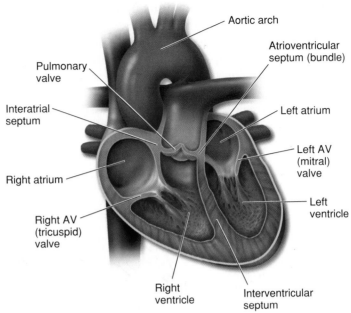

FIGURE **8-2**  The structures of the heart.

## BLOOD FLOW THROUGH THE HEART

The best way to understand how blood flows through the heart is to keep the heart's job in mind. When blood comes back to the heart after having delivered oxygen and other nutrients to the body's cells, it needs to be replenished before going out again. It re-enters the heart at the right atrium. From there it moves into the right ventricle, from which it is pumped into the lungs. After being recharged with oxygen, the blood moves back into the heart through the left atrium and into the left ventricle, from which it is pumped out for yet another trip through the body.

## HEART DISORDERS AND PROCEDURES

The heart can be compared to a mechanical device that relies on electricity for its operation. Electrical impulses emitted within the heart stimulate the heart to pump. When the electrical system malfunctions, the heart will beat too fast, too slow, at an irregular pace, or not at all, depending on the nature of the malfunction.

*Arrhythmia* is most often defined as an irregular heartbeat at any speed. When the heart pumps too fast, defined as any rate greater than 100 beats per minute, the condition is called *tachycardia*. The Greek word for "fast," *tachys*, gives us the prefix *tachy-* and also the common English word *tachometer*. A heart that is pumping too slow, which is defined as any rate less than 60 beats per minute, exhibits a condition known as *bradycardia*. The prefix *brady-* is also of Greek origin, coming from the word for "slow": *bradys*. Tachycardia is also called *tachyarrhythmia*, and bradycardia is called *bradyarrhythmia*.

Disorders of the heart are diagnosed and treated by cardiologists, who work in the field of cardiology. Table 8-2 lists common abnormal conditions related to the heart, along with some of the procedures used to diagnose and correct them.

| TABLE 8-2 | COMMON DISORDERS AND PROCEDURES ASSOCIATED WITH THE HEART |
|---|---|
| Term | Definition |
| atriomegaly | enlargement of an atrium |
| atrioseptoplasty | surgical repair of an atrial septum |
| bradycardia | also called bradyarrhythmia; abnormally slow heartbeat |
| cardiac arrest | abbreviated CA, this condition, as its name suggests, describes the sudden cessation of heart activity |
| cardiodynia | heart pain |
| cardiogram (This word and the next are often called "electrocardiogram" and "electrocardiograph," respectively; the abbreviation for both can be either EKG or ECG.) | a graphic trace of heart functions |
| cardiograph (also "myocardiograph," as well as "electrocardiograph," as noted above) | a machine to electrically measure heart functions |
| cardiomalacia | softening of the heart |
| cardiomegaly | enlargement of the heart |
| cardiomyopathy | disease of the heart muscle (myocardium) |
| cardiomyoplasty | a surgical procedure that involves engaging the latissimus dorsi muscle to stimulate the heart; please also note that the term "cardioplasty" is a surgical procedure done on the stomach, NOT the heart. |
| cardiopathy | any heart disease |
| cardiorrhaphy | suturing of the wall of the heart muscle |
| cardiorrhexis | rupture in the wall of the heart muscle |
| cardiotomy | incision into the heart OR incision into the cardia of the stomach |
| carditis | inflammation of the heart |
| endocarditis | inflammation of the endocardium |
| myocardial infarction (often abbreviated MI) | heart attack; patients suspected of having had an MI are given a blood test to measure the level of troponin in the blood (troponin is a protein that is released when an MI occurs) |
| myocarditis | inflammation of the heart muscle |
| pericardiorrhaphy | suturing of the pericardium |

| TABLE 8-2 | COMMON DISORDERS AND PROCEDURES ASSOCIATED WITH THE HEART *(continued)* |
|---|---|
| **Term** | **Definition** |
| pericardiotomy | incision into the pericardium |
| pericarditis | inflammation of the pericardium |
| tachycardia | also called tachyarrhythmia; abnormally rapid heartbeat |
| valvoplasty; also valvuloplasty | surgical repair of a heart valve |
| valvotomy; also valvulotomy | surgical removal of a blocked heart valve (stenosis of a heart valve) by cutting into it |
| valvulitis | inflammation of a heart valve |
| ventriculoplasty | surgical repair of a heart ventricle |
| ventriculoscopy | examination of a heart ventricle with an endoscope |

 **DECIPHERING MEDICAL DOCUMENTS.**

**Read the following excerpt from a cardiac catheterization report and answer the questions:**

*Left ventriculography shows the left ventricle is normal in configuration, dimensions, and segmental wall motion with ejection fraction computed at 58% by area-length method. There is no evidence of mitral regurgitation. Coronary arteriography of left anterior descending artery shows 70% focal stenosis immediately after the first septal perforator branch.*

1. What word root and suffix are contained in the term *ventriculography?* What does the term mean?
2. What does the adjective *coronary* mean?
3. What does the word *stenosis* mean?

## STUDY TABLE  THE HEART

| Term and Pronunciation | Analysis | Meaning |
|---|---|---|
| **STRUCTURE & FUNCTION** | | |
| aortic semilunar valve (ay-ORT-ik sem-ih-LOON-uhr) | *aortic* (adjectival form of aorta, the large artery leading away from the heart); *semi-* ("half"); *lunar* (English adjective from the Latin word *luna*, meaning "moon") | connects the left ventricle to the aorta |
| atria (singular: atrium) (AY-tree-ah; AY-tree-uhm) | from the Latin word *atrium* ("hall") | two of the four heart chambers, composed of the right atrium and left atrium |
| endocardium (en-doh-KAR-dee-uhm) | *endo-* ("inside"); *cardium* ("heart") | the inner surface of the heart |
| epicardium (ep-ih-KAR-dee-uhm) | *epi-* ("outside"); *cardium* ("heart") | the outer lining of the heart |
| left atrioventricular valve (ay-tree-oh ven-TRIK-yu-lahr) also known as the bicuspid or mitral valve (by-KUSS-pihd; MY-trahl) | *atri/o* ("atrium"); *ventricul* ("ventricle"); *-ar* (adjectival suffix); valve | connects the left atrium to the left ventricle |

📖 **STUDY TABLE** THE HEART *(continued)*

| Term and Pronunciation | Analysis | Meaning |
|---|---|---|
| myocardium (my-oh-KAR-dee-uhm) | *my/o* ("muscle"); *cardium* ("heart") | the heart muscle, which includes nerves and blood vessels |
| pericardial (pehr-ih-KAR-dee-ahl) | *peri-* ("around"); *cardial* (adjective for "heart") | adjective form of pericardium |
| pericardial cavity (pehr-ih-KAR-dee-ahl) | *peri-* ("around"); *cardial* (adjective for "heart"); cavity | the subcavity of the thoracic cavity in which the heart is enclosed |
| pericardial sac (pehr-ih-KAR-dee-ahl) | *peri-* ("around"); *cardial* (adjective for "heart"); *sac* (from the Latin word *saccus*, meaning "bag") | another lining of the pericardium closest to the heart |
| pericardium (pehr-ih-KAR-dee-uhm) | *peri-* ("around"); *cardium* ("heart") | serous membrane lining the pericardial cavity |
| pulmonary semilunar valve (PULL-moh-nahr-ee SEM-ee-LUN-ahr) | *pulmonary* (adjective denoting the lungs); *semi-* ("half"); *lunar* (adjective for "moon") | valve connecting the right ventricle and lungs |
| right atrioventricular valve (ay-tree-oh-ven-TRIK-yu-lahr) also known as the tricuspid valve (try-KUSS-pihd) | *atri/o* ("atrium"); *ventricul/o* ("ventricle"); *-ar* (adjectival suffix) | valve connecting the right atrium to the right ventricle |
| septa (singular septum) (SEPP-tah; SEPP-tuhm) | from the Latin *saeptum* ("partition") | thin wall that separates cavities or masses; in the heart, septa separate the right atrium from the left atrium and the right ventricle from the left ventricle |
| troponin (TROH-poh-nihn) | etymology unknown | a protein that is released into the bloodstream when a heart attack occurs |
| ventricle (VEN-trik-uhl) | *ventricle* ("cavity," from the Latin word *ventruculus*, meaning "belly") | two of the four heart chambers, composed of the right ventricle and left ventricle |
| **COMMON DISORDERS** | | |
| arrhythmia (ah-RITH-mee-ah) | the prefix *a-* ("against"); *rhythmos* (common English word derived from the Greek word *rhythmos* meaning the same thing); *-ia* ("condition") | abnormal rhythm; irregular heartbeat |
| atriomegaly (AY-tree-oh-MEG-ah-lee) | from the Latin *atrium* ("hall"); *-megaly* (suffix meaning "enlargement") | enlargement of an atrium |
| bradycardia (bray-dee-KAR-dee-ah) | *brady-* (prefix meaning "slow"); *-cardia* ("heart") | abnormally slow heartbeat |
| cardiac arrest (KAR-dee-ak) | *card/i/o* ("heart"); *-ac* (adjectival suffix); *arrest* (English word meaning "stopped") | cessation of heart activity |
| cardiodynia (kar-dee-oh-DIN-ee-ah) | *card/i/o* ("heart"); *-dynia* ("pain") | heart pain |
| cardiomalacia (kar-dee-oh-mah-LASH-ee-ah) | *card/i/o* ("heart"); *-malacia* ("softening") | softening of the heart |

## 📖 STUDY TABLE THE HEART *(continued)*

| Term and Pronunciation | Analysis | Meaning |
|---|---|---|
| cardiomegaly (kar-dee-oh-MEG-ah-lee) | *card/i/o* ("heart"); *-megaly* ("enlargement") | enlargement of the heart |
| cardiomyopathy (kar-dee-oh-my-AWP-uh-thee) | *card/i/o* ("heart"); *my/o* ("muscle"); *-pathy* ("disease") | disease of the heart muscle (myocardium) |
| cardiopathy (kar-dee-AWP-uh-thee) | *card/i/o* ("heart"); *-pathy* ("disease") | any heart disease |
| cardiorrhexis (kar-dee-oh-REX-ihs) | *card/i/o* ("heart"); *-rrhexis* ("rupture") | rupture in the wall of the heart |
| carditis (kar-DY-tiss) | *card/i/o* ("heart"); *-itis* ("inflammation") | inflammation of the heart |
| endocarditis (en-doh-kar-DY-tiss) | *endo-* ("inside"); *card/i/o* ("heart"); *-itis* ("inflammation") | inflammation of the endocardium |
| myocardial infarction (often abbreviated MI) (my-oh-KAR-dee-ahl in-FARK-shun) (Note: MI is an abbreviation, not an acronym.) | *my/o* ("muscle"); *cardi/o* ("heart"); *-al* (adjective form for heart) | heart attack |
| myocarditis (my-oh-kar-DY-tiss) | *my/o* ("muscle"); *card/i/o* ("heart"); *-itis* ("inflammation") | inflammation of the heart muscle |
| pericarditis (pehr-ih-kar-DY-tiss) | *peri-* ("around"); *card/i/o* ("heart"); *-itis* ("inflammation") | inflammation of the pericardium |
| tachycardia (tak-ih-KAR-dee-ah) | *tachy-* ("rapid"); *card/i/o* ("heart"); *-ia* ("condition") | abnormally rapid heartbeat |
| valvulitis (valv-yu-LY-tiss) | *valvul/o* ("valve"); *-itis* ("inflammation") | inflammation of a heart valve |
| **DIAGNOSIS & TREATMENT** | | |
| cardiogram (KAR-dee-oh-gram) (Note: Associated terms are "electrocardiogram" [ee LEK-troh-KAR-dee-oh-gram] and "electrocardiograph" [ee-LEK-troh-KAR-dee-oh-graf]; the abbreviation for any of them can be either EKG or ECG) | *electro-* ("electric"); *card/i/o* ("heart"); *-gram, -graph* ("writing") | a graphic trace of heart functions |
| myocardiograph (MY-oh-kar-dee-oh-graf), cardiograph (KAR-dee-oh-graf) | *my/o* ("muscle"); *card/i/o* ("heart"); *-graph* ("writing") | a machine to electrically measure heart functions |
| ventriculoscopy (ven-trik-yu-LAWS-koh-pee) | *ventricul/o* ("ventricle"); *-scopy* ("viewing") | looking at a heart ventricle with an endoscope |
| **PRACTICE & PRACTITIONERS** | | |
| cardiologist (kar-dee-AWL-oh-jist) | *card/i/o* ("heart"); *-logist* ("one who studies") | heart specialist |
| cardiology (kar-dee-AWL-oh-jee) | *card/i/o* ("heart"); *-logy* ("study of") | medical specialty dealing with the heart |

## STUDY TABLE  THE HEART  (continued)

| Term and Pronunciation | Analysis | Meaning |
|---|---|---|
| **SURGICAL PROCEDURES** | | |
| atrioseptoplasty (AY-tree-o-SEP-toh-plass-tee) | from the Latin words *atrium* ("hall") and *saeptum* ("partition"); *-plasty* (suffix meaning "surgical repair") | surgical repair of an atrial septum |
| cardiomyoplasty (kar-dee-oh-MY-oh-plass-tee) | *card/i/o* ("heart"); *my/o* ("muscle"); *-plasty* ("surgical repair") | surgical procedure that involves engaging the latissimus dorsi muscle to stimulate the heart (Note: The term "cardioplasty" [without the "my" between cardio and plasty] is a surgical procedure done on the stomach, NOT the heart.) |
| cardiorrhaphy (kar-dee-oh-RAF-fee) | *card/i/o* ("heart"); *-rrhaphy* ("suturing") | suturing of the wall of the heart |
| cardiotomy (kar-dee-AW-tuh-mee) | *card/i/o* ("heart"); *-tomy* ("cutting") | incision into the HEART or incision into the cardia of the STOMACH |
| pericardiorrhaphy (pehr-ih-KAR-dee-oh-raff-ee) | *peri-* ("around"); *card/i/o* ("heart"); *-rrhaphy* (suffix meaning "suturing") | suturing of the pericardium |
| pericardiotomy (PEHR-ih-car-dee-AW-toh-mee) | *peri-* ("around"); *card/i/o* ("heart"); *-tomy* ("cutting") | incision into the pericardium |
| valvoplasty (VALV-oh-plass-tee); also valvuloplasty (VALV-yu-loh-plass-tee) | *valv/o* or *valvul/o* ("valve"); *-plasty* ("surgical repair") | surgical repair of a heart valve |
| valvotomy (valv-AW-toh-mee); also valvulotomy (valv-yu-LAWT-oh-mee) | *valv/o* or *valvul/o* ("valve"); *-tomy* ("cutting") | surgical removal of a blocked heart valve (stenosis of a heart valve) by cutting into it |
| ventriculoplasty (ven-TRIK-yu-loh-plass-tee) | *ventricul/o* ("ventricle"); *-plasty* ("surgical repair") | surgical repair of a heart ventricle |
| **ENHANCEMENT TERMS** | | |
| atrial (AY-tree-uhl) | from the Latin word *atrium* ("hall") | adjectival form of atrium |
| cardiac (KAR-dee-ack) | adjectival form of *cardium* ("heart") | relating to the heart |
| cardiogenic (kar-dee-oh-JEN-ik) | *card/i/o* ("heart"); *-genic* ("origin") | adjective describing something originating in the heart |
| ventricular (ven-TRIK-yu-lahr) | *ventricul/o* ("ventricle"); *-ar* (adjectival suffix) | adjectival form of ventricle (Note: The brain also contains ventricles.) |

## ABBREVIATION TABLE

### COMMON ABBREVIATIONS
### The Heart

| Abbreviation | Meaning |
|---|---|
| ACV | acute cardiovascular [disease] |
| CA | cardiac arrest |
| CAD | coronary artery disease |
| CCU | cardiovascular care unit |
| CHD | cardiovascular heart disease |
| CIPS | cardiovascular imaging procedure |
| CRFS | cardiovascular risk factors |
| CSU | cardiovascular surgery unit |
| CT | cardiovascular technologist |
| CVICU | cardiovascular intensive care unit |
| CVIS | cardiovascular imaging systems |
| EKG or ECG | electrocardiogram; electrocardiograph; electrocardiography; cardiogram |
| MI | myocardial infarction |

## Exercises

### Exercise 8-1 Completing Sentences

Fill in the missing terms to complete the sentences.

1. The heart is enclosed in three linings: the _____, the _____, and the _____.

2. There are four chambers in the heart, called the _____, the _____, the _____, and the _____.

3. When blood returns to the heart from the body, it enters the heart at the _____; from there, it moves to the _____, which pumps it to the lungs to be re-oxygenated.

4. The blood moves back to the heart through the _____ and into the _____, which pumps it out to the body.

5. Cessation of heart activity is called cardiac _____.

6. _____ from within the heart stimulate it to pump.

7. When the heart malfunctions and beats too slowly, the phenomenon is called _____. Conversely, if the heart beats too fast, the condition is called _____.

8. Tachycardia and bradycardia are occasionally also referred to as _____ and _____. However, the word _____ generally refers to a heartbeat that is irregular at any speed.

9. A sufficiently higher-than-normal troponin level is an indicator of _____.

10. The abbreviation for myocardial infarction is _____.

## Exercises

### Exercise 8-2 Converting Nouns to Adjectives

Convert each of the following nouns to its adjective form by using one of the following suffixes: -al, -ar, -ic, -ous, -ated, ular.

| Noun | Adjective |
|------|-----------|
| 1. septum | Septal |
| 2. ventricle | ventricular |
| 3. oxygen | oxygenated |
| 4. atrium | atrial |
| 5. pericardium | Pericardial |
| 6. aorta | aortic |
| 7. valve | valvular |
| 8. serum | Seris |
| 9. endocardium | endocardial |
| 10. epicardium | epicardius |
| 11. membrane | Membranous |
| 12. arrhythmia | arrhythmic |
| 13. tachycardia | tachycardic |
| 14. bradycardia | bradycardic |
| 15. stenosis | Stenoic |

## Exercises

### Exercise 8-3 True, False, and Correction

Read each statement, then indicate whether you think it is true or false. If false, write the correct answer in the "Correction, if False" box at the right.

| Statement | True | False | Definition |
|-----------|------|-------|------------|
| 1. The term for inflammation of the pericardium is *valvulitis*. | ___ | ___ | ___ |
| 2. Atriomegaly is enlargement of an atrium. | ___ | ___ | ___ |
| 3. MI is the abbreviation that stands for an abnormally rapid heartbeat. | ___ | ___ | ___ |

| Statement | True | False | Definition |
|---|---|---|---|
| 4. Tachycardia is an abnormally rapid heartbeat. | ___ | ___ | _____ |
| 5. Cardiotomy is the surgical repair of an atrial septum. | ___ | ___ | _____ |
| 6. Softening of the heart is termed cardiomalacia. | ___ | ___ | _____ |
| 7. A myocardiograph is used to examine a heart ventricle. | ___ | ___ | _____ |
| 8. Cardiorrhaphy is a surgical repair of a heart valve. | ___ | ___ | _____ |
| 9. The surgical procedure that involves engaging the latissimus dorsi muscle to stimulate the heart is a pericardiotomy. | ___ | ___ | _____ |
| 10. Arrhythmia is the general term for an irregular heartbeat. | ___ | ___ | _____ |

# Exercises

## Exercise 8-4 Matching Terms with Definitions

Place the letter of the definition in the right column in the space next to the matching term in the left column.

| Term | Definition |
|---|---|
| 1. _____ myocardial infarction | A. a separation between the two ventricles of the heart |
| 2. _____ aortic semilunar valve | B. inflammation of the pericardium (the serous membrane lining the pericardial cavity) |
| 3. _____ intraventricular septum | C. the heart muscle, which includes the nerves and blood vessels |
| 4. _____ endocardium | D. the valve leading from the right atrium to the right ventricle |
| 5. _____ left ventricle | E. the serous membrane forming the outer lining of the heart |
| 6. _____ cardiologist | F. the heart's inner surface |
| 7. _____ myocardium | G. a heart specialist |
| 8. _____ epicardium | H. heart attack |
| 9. _____ pericarditis | I. the heart chamber responsible for pumping oxygenated blood out to the body |

| Term | Definition |
|---|---|
| 10. _____ right atrioventricular (tricuspid) valve | J. the valve leading out of the left ventricle |
| 11. _____ troponin | K. enlargement of the heart |
| 12. _____ septum | L. coronary artery disease, which refers to narrowing and/or blockages of the heart muscle |
| 13. _____ cardiomegaly | M. a heart rate less than 60 beats per minute |
| 14. _____ tachycardia | N. a protein released into the bloodstream when an MI occurs |
| 15. _____ stenosis | O. disease of the heart muscle |
| 16. _____ CAD | P. a thin wall that separates cavities or masses |
| 17. _____ atrioseptoplasty | Q. a heart rate over 100 beats per minute |
| 18. _____ cardiomyopathy | R. sudden cessation of heart activity, not necessarily a result of MI |
| 19. _____ bradycardia | S. surgical repair of an atrial septum |
| 20. _____ cardiac arrest | T. a narrowing and/or blockage |

# Exercises

## Exercise 8-5 Choosing from Options

Choose the term in the right column that correctly answers the question.

|  | Choices |
|---|---|
| 1. The names of two of the four heart chambers come from the Latin word for "hall." What is it? _____ | atrium; aortic; atrial |
| 2. *Epicardium* is the word for the outside of the heart. Which part of the word means "outside"? _____ | epicard; epi; cardi |
| 3. What part of the term *myocardium* refers to the muscle in the heart? _____ | myocardi; myocard; myo |
| 4. Since *cardio* refers to the heart, what does the rest of the term *cardiodynia* mean? _____ | hardening; pain; softness |
| 5. *Valvulitis* indicates that a valve is what? _____. | hardened; inflamed; infected |
| 6. The word "cardium" is the last part of what term that refers to the inside layer of the heart muscle? _____ | endocardium; epicardium; pericardium |

| | Choices |
|---|---|
| 7. What is the surgical removal of a blockage from a heart valve called? _____. | valvulitis; ventriculoplasty; valvuloplasty |
| 8. What separates the right atrium from the left atrium and the right ventricle from the left ventricle? | atria; septa; arrhythmia |
| 9. What is the name of a valve that connects the atrium to a ventricle? | aortic semilunar; atrioventricular; ventricular |
| 10. What is the name given to a graphic trace of heart functions? | cardiogram; myocardiograph; ventriculoscopy |

# Exercises

## Exercise 8-6 Identifying the Structures of the Heart

Label the following parts of the heart on Figure 8-3.

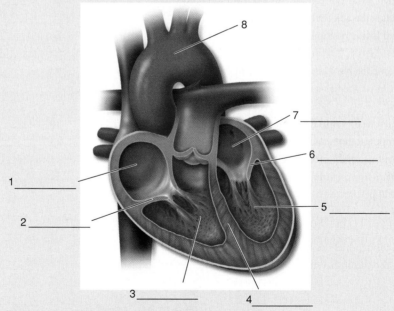

FIGURE **8-3** Selected structures of the heart (Exercise 8-6).

- ◆ aortic arch
- ◆ left atrium
- ◆ mitral valve
- ◆ right AV tricuspid valve
- ◆ intraventricular septum
- ◆ left ventricle
- ◆ right atrium
- ◆ right ventricle

## ✓ Pre-Quiz Checklist

_____ Study the word roots specific to the heart (Table 8-1).
_____ Using the study table, practice pronouncing the terms learned.
_____ Review the definitions and etymologies listed in the study table.
_____ Check the exercises with the answers in the Appendix, and consult the study table
        again to correct your errors.

## ✓ Chapter Quiz

Write the answers to the following items in the spaces provided to the right.

1. What is the abbreviation for myocardial infarction?  1. _____
2. Which valve of the heart connects the right ventricle to the lungs?  2. _____
3. What stimulates the heart to pump?  3. _____
   _____
4. Which is the lining of the pericardium that is closest to the heart?  4. _____
5. What does *arrhythmia* generally refer to?  5. _____
6. Which atrium receives the blood from the body?  6. _____
7. What is the adjectival form of ventricle?  7. _____
8. What is the function of a valve?  8 _____
   _____
9. If someone has been diagnosed with CAD, does this mean  9. _____
   that he or she has had an MI? Explain.  _____
   _____
10. Which heart ventricle would have to perform the strongest  10. _____
    pumping action, and why?  _____
11. Name a surgical procedure involving removal of a heart valve.  11. _____
12. What is a myocardial infarction, and what area of the heart  12. _____
    would be affected by it?  _____
    _____
    _____
13. If an individual has had an MI (heart attack), does  13. _____
    this also mean that he or she has had a cardiac arrest? Explain.  _____
    _____
    _____
14. Name the medical specialty dealing with the heart.  14. _____
15. What is an electrocardiogram?  15. _____
    _____
16. What would *bradycardia* and *tachycardia* indicate?  16. _____
    _____

## Chapter 9

# The Blood and Blood Vessels

CHAPTER CONTENTS

Before studying the terms commonly associated with the blood, we will consider the vessels through which it travels. The reason for doing so is that blood vessels share with the heart the job of transporting blood to all the cells in the body. This chapter introduces the terms relating to blood vessels, constituents of blood, common diseases, and methods of diagnosis and treatment.

## WORD ELEMENTS SPECIFIC TO THE BLOOD AND BLOOD VESSELS

The word elements shown in Table 9-1 are often found in terms relating to the blood and blood vessels. You will recognize them in many of the terms you will learn in this chapter.

| TABLE 9-1 | COMMON WORD ELEMENTS RELATED TO THE BLOOD AND BLOOD VESSELS | |
|---|---|---|
| Element | Type | Refers to |
| ang/i/o | root | vessel |
| arteri/o | root | artery |
| ather/o | root | gruel-like |
| -ectasis | suffix | dilation |
| -emia | suffix | blood |
| hem/o; hemat/o | root | blood |
| phleb/o | root | vein |
| thromb/o | root | clot |
| varic/o | root | dilated; from the Latin word *varix* ("a dilated vein") |
| vas/o | root | vessel |
| vascul/o | root | vessel |
| ven/o | root | vein |

## CAPILLARIES, ARTERIES, AND VEINS

### Capillaries      → microscopic Exchange

The *capillaries* (singular: *capillary*) are a good place to start in a study of the blood vessels, not because they are the largest of the vessels; on the contrary, they are the smallest. They are mentioned first, however, because they are the most numerous and because they deliver nutrients from the blood to the body's cells. The transfer of blood to the capillaries begins in large vessels and progresses through vessels of ever-diminishing size.

### Arteries      Carry Blood Away From the heart

*Arteries* (singular: *ártery*) carry blood away from the heart and, eventually, to the capillaries. Arteries contain muscle tissue, which allows them to vary their diameters. Two terms are associated with this action: they are *vasoconstriction* (a narrowing of the artery's diameter) and *vasodilation* (an enlarging of the artery's diameter). When the muscle tissue contained within an artery contracts, vasoconstriction occurs, thereby producing a resistance that increases blood pressure. When the muscle tissue relaxes, vasodilation occurs to effectively lower the blood pressure. All arteries have this capability, but in varying degrees, depending on their function.

The arteries nearest the heart must be able to accommodate the large volume of blood it pumps out with each beat. Artery diameters become smaller as they get nearer to the capillaries. The three kinds of arteries are *conducting arteries, muscular arteries,* and *arterioles.*

### Conducting Arteries

*Left Ventricle*

*Conducting arteries,* sometimes called *elastic arteries,* can have an inside diameter as great as an inch. The *aorta* is an example of a conducting artery. The *pulmonary artery* and the *aortic trunk* are examples of conducting arteries, which move blood away from the heart. Three major conducting arteries branch from the aortic arch, as shown in Figure 9-1. They are the *brachiocephalic trunk,* the *left common carotid artery,* and the *left subclavian artery.* Both the *right subclavian artery* and the *right common carotid artery* attach to the brachiocephalic trunk.

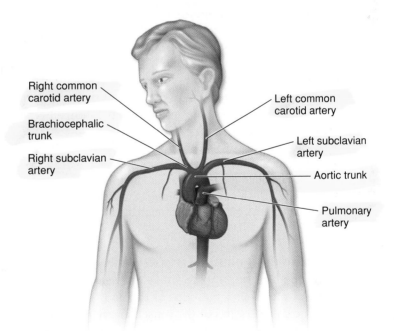

FIGURE 9-1 Conducting arteries.

### Medium-Size Arteries

Medium-size arteries, sometimes called *muscular arteries* (because they contain a lot of muscle tissue), typically have an inside diameter of about one-sixth of an inch—roughly the height of the letters *h* and *l* in this sentence. The *external carotid artery* in the neck is an example of a medium-size artery.

## Arterioles

*Arterioles* are the smallest arteries, with an average inside diameter of 0.0018 of an inch, or about 1/100 the size of a medium-size artery. Arteries and arterioles connect to the capillaries, which can be as tiny as one blood cell (or about one-fourth the size of an arteriole) in diameter (Figure 9-2).

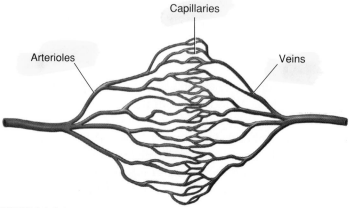

FIGURE 9-2 Schematic diagram of the arteriole-capillary-vein network.

## Veins

*Veins* carry blood back to the heart. They follow the same path as the arteries (with blood flowing in the reverse direction, of course). Also, like the arteries, they vary in diameter, becoming larger as they approach the heart because of the increasing volumes of blood they must carry.

> A fascinating fact about veins is that some of them are duplicated, one having a deep route within the body and the other running near the surface of the skin. When you are hot, the blood flows through the veins near the surface to dissipate heat, and when you are cold, it flows through the ones deeper inside the body to keep you warm.

The vein counterparts of the conducting arteries are the *superior vena cava* and the *inferior vena cava*. Together, they are known as the *venae cavae,* the Latin plurals for *vena* and *cava*. All the other large veins of the body system drain into one or the other of these. The counterparts of the muscular arteries and arterioles are the *medium veins* and *venules*. As its name implies, the superior vena cava drains blood from the upper body, including the head, neck, shoulders, and arms. The inferior vena cava, likewise, receives blood from the lower body, the dividing line being the diaphragm. Figure 9-3 shows the location of the superior and inferior venae cavae and principal connecting veins.

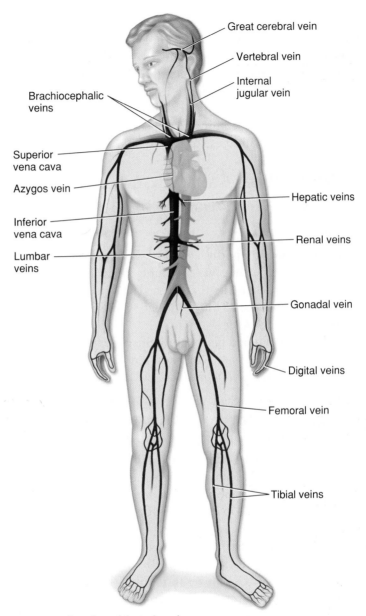

FIGURE 9-3 Locations of the major veins.

## The Superior Vena Cava

The superior vena cava collects the blood returning from the cranium from smaller veins, such as the *great cerebral vein* and the *internal jugular vein,* which runs alongside the common carotid artery. The *brachiocephalic veins* collect returning blood from the *vertebral vein* and then connects up with the *azygos vein,* which in turn connects to the superior vena cava, often referred to by its abbreviation: SVC.

The Inferior Vena Cava

Blood entering the inferior vena cava (IVC) includes that returning from the lower limbs, spinal cord, liver, kidneys, and reproductive organs. The names of these veins include the *digital, tibial, femoral,* and *lumbar* veins, all of which are familiar enough to you by now to indicate what parts of the body they serve. The *gonadal, hepatic,* and *renal* veins serve the following parts of the body: the reproductive organs, the liver, and the kidneys, respectively. You will learn more about the terminology associated with these organs in later chapters.

## TERMINOLOGY OF THE BLOOD

Whole blood is made up of *plasma* and the *formed elements* it contains.

### Blood Plasma

Blood plasma, a yellowish liquid that is 90% water, also contains proteins and other nutrients in solution, such as water-soluble vitamins and minerals. In addition, it carries the formed elements that are a part of whole blood: namely, *erythrocytes, leukocytes,* and *platelets.* Thus, although whole blood remains a fluid, it is about five times denser than water.

The three main classes of blood plasma proteins are *albumins, globulins,* and *fibrinogens.* Two other terms that name common blood proteins are *antibodies* (also known as *immunoglobulins)* and *lipoproteins.*

### Formed Elements (Erythrocytes, Leukocytes, and Platelets) *Nud to Know For test.*

*Erythrocytes* are red blood cells, abbreviated RBC, and *leukocytes* are white blood cells, abbreviated WBC. Red blood cells make up 99.9% of the formed elements in the blood. Hemoglobin, which is abbreviated Hb and binds only to RBCs, gives blood its red color. Each RBC contains approximately 280 million Hb molecules. A single drop of blood contains about 260 million red blood cells. The number of white blood cells present in a drop of blood is only 35,000 or so, although WBCs are not much larger than the RBCs.

White blood cells do not all do the same job and are not all the same size. However, all WBCs are at least slightly larger than RBCs. In fact, the WBCs of one category are double the size of RBCs. The terms naming the WBC categories are given in Figure 9-4 and are discussed further in Chapter 13.

Platelets, which are very small in comparison to both RBCs and WBCs, are formed elements that are important in the coagulation process. They are produced in the bone marrow and vary somewhat in shape (Figure 9-4).

*Nud to*

Erythrocytes  Basophil  Neutrophil  Monocyte  Eosinophil  Lymphocyte  Platelets
FIGURE 9-4 Formed elements in blood.

## BLOOD AND BLOOD VESSEL DISORDERS AND PROCEDURES

Table 9-2 lists common abnormal blood conditions, along with some of the procedures used to diagnose and correct them.

*Study this* (handwritten note, left margin)

| TABLE 9-2 | COMMON DISORDERS AND PROCEDURES ASSOCIATED WITH BLOOD AND BLOOD VESSELS |
|---|---|
| Term | Definition |
| aneurysm | a bulge in an artery (or a heart chamber) |
| angiitis (also vasculitis) | inflammation of a blood vessel |
| angiogram | the printed record obtained through angiography |
| angiography | radiography of a blood vessel after injection of a contrast medium |
| angiopathy (also vasculopathy) | any disease of blood vessels |
| angioplasty | surgical repair of a blood vessel |
| angiorrhaphy | suture of a vessel |
| angiospasm | spasm in blood vessels |
| angiostenosis | narrowing of a blood vessel |
| angiotomy | incision into a blood vessel |
| arteriolitis | inflammation of the arterioles |
| arteriopathy | any disease of the arteries |
| arterioplasty | surgical repair of an artery |
| arteriorrhexis | rupture of an artery |
| arteriorrhaphy | suturing of an artery |
| arteriosclerosis | hardening of the arteries |
| arteriospasm | spasm of an artery |
| arteriostenosis | narrowing of an artery |
| arteriotomy | an incision into an artery |
| arteriovenous | adjectival form of "arteries and veins" |
| arteritis | inflammation of an artery or arteries |
| hemolysis | change or destruction of red blood cells |
| hemopathy | any disease of the blood |
| hemophilia | congenital disorder affecting the coagulation process |
| hemorrhage | discharge of blood |
| hemorrhagic fever | category that includes a number of viral diseases, one of which is Ebola fever |
| vasculitis (also angiitis) | inflammation of a vessel |
| vasculopathy (also angiopathy) | any disease of blood vessels |
| vasoparalysis | paralysis of blood vessels |
| vasoparesis | similar to but less severe than vasoparalysis |
| vasospasm | spasm in blood vessels (angiospasm) |

*Need to know* ← (handwritten note, left margin, pointing to hemolysis)

*Breakdown of Red Cells* (handwritten note, right of hemolysis row)

## CHOLESTEROL

*Cholesterol,* a fat-soluble steroid alcohol, is manufactured in the liver and transported through the bloodstream. Cholesterol is delivered to body tissues, including arterial walls, by low-density lipoprotein (LDL), known as "bad" cholesterol.
High-density lipoprotein (HDL) is known as "good cholesterol" because it returns
LDL to the liver for excretion.

*Under 200 is Normal.* (handwritten)

## DECIPHERING MEDICAL DOCUMENTS

**Read the following excerpt from a progress note, then answer the questions.**

*Complete blood count reveals a total leukocyte count of 6,600/mm³, Hb of 8.0 g/dL, hematocrit of 23.0,
and a platelet count of 149,000/mm³. Clinical diagnosis is chronic myelomonocytic leukemia.*

1. What root and suffix combine to make up the word *leukocyte?* What does it mean?
2. What is Hb?
3. What is the suffix in *leukemia* and what does it mean?

## STUDY TABLE  THE BLOOD AND BLOOD VESSELS

| Term and Pronunciation | Analysis | Meaning |
|---|---|---|
| **STRUCTURE & FUNCTION** | | |
| albumins (al-BYU-mihns) | from the Latin *albumen* ("white of an egg") | one of the three main blood plasma proteins; globulins and fibrinogens are the other two |
| antibodies (AN-tih-bodies) | *anti-* ("against") | also called immunoglobulins; a common blood protein |
| aorta (ay-OR-tah) | from the Greek word *aeiro* ("lift up") | the main trunk of the systemic arterial system |
| arteries (AR-tuh-rees) | from the Latin word *arteria*, meaning "windpipe" (broadly, "a tube-shaped vessel") | the largest of the blood vessels |
| arterioles (ar-TEER-ee-oles) | from the Latin word *arteria*, meaning "windpipe" (broadly, "a tube-shaped vessel") | the smallest arteries that connect with the capillaries |
| azygos vein (AYZ-eye-gohs) | from the Greek prefix *a-* ("single"); and the Greek word *zygon* ("yoke") | a vein that connects the brachiocephalic veins with the superior vena cava |
| brachiocephalic trunk (BRAKE-ee-oh-seh-FALL-ik) | *brach/io* ("arm"); *cephal/o* ("head"); *-ic* (adjective suffix) | one of three major conducting arteries branching from the aortic arch |
| brachiocephalic veins (BRAKE-ee-oh-seh-FALL-ik) | *brach/io* ("arm"); *cephal/o* ("head"); *-ic* (adjective suffix) | vein connecting the azygos vein to veins of the head, neck, shoulder, and arms |

### STUDY TABLE  THE BLOOD AND BLOOD VESSELS (continued)

| Term and Pronunciation | Analysis | Meaning |
|---|---|---|
| capillaries (KAP-ih-layr-ees) | from the Latin word *capillus* ("hair") | the smallest of the blood vessels |
| cholesterol (ko-LESS-tehr-all) | from the Greek words *chole* ("bile") and *stereos* ("stiff") | a fat-soluble steroid alcohol found in animal tissues and in food; consists of both high-density (HDL) and low-density (LDL) varieties |
| conducting arteries (kon-DUCK-ting) | conducting (English word); arteries (from the Latin word *arteria*) | the largest of the arteries and nearest the heart |
| digital veins (DIJ-ih-tuhl) | *digit* (English word meaning "finger" or "toe"); *-al* (adjective suffix) | veins in the fingers and toes |
| elastic arteries (ee-LASS-tik) | *elastic* (English word); arteries (from the Latin word *arteria*) | another term for conducting arteries |
| erythrocytes (er-RITH-ro-sites) | from two Greek words *erythros* ("red"); *kytos* ("cell") | red blood cells; abbreviated RBC |
| femoral veins (FEE-mor-uhl) | from the Latin word *femur* ("thigh") | veins in the legs |
| fibrinogens (fy-BRIHN-o-jens) | from the Latin word *fibra* ("fiber") | one of the three main blood plasma proteins; globulins and albumins are the other two |
| formed elements | common English words | phrase used to refer collectively to the red blood cells, white blood cells, and platelets in the blood |
| globulins (GLAWB-yu-lins) | from the Latin word *globus* ("ball") | one of the three main blood plasma proteins; albumins and fibrinogens are the other two |
| gonadal veins (go-NAD-uhl) | from the Greek word *gone* ("seed") | veins in the reproductive system |
| great cerebral vein (seh-REEB-ruhl) | *cerebr/o* ("brain") | vein of the cranium |
| hemoglobin (hee-mo-GLO-bihn | *hem/o* ("blood"); the Latin word *globus* ("ball") | the protein that gives blood its red color; abbreviated Hb |
| hepatic veins (heh-PAT-ik) | *hepat/o* ("liver"); *-ic* (adjective suffix) | veins that drain the liver |
| immunoglobulins (IM-yu-no-GLOB-yu-lins) | from the Latin words *immunis* ("tax exempt") and *globus* ("ball") | also called antibodies; a common blood protein |
| inferior vena cava (VEE-nah KAV-ah) | from the Latin words *vena* ("vein") and *cavus* ("hollow") | large vein that collects blood from the smaller veins of the lower body |
| internal jugular vein (JUG-yu-lahr) | from the Latin word *jugulum* ("throat") | a vein in the neck that runs alongside the common carotid artery |
| left common carotid artery (kah-ROT-ihd) | from the Greek word *karotides* | one of three major conducting arteries branching from the aortic arch |
| left subclavian artery (SUB-klay-vee-ahn) | *sub-* ("beneath"); *clavian* (adjective related to the clavicle) | one of three major conducting arteries branching from the aortic arch |

## STUDY TABLE THE BLOOD AND BLOOD VESSELS (continued)

| Term and Pronunciation | Analysis | Meaning |
|---|---|---|
| leukocytes (LUKE-o-sytes) | *leuk/o* ("white"); and the Greek word *kytos* ("cell") | white blood cells; abbreviated WBC |
| lipoproteins (lip-o-PRO-teens) | *lip/o* ("fatty"); proteins (common word) | a common blood protein |
| lumbar veins (LUM-bar) | from the Latin word *lumbus* ("loin") | veins in the lower back |
| muscular arteries | muscular (English adjective); arteries (from the Latin word *arteria*) | medium-size arteries that connect the conducting arteries and the arterioles |
| plasma (PLAZ-muh) | from the Latin word *plasticus* ("molded") | as differentiated from its non-medical context, the yellow fluid that makes up a bit more than half of whole blood by volume |
| platelets (PLATE-lets) | from the English word *plate* or the Greek work *platys* ("flat") | smallest of the formed elements; important in the coagulation process |
| renal veins | *ren/o* ("kidney"); -*al* (adjective suffix) | veins in the kidneys |
| right common carotid artery (kah-ROT-ihd) | from the Greek word *karotides* | one of two conducting arteries attached to the brachiocephalic trunk |
| right subclavian artery (SUB-klay-vee-ahn) | *sub-* ("beneath"); *clavian* (adjective related to the clavicle) | one of two conducting arteries attached to the brachiocephalic trunk |
| superior vena cava (VEE-nah KAV-ah) | from the Latin words *vena* ("vein") and *cavus* ("hollow") | large vein that collects blood from the smaller veins of the upper body |
| tibial veins | from the Latin word *tibia* ("shin bone") | veins in the legs |
| venae cavae (VEE-nay KA-vay) | plural form of vena cava | the superior vena cava and the inferior vena cava, taken together |
| veins (VAYNS) | English word | the blood vessels that return blood from the tissues to the heart |
| vertebral veins (VURT-eh-bruhl) | *vertebra* ("spinal column"); -*al* (adjective suffix) | veins flowing from the upper spinal area into the brachiocephalic veins |
| **COMMON DISORDERS** | | |
| aneurysm (AN-yur-iz-um) | from the Greek word *aneurysma* ("dilation") | a localized dilation of an artery, cardiac chamber, or other vessel |
| angiitis (an-jee-EYE-tiss); also called vasculitis | *angi/o* ("vessel"); -*itis* ("inflammation") | inflammation of a vessel |
| angiopathy (an-jee-AWP-uh-thee); also vasculopathy | *ang/io* ("vessel"); -*pathy* ("disease") | any disease of blood vessels |
| angiospasm (AN-jee-o-spaz-uhm) | *angi/o* ("vessel"); -*spasm* ("involuntary muscle contraction") | spasm in blood vessels |

## STUDY TABLE THE BLOOD AND BLOOD VESSELS *(continued)*

| Term and Pronunciation | Analysis | Meaning |
|---|---|---|
| angiostenosis (AN-jee-o-steh-NO-siss) | *angi/o* ("vessel"); *-stenosis* ("narrowing") | narrowing of a blood vessel |
| arteriolitis (ar-TEER-ee-oh-LY-tihs) | *arteriol/o* (the arterioles); *-itis* ("inflammation") | inflammation of an arteriole |
| arteriopathy (ar-teer-ee-OP-ah-thee) | *arteri/o* (artery); *-pathy* ("disease") | any disease of the arteries |
| arteriorrhexis (ar-TEER-ee-oh-REK-sihs) | *arteri/o* (artery); *-rrhexis* ("rupture") | rupture of an artery |
| arteriosclerosis (ar-TEER-ee-o-sklu-RO-sis) | *arteri/o* (artery); *-sclerosis* ("hardening") | hardening of the arteries |
| arteriospasm (ar-TEER-ee-o-spaz-uhm) | *arteri/o* (artery); *-spasm* ("involuntary muscle contraction") | spasm of an artery |
| arteriostenosis (ar-TEER-ee-oh-steh-NO-sihs) | *arteri/o* (artery); *-stenosis* ("narrowing") | narrowing of an artery |
| arteritis (ar-tur-EYE-tihs) | *arteri/o* (artery); *-itis* ("inflammation") | inflammation of an artery or arteries |
| hemolysis (hee-MAWL-ih-sihs) | *hem/o* ("blood"); *-lysis* ("destruction") | change or destruction of red blood cells |
| hemopathy (hee-MAWP-uh-thee) | *hem/o* ("blood"); *-pathy* ("disease") | any disease of the blood |
| hemophilia (hee-mo-FEEL-ee-ya) | *hem/o* ("blood"); *-philia* (from the Greek word *philos*), meaning "love" | congenital disorder affecting the coagulation process |
| hemorrhage (HEM-o-rij) | *hem/o* ("blood"); *-rrhage* ("flow") | discharge of blood |
| hemorrhagic fever (hem-o-RAJ-ik) | *hem/o* ("blood"); *-rrhage* ("flow"); *-ic* (adjective suffix) | category of diseases that include a number of viral diseases, one of which is Ebola fever |
| vasculitis (also angiitis) | *vascul/o* ("vessel"); *-itis* ("inflammation") | inflammation of a vessel |
| vasculopathy (vass-cue-LOP-ah-thee) (also angiopathy) | *vascu/lo* ("vessel"); *-pathy* ("disease") | any disease of blood vessels |
| vasoconstriction (VAZE-o-kon-STRIK-shun) | *vas/o* ("vessel"); *constriction* (English word meaning "narrowing") | narrowing of the arteries |
| vasodilation (VAZE-o-dy-LAY-shun) (also sometimes vasodilatation) | *vas/o* ("vessel"); *dilation* (widening) | the widening of the arteries |
| vasoparalysis (VAZE-o-pah-RAL-ih-sis) | *vas/o* ("vessel"); *paralysis* (immobility) | paralysis of blood vessels |
| vasoparesis (VAZE-o-pah-REE-sis) | *vas/o* ("vessel"); *paresis* ("weakness") | similar to but less severe than vasoparalysis |
| vasospasm (VAYZE-o-spaz-uhm) | *vas/o* ("vessel"); *-spasm* ("involuntary muscle contraction") | spasm in blood vessels (angiospasm) |
| **DIAGNOSIS & TREATMENT** | | |
| angiogram (AN-jee-o-gram) | *angi/o* ("vessel"); *-gram* ("record") | printed record obtained through angiography |
| angiography (an-jee-AWG-ruff-ee) | *angi/o* ("vessel"); *-graphy* ("process of recording") | radiography of a blood vessel after injection of a contrast medium |

## STUDY TABLE THE BLOOD AND BLOOD VESSELS (continued)

| Term and Pronunciation | Analysis | Meaning |
|---|---|---|
| **SURGICAL PROCEDURES** | | |
| angioplasty (AN-jee-o-plass-tee) | angi/o ("vessel"); -plasty ("surgical repair") | surgical repair of a blood vessel |
| angiorrhaphy (an-jee-OR-ah-fee) | angi/o ("vessel"); -rrhaphy ("suturing") | suturing of a vessel |
| angiotomy (an-jee-AWT-uh-mee) | angi/o ("vessel"); -tomy ("cutting into") | incision into a blood vessel |
| arterioplasty (ar-TEER-ee-oh-plass-tee) | arteri/o ("artery"); -plasty ("surgical repair") | surgical repair of an artery |
| arteriorrhaphy (ar-teer-ee-OR-ah-fee) | arteri/o ("artery"); -rrhaphy ("suture") | suturing of an artery |
| arteriotomy (ar-teer-ee-OT-oh-mee) | arteri/o ("artery"); -tomy ("incision") | incision of an artery |
| **ENHANCEMENT TERMS** | | |
| angiogenic (an-jee-o-JENN-ik) | angi/o ("vessel"); -genic ("origin") | originating in a blood vessel |
| angioid (AN-jee-oyd) | angi/o ("vessel"); -oid ("similarity") | resembling blood vessels |
| angina pectoris (an JY-nah-pek-TOR-ihs) | angina from the Latin verb ango ("to press tightly"); pectoris from the Latin word pectus ("breastbone") | pain in the chest (Note: Some believe that angi/o (vessel) is the root of angina; such is probably not the case, since angina once meant "sore throat.") |
| arteriovenous (ar-TEER-ee-o-VANE-uhs) | arteri/o ("artery"); venous (adjectival form of vein) | adjectival form of "arteries and veins" |
| atherosclerosis (ATH-ah-roh-skleh-ROH-sihs) | from the Greek word athere ("gruel"); -sclerosis ("hardening") | the most common form of arteriosclerosis |
| basophil (BAY-soh-fil) | bas/o ("base"); -phil ("love") | a white blood cell with granules that stain with basic dyes |
| eosinophil (ee-oh-SIHN-oh-fil) | eosin (a fluorescent dye); -phil ("love") | a white blood cell that stains with certain dyes |
| hemolytic (hee-mo-LIH-tik) | hem/o ("blood"); -lysis ("destruction") | adjective form of hemolysis |
| lymphocyte (LIM-foh-site) | lymph/o ("lymph"); -cyte ("cell") | a white blood cell formed in lymphatic tissue |
| monocyte (MON-oh-site) | mon/o ("single"); -cyte ("cell") | a relatively large white blood cell |
| neutrophil (NU-troh-fil) | neutr/o ("neutral"); -phil ("love") | a mature white blood cell normally constituting more than half of the total number of leukocytes |
| phagocyte (FAG-oh-site) | phag/o ("eat") -cyte ("cell") | a white blood cell capable of ingesting bacteria and other foreign matter |
| vascular (VASS-cue-lahr) | vascul/o ("vessel"); -ar (adjective suffix) | adjectival form of vessel |
| venous (VEE-nuhs) | ven/o ("vein"); -ous (adjective suffix) | adjectival form of vein |

## ABBREVIATION TABLE

### COMMON ABBREVIATIONS:
**The Blood and Blood Vessels**

| Abbreviation | Meaning |
| --- | --- |
| Hb | hemoglobin |
| HDL | high-density lipoprotein |
| IVC | inferior vena cava |
| LDL | low-density lipoprotein |
| RBC | red blood cells |
| SVC | superior vena cava |
| WBC | white blood cell |

# 🐟 Exercises

## Exercise 9-1 Choosing the Correct Term

Fill in the missing terms to complete the sentences.

1. Arteries carry blood away from the heart through the _Conducting Arteries_, also called the elastic arteries, to the medium-size arteries, sometimes called muscular arteries.

2. Blood then flows to the _Arterioles_, which are the smallest arteries, connecting with the _Capillaries_ which transfer nutrients directly to the body's cells.

3. _Veins_ carry blood back to the heart.

4. The _Superior Vena Cava_ drains blood from the upper body, and the _inferior Vena Cava_ receives blood from the lower body.

5. Cholesterol is delivered to body tissues, including arterial walls, by low-density lipoprotein (LDL), also known as _Bad_ cholesterol.

6. Cholesterol is manufactured in the liver and transported through the _Bloodstream_.

7. High-density lipoprotein (HDL) is known as "good cholesterol" because it returns LDL to the _Liver_ for excretion.

8. Narrowing of artery walls from cholesterol causes _Vaso Constri_ in the vessel.

9. Arteriosclerosis is diagnosed by a radiographic procedure called angiography, and a surgical repair to the vessel called _Angioplasty_ may be carried out.

10. If not repaired, the vessel could become completely blocked, cutting off oxygen to the heart, causing a myocardial infarction, commonly called a _Heart Attack_.

## Exercises

### Exercise 9-2 Converting Nouns to Adjectives

Convert each of the following nouns to its adjective form using one of the following suffixes: -al, -ar, -ous, ic.

| Noun | Adjective |
|---|---|
| 1. artery | _____ |
| 2. vein | _____ |
| 3. vessel | _____ |
| 4. sclerosis | _____ |
| 5. hemolysis | _____ |
| 6. hemorrhage | _____ |
| 7. stenosis | _____ |
| 8. vasospasm | _____ |
| 9. vasculopathy | _____ |
| 10. angina | _____ |

## Exercises

### Exercise 9-3 Matching Terms with Definitions

Place the letter of the definition in the right column in the space next to the matching term in the left column.

| Noun | Definition |
|---|---|
| 1. _____ hemoglobin | A. carries blood back to the heart |
| 2. _____ arteriole | B. the smallest but most numerous of the blood vessels, responsible for transferring nutrients directly to the cells |
| 3. _____ erythrocytes | C. the blood plasma proteins that are also known as antibodies |
| 4. _____ capillary | D. contains muscle tissue and carries blood away from the heart |
| 5. _____ leukocytes | E. the protein that gives blood its red color |
| 6. _____ platelets | F. a large venous vessel that drains blood from the upper body to be transported to the heart |
| 7. _____ immunoglobulin | G. red blood cells |
| 8. _____ vein | H. the smallest of the arteries, connecting with the capillaries |

9. _____ superior vena cava (SVC)

10. _____ artery

11. _____ angiostenosis

12. _____ vasculopathy

13. _____ aneurysm

14. _____ angioplasty

15. _____ HDL

16. _____ angiography

17. _____ LDL

18. _____ arteriosclerosis

19. _____ hemorrhage

20. _____ hemophilia

I. white blood cells

J. a formed element found in whole blood, which is important in the coagulation process

K. surgical repair of a blood vessel

L. discharge of blood

M. a congenital disorder affecting the coagulation process, causing excessive bleeding

N. "hardening" of the arteries

O. the narrowing of a blood vessel

P. a bulge in an artery or a heart chamber

Q. radiography of a blood vessel after injection of a contrast medium

R. any disease of the blood vessels

S. "good cholesterol"; picks up "dead" cholesterol from cells and removes it

T. "bad cholesterol"; delivers cholesterol to the body

# Exercises

## Exercise 9-4 True, False, and Correction

Read each statement, then indicate whether you think it is true or false. If False, fill in the correct answer in the "Correction, if False" box at the right.

| Statement | True | False | Correction, if False |
|---|---|---|---|
| 1. A vein that connects brachiocephalic veins with the superior vena cava is the renal vein. | ___ | ___ | _____ |
| 2. Conducting arteries are the largest of the arteries and nearest the heart. | ___ | ___ | _____ |
| 3. Vasoparalysis is the paralysis of blood vessels. | ___ | ___ | _____ |
| 4. Vasculitis is any disease of blood vessels. | ___ | ___ | _____ |
| 5. Hemopathy is any disease of the blood. | ___ | ___ | _____ |
| 6. Erythrocytes are white blood cells. | ___ | ___ | _____ |
| 7. The vein in the neck that runs alongside the common carotid artery is the vertebral vein. | ___ | ___ | _____ |
| 8. Lumbar veins are in the kidneys. | ___ | ___ | _____ |
| 9. The great cerebral vein is in the cranium. | ___ | ___ | _____ |
| 10. The three main blood plasma proteins include the femorals, globulins, and albumins. | ___ | ___ | _____ |

## Exercises

### Exercise 9-5 Choosing from Options

Choose the term in the right column that correctly completes the sentence.

| Sentence | Origin |
| --- | --- |
| 1. _____ is the inflammation of a vessel. | angiitis; angina pectoris; arteriosclerosis; arteriospasm |
| 2. Hardening of the arteries is referred to as _____. | angiitis; angina pectoris; arteriosclerosis; arteriospasm |
| 3. The phrase _____ means a pain in the chest. | angiitis; angina pectoris; arteriosclerosis; arteriospasm |
| 4. A change in or destruction of red blood cells is known as _____. | hemolysis; hemopathy; hemophilia; hemorrhage |
| 5. _____ is a congenital disorder affecting the coagulation process. | hemolysis; hemopathy; hemophilia; hemorrhage |
| 6. Any disease of the blood may be referred to as _____. | hemolysis; hemopathy; hemophilia; hemorrhage |
| 7. An incision into a blood vessel is called _____. | angiography; angioplasty; angiorrhaphy; angiotomy |
| 8. X-raying a blood vessel after injection of a contrast medium is called _____. | angiography; angioplasty; angiorrhaphy; angiogram |
| 9. _____ is the surgical repair of a blood vessel. | angiography; angioplasty; angiorrhaphy; angiotomy |
| 10. A printed record obtained through angiography is an _____. | angiography; angioplasty; angiorrhaphy; angiogram |

## Exercises

### Exercise 9-6 Misspelled Terms

Check the terms below and correct all misspellings that you find.

| Term | Correction |
| --- | --- |
| 1. angiojenic | _____ |
| 2. anjoid | _____ |
| 3. arteriovenous | _____ |
| 4. capillarys | _____ |
| 5. erythrocites | _____ |
| 6. gobulins | _____ |
| 7. hemolytic | _____ |
| 8. immunogobulins | _____ |
| 9. leukocytes | _____ |

10. platilets          _____
11. tibial veins       _____
12. venos              _____
13. angiostenosys      _____
14. angitis            _____
15. vasseldilation     _____
16. vasoparesis        _____
17. angiotomii         _____
18. angiorhaphy        _____
19. lipoprotenes       _____
20. inferior venae cava _____

# Exercises

## Exercise 9-7 Identifying the Conducting Arteries

Label the conducting arteries on Figure 9-5.

- aortic trunk
- brachiocephalic
- left common carotid
- left subclavian
- pulmonary artery
- right common carotid
- right subclavian

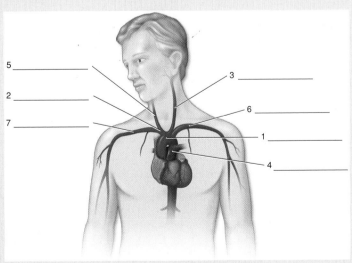

FIGURE 9-5 Identifying the conducting arteries (Exercise 9-7).

## Pre-Quiz Checklist

_____  Study the word roots specific to the blood and blood vessels (Table 9-1).
_____  Review the definitions and etymologies listed in the study table.
_____  Check the exercises with the answers in the Appendix, and consult the review
         table again to correct your errors.
_____  Complete the quiz, and check your answers.

## Chapter Quiz

Write the answers in the spaces provided to the right of each item.

1. What is an aneurysm?                                          1. _____
                                                                   _____
                                                                   _____
                                                                   _____

2. What is vasoconstriction?                                    2. _____
                                                                   _____
                                                                   _____

3. What effect does vasoconstriction have on blood             3. _____
   pressure and why?                                               _____
                                                                   _____

4. What are the three major conducting arteries branching      4. _____
   from the aortic arch?                                           _____
                                                                   _____

5. Name five veins draining into the superior vena cava.       5. _____
                                                                   _____
                                                                   _____
                                                                   _____

6. What are the three formed elements in whole blood?          6. _____
                                                                   _____
                                                                   _____

7. Name the three main classes of blood plasma proteins.       7. _____
                                                                   _____

8. What happens to blood pressure with vasodilation of         8. _____
   arteries and why?                                               _____
                                                                   _____

9. What are the three main types of arteries?                  9. _____
                                                                   _____
                                                                   _____

## ✓ Chapter Quiz  (continued)

10. Name five veins draining into the inferior vena cava.

10. _____
_____
_____

11. What is the medical term for heart attack?

11. _____
_____
_____
_____
_____
_____

12. What does the abbreviation SVC stand for?

12. _____
_____
_____
_____
_____

13. What does the abbreviation Hb stand for?

13. _____

14. Name two possible terms for inflammation of a blood vessel.

14. _____

15. What is the medical name for a person who has a congenital disorder characterized by excessive bleeding?

15. _____

16. Hemorrhagic fever is a category of viral diseases; what two symptoms are suggested by the etymology of the term?

16. _____
_____

17. What word signifies a change in red blood cells?

17. _____

18. Name a common medical disorder that is characterized by pain in the heart or chest pain resulting from sclerotic or narrowed coronary vessels, but that is not a heart attack or MI.

18. _____

19. What is the one-word term for any disease of the blood?

19. _____

20. What is the one-word term for any disease of the blood vessels?

20. _____

## Chapter 10

# The Respiratory System

Y ou have already learned that the heart pumps blood through the circulatory vessels, from which it delivers oxygen and other important nutrients to all parts of the body. For the blood to obtain the oxygen it carries, our lungs must first make it available by extracting it from the air we breathe. That is the job of the respiratory system. Most of the oxygen (98.5%) goes into hemoglobin and the rest is absorbed by plasma. The process has to be continuous because the body's tissues cannot store oxygen. Because the respiratory system is the source of oxygen for the whole body, one can hardly overestimate the importance of keeping it in good working order. In this chapter, you will learn terminology associated with the respiratory system and its common disorders, along with terms that name some of the procedures currently available for diagnosis and treatment.

## WORD ELEMENTS SPECIFIC TO THE RESPIRATORY SYSTEM

The roots and suffixes shown in Table 10-1 are often found in terms related to the respiratory system. You will recognize them in many of the terms you will learn in this chapter.

| TABLE 10-1 | COMMON WORD ELEMENTS RELATED TO THE RESPIRATORY SYSTEM |
|---|---|
| Root or Suffix | Refers to |
| bronchi/o | bronchus |
| laryng/o | larynx |
| nas/o, rhin/o | nose |
| pharyng/o | pharynx |
| phren/o | diaphragm |
| -pnea (suffix) | breathing (a suffix used in such terms as *dyspnea*, which means "difficulty in breathing") |
| pneum/o, pneumon/o, pulmon/o | lung |
| sinus/o | sinus cavity |
| trache/o | trachea |

*Phren/o* is a word root that can signify more than the diaphragm. It may also mean the heart, breast, emotions, instinct (in animals), and even life itself. The fairly common medical adjective *phrenic* can refer either to the mind or the diaphragm. When you have the option, you might choose the adjective *diaphragmatic* instead of *phrenic* when speaking or writing about the diaphragm.

## BREATHING

Our lungs are the biggest of our respiratory organs. Air flows into the lungs through the nose, *nasal passage, pharynx, larynx, trachea,* and *bronchi.* The *diaphragm* also figures prominently in the overall breathing process. The best way to understand the whole system, and thus remember its terminology, is to divide it into two parts: the upper respiratory system and the lower respiratory system (Figure 10-1).

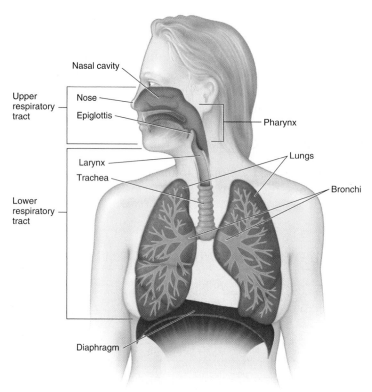

FIGURE **10-1** The respiratory system.

## THE UPPER RESPIRATORY SYSTEM

The upper respiratory system is composed of the nose, nasal cavity, and pharynx, which together act as a series of passageways to move air toward the lungs.

### The Nose

Air that enters through the nose encounters the body's first line of defense against contaminants in the air. Any large particulate matter contained in air entering the nose is filtered out by the hairs inside the nose.

### The Nasal Cavity

The nasal cavity is the second line of defense against any foreign material trying to get into the respiratory system. The mucus that coats the lining of the nasal cavity filters out particles that are too small to be picked up by the hairs in the nose.

Also, incoming air is warmed and moistened as it passes through the nasal cavity, while outgoing air gives up its heat and water vapor. To maintain good health, it is essential to keep the lower respiratory system warm and humidified.

### The Pharynx

Incoming air passes out of the nasal cavity into the pharynx, where it is further purified and filtered to eliminate germs and unwanted chemicals.

## THE LOWER RESPIRATORY SYSTEM

### The Larynx

The larynx marks the beginning of the lower respiratory system. Its job, apart from its other major task of providing us with a means of speech, is to pass the now purified air into the trachea. Along with the *epiglottis,* which is technically part of the digestive system, the larynx also prevents food and drink from entering the trachea.

### The Trachea and Bronchi

The trachea is often called the *windpipe* because air flows through it into the bronchi. Leaving the bronchi, incoming air passes into the lungs. The trachea is a bit more than 4 inches long, and the bronchi start at about shoulder level.

The bronchi become smaller and smaller as they move into the lungs, and both *secondary* (second-order) and *tertiary* (third-order) bronchi are terms you should become familiar with, along with *bronchioles,* which are somewhat like the capillaries in the cardiovascular system. That is, they get smaller and smaller as they extend deeper into the lungs, eventually reaching a diameter of about half a millimeter.

### The Lungs

The right lung looks something like half of a bigger-than-normal football with the tip, called the *apex,* pointing upward and the bottom part, called the *base,* resting on top of the diaphragm. The left lung looks almost the same except for an indentation on its inner side to accommodate the heart.

As air flows deep inside the lungs, it branches off from the bronchioles into tiny passageways and sacs called *alveoli* (singular: *alveolus*). The alveoli contained in the lungs receive oxygen from the air so that it can be picked up by the blood in the capillaries associated with them. Since alveoli occur in other parts of the body, you should use the adjective *pulmonary* when speaking or writing of those in the lungs. The lungs also contain arteries and veins, which are preceded by the adjective *pulmonary* to indicate their location in the lungs (Figure 10-2).

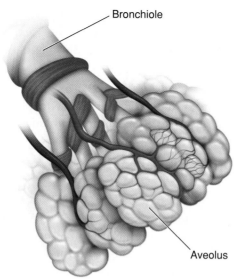

FIGURE **10-2** Location of the bronchioles and alveoli.

## The Diaphragm

Although the diaphragm is located at the very bottom of the respiratory system, it initiates the breathing process. When the diaphragm moves downward, the partial vacuum thus formed draws air into the lungs. When it pushes upward, air is expelled from the lungs.

## ABBREVIATION TABLE

### COMMON ABBREVIATIONS:
### The Respiratory System

| Abbreviation | Meaning |
| --- | --- |
| AARC | American Association for Respiratory Care |
| AART | American Association for Respiratory Therapy |
| AIURT | acute infections of the upper respiratory tract |
| ALR | acute lower respiratory infection |
| CNRD | chronic nonspecific respiratory diseases |
| ERV | expiratory reserve volume (as measured with test equipment) |
| IRV | inspiratory reserve volume (as measured with test equipment) |
| PFT | pulmonary function test |
| RV | residual volume (as measured with test equipment) |
| T&A | tonsils and adenoids (also tonsillectomy and adenoidectomy) |
| TLC | total lung capacity (as measured with test equipment) |
| TV | tidal volume (as measured with test equipment) |
| SOB | shortness of breath |
| COPD | chronic obstructive pulmonary disease |

## DECIPHERING MEDICAL DOCUMENTS

**Read the following excerpt from an admitting statement, and answer the questions that follow.**

*A 68-year-old woman is admitted from her home with acute SOB due to exacerbated COPD, decompensated congestive heart failure, and pneumonia. Taken by the attending physician, her history reveals a former 40-year smoking history, and she is status post–previous stroke with residual dysphagia. During her hospital stay, the patient received intravenous steroids for COPD exacerbation and ALR, diuretics for decompensated CHF, and antibiotics for pneumonia.*

1. What prefix, root, and suffix combine to make up the word *dysphagia*? What does it mean?
2. What is COPD?
3. What is ALR?

## RESPIRATORY SYSTEM DISORDERS AND PROCEDURES

Table 10-2 lists common abnormal respiratory conditions, along with some of the procedures used to diagnose and correct them.

| TABLE 10-2 | COMMON DISORDERS AND PROCEDURES ASSOCIATED WITH THE RESPIRATORY SYSTEM |
|---|---|
| Term | Definition |
| apnea | absence of breathing |
| asthma | a lung disease characterized by reversible inflammation and constriction |
| bronchial pneumonia (also called *bronchopneumonia*) | inflammation of the smaller bronchial tubes |
| bronchiolitis | inflammation of the bronchioles |
| bronchiostenosis (note the difference in meaning between this word and *bronchostenosis*) | narrowing of the bronchial tubes |
| bronchitis | inflammation of the mucous membrane of the bronchial tubes |
| bronchomalacia | degeneration or softening of the bronchi |
| bronchoplasty | surgical repair of a bronchus |
| bronchopneumonia (also called *bronchial pneumonia*) | inflammation of the smaller bronchial tubes |
| bronchorrhaphy | suturing of a bronchus |
| bronchorrhea | excessive mucus production by a bronchus |
| bronchoscope | a device used for visual inspection of the interior of a bronchus |
| bronchoscopy | inspection with a bronchoscope |
| bronchospasm | abnormal contraction of bronchi |
| bronchostenosis (note the difference in meaning between this word and *bronchiostenosis*) | chronic narrowing of a bronchus |
| bronchotomy | incision into a bronchus |
| dyspnea | difficult breathing |

| TABLE 10-2 | COMMON DISORDERS AND PROCEDURES ASSOCIATED WITH THE RESPIRATORY SYSTEM *(continued)* |
|---|---|

| Term | Definition |
|---|---|
| emphysema | condition in which the alveoli are inefficient because of distension |
| laryngectomy | excision of the larynx |
| laryngitis | inflammation of the larynx |
| laryngology | study of the larynx and its abnormalities |
| laryngoplasty | surgical repair of the larynx |
| laryngoscope | instrument with a light at the tip to aid in visual inspection of the larynx |
| laryngoscopy | visual inspection of the larynx with the aid of a laryngoscope |
| laryngospasm | involuntary contraction of the larynx |
| laryngostenosis | a narrowing of the larynx |
| laryngotomy | incision into the larynx |
| pharyngitis | inflammation of the pharynx |
| pharyngocele | a hernia or diverticulum in the pharynx |
| pharyngoplasty | surgical repair of the pharynx |
| pharyngoplegia | paralysis of the pharynx |
| pharyngoscope | instrument with a light at the tip to aid in the visual inspection of the pharynx |
| pharyngoscopy | visual inspection of the pharynx with the aid of a pharyngoscope |
| pharyngospasm | involuntary contraction of the pharynx |
| pharyngostenosis | narrowing of the pharynx |
| pharyngotomy | surgical incision into the pharynx |
| phrenalgia | pain in the diaphragm |
| phrenoplegia | paralysis of the diaphragm |
| pneumolith | calculus in a lung |
| pneumonectomy | removal of pulmonary lobes from a lung |
| pneumonia, pneumonitis | inflammation of a lung caused by infection, chemical inhalation, or trauma |
| pneumonopexy | surgical fixation of a lung |
| pneumonorrhaphy | suturing of a lung |
| pneumonotomy | incision into a lung |
| rhinalgia | pain in the nose |
| rhinitis | inflammation of the inner lining of the nasal cavity |
| rhinodynia | rhinalgia; pain in the nose |
| rhinology | study of the nose and its abnormalities |
| rhinopathy | any disease of the nose |
| rhinoplasty | surgery performed on the nose |
| rhinorrhea | discharge from the rhinal mucous membrane |
| rhinoscope | a small mirror with a thin handle; used in rhinoscopy |
| rhinoscopy | visual inspection of the nasal areas |
| rhinostenosis | narrowing or obstruction occurring in the nasal passages |

| TABLE 10-2 | COMMON DISORDERS AND PROCEDURES ASSOCIATED WITH THE RESPIRATORY SYSTEM *(continued)* |
|------------|------------------------------------------------------------------------------------|

| Term | Definition |
|------|------------|
| rhinotomy | surgical incision into the nose |
| sinusitis | inflammation of the sinuses |
| sinusotomy | incision into a sinus |
| tracheitis | inflammation of the trachea |
| tracheomalacia | softening (degeneration) of tracheal tissue |
| tracheomegaly | abnormal dilation of the trachea |
| tracheoplasty | surgical repair of the trachea |
| tracheorrhagia | hemorrhage of the trachea |
| tracheostenosis | abnormal narrowing of the trachea |
| tracheotomy | incision into the trachea |

Blood tests are commonly used not only as an aid in diagnosing heart attacks, as you learned in Chapter 8, but in determining respiratory disorders. Blood gas analysis can tell the physician whether a patient has an abnormal respiratory condition and is particularly useful in the diagnosis of emphysema, asthma, and other disorders caused by obstructed airways.

## STUDY TABLE  THE RESPIRATORY SYSTEM

| Term and Pronunciation | Analysis | Meaning |
|------------------------|----------|---------|
| **STRUCTURE & FUNCTION** | | |
| alveoli (al-VEE-oh-lee); singular: alveolus | From the Latin word *alveus* ("trough") | small cavities in which oxygen is removed from the air delivered by the bronchioles (Note: Alveoli are also found in other body systems.) |
| apex (AY-pex) | Latin ("tip") | word used to describe the upper tip of each lung |
| base | common English word | word used to describe the bottom of each lung |
| bronchi (BRON-kee); singular: bronchus (BRON-kuss) | Latin ("windpipe") | tubes (right and left) branching off from the trachea and into the lungs |
| bronchiole (BRAWN-kee-ole) | from the Latin word *bronchiolus* ("small windpipe") | very small branches of bronchi that extend into the lungs |
| diaphragm (DY-uh-fram) | from the Greek *diaphragma* ("partition") | muscular partition at the base of the thoracic cavity |
| epiglottis (ep-ih-GLOT-ihs) | *epi-* ("outside"); *glottis* ("opening of the windpipe") | a mucous membrane–covered, leaf-shaped piece of cartilage at the root of the tongue |
| larynx (LAYR-inx) | from a Greek word meaning "larynx" | vocal cords, voice box |

## 📖 STUDY TABLE THE RESPIRATORY SYSTEM *(continued)*

| Term and Pronunciation | Analysis | Meaning |
|---|---|---|
| nasal (NAY-zuhl) | *nas/o* ("nose"); *-al* (adjective suffix) | adjective referring to the nose |
| pharynx (FAYR-inx) | Greek word meaning "throat" | passageway just below the nasal cavity and mouth |
| phrenic (FREN-ik) | *phren/o* ("diaphragm")' *-ic* (adjective suffix) | adjective referring to the diaphragm; synonymous with diaphragmatic |
| pulmonary (PULL-muhn-ayr-ee) | from the Latin word *pulmo* ("lung") | adjective frequently used to modify another term in or associated with the lungs |
| trachea (TRAY-kee-uh) | from the Greek word *tracheia,* meaning "rough" (this usage may have originated because the trachea is composed of cartilage rings) | windpipe |
| **COMMON DISORDERS** | | |
| apnea (APP-nee-uh) | *a-* ("not"); *pnea* ("breathing") | absence of breathing |
| asthma (AZ-mah) | Greek word meaning "breathless" | a lung disease characterized by reversible inflammation and constriction |
| bronchial pneumonia (BRAWN-kee-uhl nu-MO-nee-ah); also called *bronchopneumonia* | *bronch/i/o* ("bronchus"); *-al* (adjective suffix); *pneumon/o* ("lung"); *-ia* ("condition") | inflammation of the smaller bronchial tubes |
| bronchiolitis (brawn-kee-oh-LY-tihs) | *bronchiol* ("bronchiole"); *-itis* ("inflammation") | inflammation of the bronchioles |
| bronchiostenosis (BRAWN-kee-oh-steh-NOH-sis) (Note the difference in meaning between this word and *bronchostenosis.*) | *bronch/i/o* ("bronchus"); *-stenosis* ("narrowing") | narrowing of the bronchial tubes |
| bronchitis (brawn-KY-tihs) | *bronch/i/o* ("bronchus); *-itis* ("inflammation") | inflammation of the mucous membrane of the bronchial tubes |
| bronchomalacia (BRAWN-koh-mah-LAW-she-uh) | *bronch/i/o* ("bronchus"); *-malacia* ("softening") | degeneration or softening of the bronchi |
| bronchopneumonia (BRAWN-koh-nu-MO-nee-uh); also called *bronchial pneumonia* | *bronch/i/o* ("bronchus"); *pneumon/o* ("lung"); *-ia* ("condition") | inflammation of the smaller bronchial tubes |
| bronchorrhea (BRAWN-kor-ee-ah) | *bronch/i/o* ("bronchus"); *-rrhea* ("flow") | excessive mucus production by a bronchus |
| bronchospasm (BRAWN-ko-spaz-uhm) | *bronch/i/o* ("bronchus"); *-spasm* ("involuntary contraction") | abnormal contraction of bronchi |
| bronchostenosis (BRAWN-ko-steh-NO-sihs) (Note the difference in meaning between this word and *bronchiostenosis.*) | *bronch/i/o* ("bronchus"); *-stenosis* ("narrowing") | chronic narrowing of a bronchus |
| dyspnea (DISP-nee-uh) | *dysp-* ("faulty"); *pnea* ("breathing") | difficult breathing |

## STUDY TABLE  THE RESPIRATORY SYSTEM *(continued)*

| Term and Pronunciation | Analysis | Meaning |
|---|---|---|
| emphysema (ehm-fih-SEE-mah) | from a Greek word meaning "inflate" | condition in which the alveoli are inefficient because of distension |
| laryngitis (LAYR-ihn-jy-this) | *laryng/o* ("larynx"); *-itis* ("inflammation") | inflammation of the larynx |
| laryngospasm (lah-RIHN-go-spaz-uhm) | *laryng/o* ("larynx"); *-spasm* ("involuntary contraction") | involuntary contraction of the larynx |
| laryngostenosis (lah-RIHN-go-steh-NO-sihs) | *laryng/o* ("larynx"); *-stenosis* ("narrowing") | a narrowing of the larynx |
| pharyngitis (fair-in-JY-tihs) | *pharyng/o* ("pharynx"); *-itis* ("inflammation") | inflammation of the pharynx |
| pharyngocele (fah-RIHN-go-seel) | *pharyng/o* ("pharynx"); *-cele* ("hernia") | a hernia or diverticulum in the pharynx |
| pharyngoplegia (fah-RIHN-go-PLEE-jee-ah) | *pharyng/o* ("pharynx"); *-plegia* ("paralysis") | paralysis of the pharynx |
| pharyngospasm (fah-RIN-goh-spas-uhm) | *pharyng/o* ("pharynx"); *-spasm* ("involuntary contraction") | involuntary contraction of the pharynx |
| pharyngostenosis (fah-RIN-goh-steh-NO-sihs) | *pharyng/o* ("pharynx"); *-stenosis* ("narrowing") | narrowing of the pharynx |
| phrenalgia (freh-NAL-jee-ah) | *phren/o* ("diaphragm"); *-algia* ("pain") | pain in the diaphragm |
| phrenoplegia (freh-no-PLEE-jee-ah) | *phren/o* ("diaphragm"); *-plegia* ("paralysis") | paralysis of the diaphragm |
| pneumolith (NOO-mo-lith) | *pneum/o* ("lung"); *-lith* ("stone") | calculus in a lung |
| pneumonia (noo-MONE-yah) (synonym for *pneumonitis*) | *pneumon/o* ("lung"); *-ia* ("condition") | inflammation of a lung caused by infection, chemical inhalation, or trauma |
| pneumonitis (noo-mo-NY-tihs) (synonym for *pneumonia*) | *pneumon/o* ("lung"); *-itis* ("inflammation") | inflammation of a lung caused by infection, chemical inhalation, or trauma |
| rhinalgia (ry-NAL-jee-ah) | *rhin/o* ("nose"); *-algia* ("pain") | pain in the nose |
| rhinitis (ry-NY-tihs) | *rhin/o* ("nose"); *-itis* ("inflammation") | inflammation of the inner lining of the nasal cavity |
| rhinodynia (ry-no-DIHN-ee-ah) | *rhin/o* ("nose"); *-dynia* ("pain") | rhinalgia; pain in the nose |
| rhinopathy (ry-NAW-pah-thee) | *rhin/o* ("nose"); *-pathy* ("disease") | any disease of the nose |
| rhinorrhea (ry-no-REE-ah) | *rhin/o* ("nose"); *-rrhea* ("flow") | discharge from the rhinal mucous membrane |
| rhinostenosis (RY-no-steh-NO-siss) | *rhin/o* ("nose"); *-stenosis* ("narrowing") | narrowing or obstruction occurring in the nasal passages |
| sinusitis (sy-nuh-SY-tihs) | from the Latin word *sinus* ("cavity"); *-itis* ("inflammation") | inflammation of the respiratory sinuses |
| tracheitis (tray-kee-EYE-tihs) | *trache/o* ("trachea"); *-itis* ("inflammation") | inflammation of the trachea |
| tracheomalacia (TRAY-kee-o-mah-LAH-she-ah) | *trache/o* ("trachea"); *-malacia* ("softening") | softening (degeneration) of tracheal tissue |

📖 **STUDY TABLE** THE RESPIRATORY SYSTEM *(continued)*

| Term and Pronunciation | Analysis | Meaning |
| --- | --- | --- |
| tracheomegaly (TRAY-kee-oh-MEG-ah-lee) | *trache/o* ("trachea"); *-megaly* ("enlargement") | abnormal dilation of the trachea |
| tracheorrhagia (tray-kee-oh-RAHJ-ee-ah) | *trache/o* ("trachea"); *-rrhagia* ("hemorrhage") | hemorrhage of the trachea |
| tracheostenosis (TRAY-kee-oh-steh-NO-sihs) | *trache/o* ("trachea"); *-stenosis* ("narrowing") | abnormal narrowing of the trachea |
| **DIAGNOSIS & TREATMENT** | | |
| angiogram (AN-jee-o-gram) | *angi/o* ("vessel"); *gram* ("record") | printed record obtained through angiography |
| bronchoscope (BRAWN-ko-skope) | *bronchi/o* ("bronchus"); *-scope* ("view") | a device for visually inspecting the interior of a bronchus |
| bronchoscopy (brawn-KOSS-ko-pee) | *bronchi/o* ("bronchus"); *-scopy* ("viewing") | inspection using a bronchoscope |
| laryngoscope (lah-RIHN-go-skope) | *laryng/o* ("larynx"); *-scope* ("view") | instrument with a light at the tip to aid in visual inspection of the larynx |
| laryngoscopy (LAYR-ihn-GOSS-koh-pee) | *laryng/o* ("larynx"); *-scopy* ("viewing") | visual inspection of the larynx with the aid of a laryngoscope |
| pharyngoscope (fah-RIN-goh-skope) | *pharyng/o* ("pharynx"); *-scope* ("view") | instrument with a light at the tip to aid in the visual inspection of the pharynx |
| pharyngoscopy (FAH-rihn-GAW-skoh-pee) | *pharyng/o* ("pharynx"); *-scopy* ("viewing") | visual inspection of the pharynx with aid of a pharyngoscope |
| rhinoscope (RY-noh-skope) | *rhin/o* ("nose"); *-scope* ("view") | a small mirror with a thin handle; used in rhinoscopy |
| rhinoscopy (ry-NAW-skoh-pee) | *rhin/o* ("nose"); *-scopy* ("viewing") | visual inspection of the nasal areas |
| **SURGICAL PROCEDURES** | | |
| bronchoplasty (BRAWN-koh-plass-tee) | *bronchi/o* ("bronchus"); *-plasty* ("surgical repair") | surgical repair of a bronchus |
| bronchorrhaphy (brawn-KOR-ah-fee) | *bronchi/o* (bronchus"); *-rrhaphy* ("suturing") | suturing of a bronchus |
| bronchotomy (brawn-KAW-tuh-mee) | *bronchi/o* ("bronchus"); *-tomy* ("incision") | incision into a bronchus |
| laryngectomy (LAYR-ehn-JEK-toh-mee) | *laryng/o* ("larynx"); *-ectomy* ("excision") | excision of the larynx |
| laryngoplasty (lah-RIHN-go-plass-tee) | *laryng/o* ("larynx"); *-plasty* ("surgical repair") | surgical repair of the larynx |
| laryngotomy (layr-ihn-GOT-oh-mee) | *laryng/o* ("larynx"); *-tomy* ("incision") | incision into the larynx |
| pharyngoplasty (fah-RIHN-go-plass-tee) | *pharyng/o* ("pharynx"); *-plasty* ("surgical repair") | surgical repair of the pharynx |
| pharyngotomy (FAYR-ihn-GOT-oh-mee) | *pharyng/o* ("pharynx"); *-tomy* ("incision") | surgical incision into the pharynx |

📖 **STUDY TABLE** THE RESPIRATORY SYSTEM *(continued)*

| Term and Pronunciation | Analysis | Meaning |
|---|---|---|
| pneumonectomy (NOO-mo-NEK-toh-mee) | *pneumon/o* ("lung"); *-ectomy* ("excision") | removal of pulmonary lobes from a lung |
| pneumonopexy (NOO-mo-no-pek-see) | *pneumon/o* ("lung"); *-pexy* ("fixation") | surgical fixation of a lung |
| pneumonorrhaphy (noo-mo-NOR-ah-fee) | *pneumon/o* ("lung"); *-rrhaphy* ("suturing") | suturing of a lung |
| pneumonotomy (noo-mo-NOT-ah-mee) | *pneumon/o* ("lung"); *-tomy* ("incision") | incision into a lung |
| rhinoplasty (RY-no-plass-tee) | *rhin/o* ("nose"); *-plasty* ("surgical repair") | surgery performed on the nose |
| rhinotomy (ry-NAW-toh-mee) | *rhin/o* ("nose"); *-tomy* ("incision") | surgical incision into the nose |
| sinusotomy (sy-nuh-SOT-oh-mee) | from the Latin word *sinus* ("cavity"); *-tomy* ("incision") | incision into a sinus |
| tracheoplasty (TRAY-kee-oh-plass-tee) | *trache/o* ("trachea"); *-plasty* ("surgical repair") | surgical repair of the trachea |
| tracheotomy (tray kee-AW-toh-mee) | *trache/o* (trachea"); *-tomy* ("incision") | incision into the trachea for the purpose of restoring airflow to the lungs |
| **PRACTICE & PRACTITIONERS** | | |
| laryngology (LAYR-ihn-GAW-loh-jee) | *laryng/o* ("larynx"); *-logy* ("study") | branch of medical study concerned with the larynx and diagnosis and treatment of its diseases |
| rhinologist (ry-NAW-loh-jist) | *rhin/o* ("nose"); *-logist* ("practitioner") | one who specializes in the study, diagnosis, and treatment of abnormal conditions of the nose |
| rhinology (ry-NAW-loh-jee) | *rhin/o* ("nose"); *-logy* ("study") | branch of medical study concerned with the nose and diagnosis and treatment of its diseases |
| **ENHANCEMENT TERMS** | | |
| atelectasis (at-eh-LEK-tah-sihs) | from the Greek word *ateles* ("incomplete"); *-ectasis* ("extension") | reduction or absence of air in part or all of a lung, resulting in loss of lung volume |
| pertussis (per-TUSS-ihs) | *per-* ("intense"); *tussis* (Latin word for "cough") | an acute infectious inflammation of the larnyx, trachea, and bronchi caused by *Bordetella pertussis* |
| tuberculosis (tu-BURK-yu-loh-sihs) | *tuber* (Latin word for "swelling"); *-osis* ("condition") | disease caused by presence of *Mycobacterium tuberculosis*, most commonly affecting the lungs |

# 🖏 Exercises

## Exercise 10-1 Choosing the Correct Term

Fill in the blanks.

The 1)_____ is responsible for initiating the breathing process. When it moves downward, the partial vacuum created draws air through the 2)_____ and into the 3)_____ where it is filtered, warmed, and humidified. The incoming air then passes through the 4)_____, which filters out yet more impurities, to the 5)_____ or "voice box" and next to the 6)_____ or "windpipe." Air flows through the trachea into the 7)_____, which branches out into tiny 8)_____. The bronchioles pass oxygen to tiny sacs called 9)_____, which then transfer it to the 10)_____.

There are many disease processes that can cause difficulty breathing or 11)_____. To determine the type and extent of respiratory disorders, a common blood test is used, called 12)_____. This test measures the ratio of 13)_____ to 14)_____ in the 15)_____. Typically, the first intervention for an abnormality in this ratio is to administer 16)_____, but other treatments are often required. For example, if narrowing of bronchial tubes or 17)_____ is present, the oxygen administered would still have difficulty reaching the lungs. Therefore, shortness of breath or 18)_____ would still be present, unless other interventions were utilized.

# Exercises

## Exercise 10-2 Converting Nouns to Adjectives

Convert each of the following nouns to an adjectival form using one of the following suffixes: *al, ar, ic.*

| Noun | Adjective Form |
|---|---|
| 1. bronchus | _____ |
| 2. larynx | _____ |
| 3. pharynx | _____ |
| 4. diaphragm | _____ |
| 5. trachea | _____ |
| 6. nose | _____ |
| 7. base | _____ |
| 8. alveolus | _____ |
| 9. apex | _____ |
| 10. stenosis | _____ |
| 11. apnea | _____ |
| 12. dyspnea | _____ |
| 13. asthma | _____ |

# Exercises

## **Exercise 10-3** Matching Terms with Definitions

Match the numbers in Column 1 with the letters in Column 2 according to the corresponding terms and definitions they designate.

| Term | Definition |
|---|---|
| 1. _____ pulmonary alveoli | A. the "indentation" in the right lung that makes way for the heart |
| 2. _____ diaphragm | B. this helps prevent food and drink from entering the trachea, and acts as the "voice box" |
| 3. _____ pulmonary | C. referring to the upper tip of each lung |
| 4. _____ trachea | D. accomplishes the mechanical process of breathing by means of its upward and downward movements |
| 5. _____ cardiac arch | E. tiny "sacs" in the lungs that receive oxygen from the bronchioles and transfer it to the capillaries |
| 6. _____ base | F. the "windpipe"; air flows through it to the bronchi |
| 7. _____ larynx | G. its epithelium purifies air coming from the nasal cavity |
| 8. _____ bronchioles | H. referring to the bottom of each lung |
| 9. _____ apex | I. indicating something in or associated with the lungs |
| 10. _____ pharynx | J. the smallest extensions of the bronchi, which pass air directly to the alveoli |
| 11. _____ emphysema | K. a lung disease characterized by reversible inflammation and constriction |
| 12. _____ bronchitis | L. surgery performed on the nose |
| 13. _____ dyspnea | M. narrowing of a bronchial tube |
| 14. _____ tracheotomy | N. inflammation of the mucous membrane of the bronchial tubes |
| 15. _____ bronchiostenosis | O. inflammation of a lung, caused by infection, chemical inhalation, or trauma |
| 16. _____ apnea | P. inspection using a bronchoscope |
| 17. _____ rhinoplasty | Q. absence of breathing |
| 18. _____ bronchoscope | R. condition in which the alveoli are inefficient due to distension |
| 19. _____ asthma | S. incision into the trachea |
| 20. _____ pneumonia, pneumonitis | T. difficult breathing |

# Exercises

## Exercise 10-4 Building Medical Terms

Build terms to satisfy the following definitions, and then analyze each term by identifying its word elements.

| Definition | Term | Analysis |
|---|---|---|
| 1. inflammation of the bronchioles | _____ | _____ |
|  |  | _____ |
| 2. excessive mucus production by a bronchus | _____ | _____ |
|  |  | _____ |
| 3. muscular partition at the base of the thoracic cavity | _____ | _____ |
|  |  | _____ |
| 4. excision of the larynx | _____ | _____ |
|  |  | _____ |
| 5. hernia or diverticulum in the pharynx | _____ | _____ |
|  |  | _____ |
| 6. pain in the diaphragm | _____ | _____ |
|  |  | _____ |
| 7. paralysis of the diaphragm | _____ | _____ |
|  |  | _____ |
| 8. inflammation of the inner lining of the nasal cavity | _____ | _____ |
|  |  | _____ |
| 9. incision into a sinus | _____ | _____ |
|  |  | _____ |
| 10. surgical repair of the trachea | _____ | _____ |
|  |  | _____ |

## Exercises

### Exercise 10-5 Assembling and Defining Terms

Using the Term Analysis, assemble and define each term.

| Term Analysis | Term | Definition |
|---|---|---|
| 1. a- (not); -pnea (breathing) | _____ | _____ |
| 2. bronchi/o (bronchus); -stenosis (narrowing) | _____ | _____ |
| 3. dys- (faulty or difficult); -pnea | _____ | _____ |
| 4. laryng/o (larynx); -spasm (involuntary contraction) | _____ | _____ |
| 5. pharyng/o (pharynx); -plegia (paralysis) | _____ | _____ |
| 6. pneum/o (lung); -lith (stone) | _____ | _____ |
| 7. rhin/o (nose); -algia (pain) | _____ | _____ |
| 8. rhin/o (nose); -rrhea (flow) | _____ | _____ |
| 9. rhin/o (nose); -stenosis (narrowing) | _____ | _____ |
| 10. trache/o (trachea); -megaly (enlargement) | _____ | _____ |

## Exercises

### Exercise 10-6 Identifying Parts of the Respiratory System

Label the following parts on Figure 10-3.

- bronchi
- diaphragm
- epiglottis
- larynx
- lower respiratory tract
- lungs

- nasal cavity
- nose
- pharynx
- trachea
- upper respiratory tract

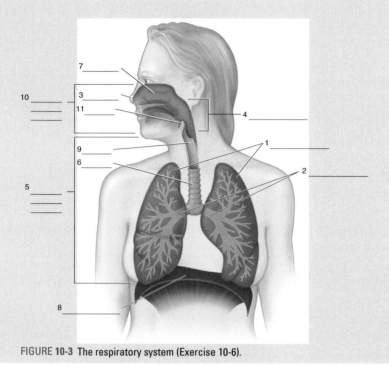

FIGURE **10-3** The respiratory system (Exercise 10-6).

---

☑ **Pre-Quiz Checklist**

_____ Study the word roots specific to the respiratory system listed in Table 10-1.
_____ Carefully review the definitions and etymologies listed in the Study Table to make certain you can define all the terms.
_____ Re-check your answers to the exercises with the answers in the Appendix, paying special attention to any you missed the first time.

## ✓ Chapter Quiz

Write the answers to the following items in the spaces provided to the right.

1. What part of the blood absorbs most of the oxygen from the air we breathe?

1. _____

2. What are the three parts of the upper respiratory system?

2. _____
_____

3. Which part of the respiratory system provides us with the means of speech?

3. _____

4. What keeps us from inhaling food or drink?

4. _____

5. What is bronchiostenosis, and according to its definition, what major symptom might it cause?

5. _____
_____

6. What parts make up the lower respiratory system?

6. _____

7. Where is the diaphragm?

7. _____
_____

8. What is laryngitis?

8. _____
_____

9. Why are the left and right lungs different shapes?

9. _____
_____

10. What characteristic of the body's cells requires the respiratory system to function continuously?

10. _____
_____

11. What respiratory organs are the biggest?

11. _____
_____

12. List terms for the narrowing of each of the following: the larynx, the pharynx, and the trachea.

12. _____
_____
_____

13. Why does laryngitis cause loss of voice?

13. _____
_____

14. What is the name of the disease characterized by the alveoli being inefficient because of distension?

14. _____
_____

15. Explain the difference between bronchiostenosis and bronchostenosis.

15. _____
_____
_____
_____
_____

16. What is a synonym for pneumonia?

16. _____

✓ **Chapter Quiz** *(continued)*

17. Give terms for the surgical repair of the following areas: bronchus, larynx, pharynx, nose, and trachea.

17. _____

_____

_____

_____

_____

18. What is the purpose of a tracheotomy?

18. _____

19. What is a synonym for *bronchial pneumonia*?

19. _____

20. What is the difference between apnea and dyspnea?

20. _____

_____

_____

# The Digestive System

CHAPTER CONTENTS

I n Chapter 9, you learned how blood transports oxygen to all the body's cells. You may also recall that, besides oxygen, the blood transports nutrients to the cells, which use the food we eat as fuel to do all their various jobs. But before that can happen, the food must be converted into a usable form. The digestive system does this job in somewhat the same way that a refinery converts crude oil into special carbon molecules that can fuel a car engine. The difference is that the digestive system's products are proteins, fats, and carbohydrates.

The digestive system may be considered according to the functions of its parts. The first part consists of the muscular apparatus that food travels through to become converted into usable form, and the second includes the various glands and organs that provide the chemicals needed for the process. Like the heart and respiratory system, the digestive system operates continuously.

Since the digestive system is essential in two ways—moving the food we eat through the alimentary canal and providing the chemicals needed for processing it—disorders can affect either function. That is to say, the muscular part of the system can become diseased and malfunction, or the organs that produce the chemicals can fail. This chapter introduces the terms associated with the anatomy and physiology of the digestive system, along with those of its common disorders, diagnostic tests, and treatments.

## WORD ROOTS SPECIFIC TO THE DIGESTIVE SYSTEM

The word roots shown in Table 11-1 are often found in terms related to the digestive system. You will recognize them in many of the terms you will learn in this chapter.

**TABLE 11-1** COMMON WORD ELEMENTS RELATED TO THE DIGESTIVE SYSTEM

| Root or Suffix | Refers to |
|---|---|
| cholecyst/o | gallbladder |
| colon/o | colon |
| duoden/o | duodenum |
| enter/o | small intestine |
| esophag/o | esophagus |
| gastr/o | stomach |
| hepat/o | liver |
| ile/o | ileum |
| jejun/o | jejunum |
| pancreat/o | pancreas |
| phag/o | eating; swallowing |
| sial/o | salivary glands; since the root for gland is *aden/o*, it may be added onto *sial/o*; you will recall that the root *angi/o* refers to vessels, which include salivary ducts, and that may also appear with *sial/o*. |
| -scope | suffix meaning "device for visual examination" |
| -scopy | suffix meaning "visual examination" |

## THE MUSCULAR APPARATUS OF THE DIGESTIVE SYSTEM

Digestion starts in the mouth and proceeds through the *pharynx, esophagus, stomach, small intestine,* and *large intestine.* The "apparatus" as a whole has several names: *alimentary canal, digestive tract,* and *gastrointestinal* (abbreviated GI) *tract* (Figure 11-1).

The operation of the digestive tract has two terms that describe how it moves its contents along from one part to the next. The process begins with swallowing, the technical word for which is *deglutition. Peristalsis,* which refers to the involuntary muscle contractions within the rest of the tract, takes over after we swallow.

### The Pharynx

You encountered the pharynx in the respiratory system (Chapter 10), but the pharynx has "dual citizenship." It belongs to both the respiratory and digestive

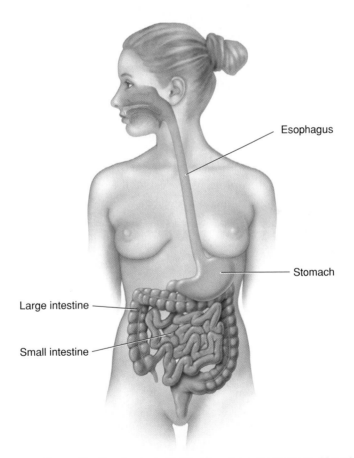

FIGURE **11-1**  The digestive tract. *Modified from:* Cohen BJ, Taylor JJ,  Memmler RL, eds. *Memmler's The Structure and Function of the Human Body.* 8th ed. Baltimore, MD: Lippincott Williams & Wilkins; 2005.

systems because it is a passageway for both air *and* for food and drink. Liquid and chewed (masticated) food enters the pharynx from the oral cavity, and muscular action sends it on to the esophagus.

### The Esophagus

Because the esophagus is about a foot long, it has to get through the diaphragm (Chapter 10) to reach the stomach. It does so by passing through an opening called the *esophageal hiatus* in the diaphragm. That opening is properly part of the diaphragm and not the esophagus, and the term is mentioned here only because of its name.

### The Stomach

The stomach is the center of the system, both physically and functionally. Its four main areas are the *fundus, cardia, body,* and *antrum.* The stomach's first job is to act as a temporary storage place for the food we eat, which allows time for its second job: secreting acid and enzymes to help break down proteins, fats, and carbohydrates. Digestion thus includes not only mechanical changes, such as the reduction of particle size and liquefaction (converting solids to liquids), but also the chemical changes needed to produce fuel for the body's cells. After 3 or 4 hours, the contents of the stomach, which by that stage is a liquid called *chyme* (pronounced kyme), begin to enter the small intestine (Figure 11-2).

### The Small Intestine

Ninety percent of nutrient absorption occurs in the small intestine, and the other 10% occurs in the large intestine.

The first 10 inches of the small intestine is called the *duodenum,* which comes from the Latin word *duodeni,* meaning "twelve each," the reference being to its length

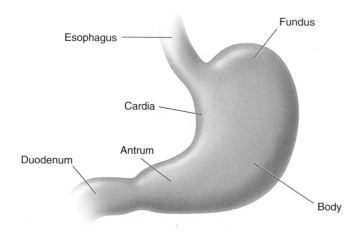

FIGURE **11-2** The stomach.

of 12 finger-breadths. The adjective *duodenal* may already be familiar to you since the phrase *duodenal ulcer* is fairly common. Even though the duodenum is attached to the stomach, a duodenal ulcer is technically a condition of the small intestine.

The segment coming right after the duodenum is the *jejunum,* which is about 8 feet long. That name comes from the Latin word *jejunus,* which means "fasting" (i.e., abstaining from taking in food and thereby becoming empty). The jejunum is the segment from which most nutrients are emptied into the bloodstream. The final segment of the small intestine is called the *ileum,* which is about 12 feet long (Figure 11-3).

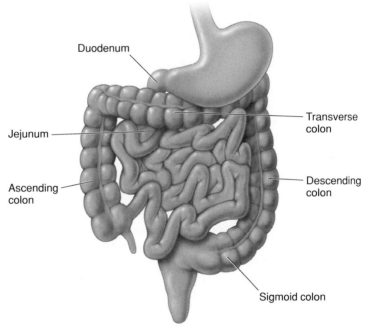

FIGURE **11-3** The small and large intestines. *Modified from:* Cohen BJ, Taylor JJ, Memmler RL, eds. *Memmler's The Structure and Function of the Human Body.* 8th ed. Baltimore, MD: Lippincott Williams & Wilkins; 2005.

### The Large Intestine

Besides absorbing 10% of nutrients, the large intestine compacts waste material for elimination. The term *colon* is sometimes used as a synonym for the large intestine, which can be subdivided into the *ascending colon, transverse colon, descending colon,* and *sigmoid colon* (Figure 11-3).

## OTHER ORGANS OF DIGESTION

To enable the digestive tract to complete its work, many chemicals are needed. Some of these come from the stomach, of course, but they are also supplied by the *salivary glands,* the *pancreas,* the *liver,* and the *gallbladder* (Figure 11-4).

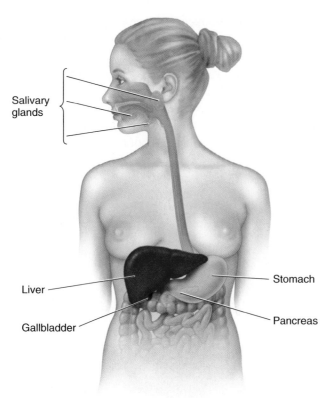

Salivary glands

Liver

Gallbladder

Stomach

Pancreas

FIGURE 11-4 The organs of digestion. *From:* Smeltzer SC, Bare BG, eds. *Brunner & Suddarth's Textbook of Medical-Surgical Nursing.* 9th ed. Philadelphia: Lippincott Williams & Wilkins; 2005.

## The Salivary Glands

As mentioned earlier, digestion starts in the mouth, where it is aided by the *salivary glands*, so-called because they produce saliva. There are three separate pairs of salivary glands, located in different parts of the oral cavity. They are called the *parotid, sublingual,* and *submandibular* salivary glands. Although saliva is more than 99% water, it contains essential enzymes that break down complex carbohydrates. Saliva also contains antibodies that kill bacteria (Figure 11-5).

## The Pancreas

The pancreas acts as both an endocrine and an exocrine gland. The pancreas provides *insulin* directly to the bloodstream (endocrine function) and secretes a fluid containing enzymes into the small intestine (exocrine function) (Figure 11-4). Both of these pancreatic secretions are essential to digestion.

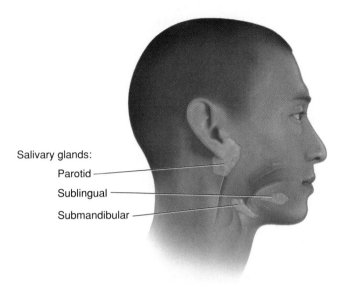

Salivary glands:
   Parotid
   Sublingual
   Submandibular

FIGURE **11-5** The salivary glands. *Modified from:* Cohen BJ, Taylor JJ, Memmler RL, eds. *Memmler's The Structure and Function of the Human Body.* 8th ed. Baltimore, MD: Lippincott Williams & Wilkins; 2005. [AU6]

The adjective *endocrine* indicates that a particular gland's secretions are internal, rather than external; that is, secretions are not expelled through a duct. Glands that do expel their secretions through a duct are called *exocrine* glands. You will learn more about the endocrine system in Chapter 12. Recalling (from Chapter 3) that *endo-* means "inside" and *exo-* means "outside" will help you remember the differences between endocrine and exocrine secretions.

## The Liver

Although nearly all nutrients are absorbed in the small and large intestines, blood from the digestive tract also absorbs some of those nutrients, which are then passed on to the liver. The liver extracts and stores these nutrients for later use. In this way, the liver keeps the body's metabolism balanced and promotes good health by releasing fat-soluble vitamins, such as A and D, when the body needs them.

The liver also produces *bile*, which helps in breaking down the *lipids* (fats) so that they will mix with the other liquids. After bile does its work in the small intestine, it goes back to the liver where it is recycled and used again.

## The Gallbladder

Although the liver produces and recycles bile, the *gallbladder*, which is located in a depression under the liver, stores, condenses, and delivers the bile to the small intestine (Figure 11-4). The gallbladder is also sometimes referred to as the *cholecystis* or *cholecyst*, yielding the word root *cholecyst/o*.

## DISORDERS OF THE MUSCULAR APPARATUS

*Enterology* is the medical specialty concerned with the intestinal tract. Therefore, *enterologists* discover and treat many ailments of the digestive system, including those with names that include *enter/o* as a root. Among those ailments are *enteralgia (enterodynia), enteritis, enterorrhagia, enterospasm,* and *enterostenosis.* By now, you should be able to define those terms without looking them up. The term that encompasses all of them is *enteropathy.*

You might even be able to surmise that an instrument called an *enteroscope* exists, the purpose of which is *enteroscopy,* and that it would be used to diagnose some of the conditions named. By considering the other roots contained in Table 11-1, you should also be able to define terms such as *gastritis* and *gastrocele.*

### 🔖 DECIPHERING MEDICAL DOCUMENTS

**Read the following excerpt from an operative report, and answer the questions that follow.**

*The patient in the oblique position, the scope was advanced without difficulty. Retroflexing the scope in the stomach, a hiatal hernia was noted of moderate size. The scope was advanced to the antrum, which was unremarkable. The second portion of the duodenum appeared normal. The tube was straightened into the straight position. A standard catheter was used and initially I injected the pancreatic duct and filled it to its tail that was unremarkable. There was no filling of any secondary branches.*

1. The antrum is a part of which digestive organ?
2. What is the duodenum?
3. What word in the first sentence tells you what this procedure is?
4. What kind of procedure is it?

## DISORDERS OF THE SALIVARY GLANDS, PANCREAS, AND LIVER

The same conditions that affect other parts of the body can affect glands such as the salivary glands. Therefore, *sialostenosis, sialorrhea,* and *sialography* are terms you can most likely define without looking them up.

 Since the salivaries are glands, the root *aden/o* is sometimes added to *sial/o,* giving us such terms as *sialoadenotomy* and *sialoadenectomy.* The salivaries have ductwork as part of their makeup as well, so you may encounter the term *sialoangiitis,* which means inflammation of a salivary duct.

The general term referring to diseases of the pancreas is *pancreatopathy.* When the pancreas fails to produce insulin in the required amounts, a condition known as *diabetes* occurs. There are many subcategories of this condition, the best known of which is *diabetes mellitus.*

The root *hepat/o* (see Table 11-1) will serve you well in your efforts to decipher liver abnormalities. Simply begin with *hepatopathy,* which includes all abnormal conditions, and then apply your knowledge of the many other suffixes you now know. Likewise, *cholecyst/o* is the root you will encounter in the names of many abnormal gallbladder conditions.

Table 11-2 lists common abnormal conditions and procedures, along with short definitions.

| TABLE 11-2 | COMMON DISORDERS AND PROCEDURES ASSOCIATED WITH THE DIGESTIVE SYSTEM |
|---|---|
| Term | Definition |
| cholecystectomy | excision of the gallbladder |
| cholecystitis | inflammation of the gallbladder |
| cholecystopathy | any disease of the gallbladder |
| cholecystotomy | incision into the gallbladder |
| colectomy | excision of all or part of the colon |
| colitis | inflammation of the colon |
| colonoscope | device used in colonoscopy |
| colonoscopy | visual inspection of the colon with a colonoscope |
| colopexy | fixation of the colon |
| colorrhagia | abnormal discharge from the colon |
| colostomy | surgical establishment of an opening into the colon |
| colotomy | incision into the colon |
| duodenectomy | excision of the duodenum |
| duodenitis | inflammation of the duodenum |
| duodenorrhaphy | suture of the duodenum |
| duodenoscopy | visual inspection of the duodenum with the aid of an endoscope |
| duodenostomy | surgical establishment of an opening in the duodenum |
| duodenotomy | incision of the duodenum |
| enteralgia | abdominal pain |
| enterectomy | excision of part of the intestine |
| enteritis | inflammation of the intestine |
| enterodynia | abdominal pain |
| enterogastritis | inflammation of the intestine and stomach |
| enterohepatitis | inflammation of the intestine and liver |
| enteropathy | any intestinal disease |
| enteropexy | surgical fixation of part of the intestine |
| enterorrhagia | bleeding in the intestinal tract |
| enterorrhaphy | suturing of the intestine |
| enterospasm | painful peristalsis |
| enterostenosis | narrowing within the intestinal tract |
| esophagology | study of the structure and diseases of the esophagus |

**TABLE 11-2** COMMON DISORDERS AND PROCEDURES ASSOCIATED WITH THE DIGESTIVE SYSTEM *(continued)*

| Term | Definition |
| --- | --- |
| gastrectomy | excision of part of the stomach |
| gastritis | inflammation of the stomach |
| gastrocele | hernia of the stomach |
| gastrocolitis | inflammation of the stomach and colon |
| gastroduodenitis | inflammation of the stomach and duodenum |
| gastroenteritis | inflammation of the stomach and intestine |
| hepatitis | inflammation of the liver |
| hepatocele | protrusion of a part of the liver through an adjacent structure |
| hepatopathy | any disease of the liver |
| hepatopexy | fixation of the liver |
| hepatorrhaphy | suturing of the liver |
| hepatorrhexis | rupture of the liver |
| hepatoscopy | examination of the liver |
| ileopexy | surgical fixation of the ileum |
| jejunectomy | excision of all or part of the jejunum |
| jejunitis | inflammation of the jejunum |
| jejunoplasty | surgical repair of the jejunum |
| jejunotomy | incision into the jejunum |
| pancreatalgia | pain in the general area of the pancreas |
| pancreatitis | inflammation of the pancreas |
| pancreatopathy | any disease of the pancreas |
| pancreatotomy | incision into the pancreas |
| sialoadenitis | inflammation of a salivary gland |
| sialoadenectomy | excision of a salivary gland |
| sialoadenotomy | incision of a salivary gland |
| sialoangiitis | inflammation of a salivary duct |
| sialography | radiography of the salivary glands and ducts |
| sialorrhea | excessive production of saliva |
| sialostenosis | an narrowing of a salivary duct |

## 📖 STUDY TABLE THE DIGESTIVE SYSTEM

| Term and Pronunciation | Analysis | Meaning |
|---|---|---|
| **STRUCTURE & FUNCTION** | | |
| alimentary canal (al-ih-MEN-tah-ree) | from the Latin word *alimentum* ("food") | the digestive tract, the gastrointestinal (GI) tract |
| antibody (AN-tih-body) | *anti-* ("against") + body | antibodies contained in saliva that act as antibacterial agents |
| antrum (AN-truhm) | a Latin word meaning "cave" | the part of the stomach nearest the entrance to the duodenum |
| cardia (KAR-dee-uh) | from the Latin adjective *cardiacus,* which is used to refer to the heart or the stomach | the area of the stomach between the fundus and its main body |
| cholecystis (koh-lee-SIHS-tihs); cholecyst (KOH-leh-sihst) | from the two Greek words for "gall" and "bladder" | gallbladder |
| chyme (KYME) | from a Greek word meaning "juice" | name given to the liquefied food entering the duodenum |
| colon (KOH-luhn); also called the *large intestine* | from the Greek word *kolon* | the large intestine, divisible into the ascending, transverse, descending, and sigmoid colons |
| deglutition (dee-glu-TISH-uhn) | from the Latin word *deglutio* ("to swallow") | swallowing |
| duodenal (doo-ODD-eh-nuhl) | *duoden/o* ("duodenum"); *-al* (adjective suffix) | adjective form of duodenum used in the terms naming some digestive system disorders |
| duodenum (doo-ODD-eh-num) | from the Latin word *duodeni* ("twelve") | segment of the small intestine connecting with the stomach |
| esophagus | from the Greek word *oisophagos* ("gullet") | the part of the digestive tract between the pharynx and stomach |
| fundus (FUN-duhs) | Latin for "bottom" | part of the stomach |
| gastric (GAS-trik) | *gastr/o* ("stomach"); *-ic* (adjective suffix) | adjectival form of stomach |
| hepatoid (HEH-pah-toyd) | *hepat/o* ("liver"); *-oid* ("resembling") | resembling the liver |
| ileum (ILL-ee-uhm) | Latin word ("lower part of the abdomen") | the longest segment of the small intestine, which leads into the large intestine |
| intestine (ihn-TESS-tin); the term includes the small intestine and the large intestine, also called the *colon* | from the Latin word *intestinum* ("gut") | the small intestine is divisible into the duodenum, jejunum, and ileum; the large intestine comprises the cecum, colon, rectum, and anus |
| jejunum (jeh-JOO-nuhm) | from the Latin word *jejunus* ("empty") | eight-foot-long segment of the small intestine between the duodenum and the ileum |
| pancreatic (pan-kree-AT-ik) | *pancreat/o* (pancreas"); *-ic* (adjective suffix) | adjective for pancreas |
| salivary glands (SAL-ih-vahr-ee) | adjective for saliva ("spittle") | collectively, the parotid, sublingual, and submandibular salivary glands |

📖 **STUDY TABLE** THE DIGESTIVE SYSTEM (*continued*)

| Term and Pronunciation | Analysis | Meaning |
|---|---|---|
| stomach (STUM-uhk) | from the Latin word *stomachus* ("stomach") | digestive organ composed of four parts: the fundus, the cardia, the body, and the antrum |
| **COMMON DISORDERS** | | |
| cholecystitis (KOH-lee-siss-TY-tiss) | *cholecyst/o* ("gallbladder"); *-itis* ("inflammation") | inflammation of the gallbladder |
| cholecystopathy (KOH-lee-siss-TOP-ah-thee) | *cholecyst/o* ("gallbladder"); *-pathy* ("disease") | any disease of the gallbladder |
| colitis (ko-LY-tihs) | *col/o/n/o* ("colon"); *-itis* ("inflammation") | inflammation of the colon |
| colorrhagia (ko-loh-RAY-jee-uh) | *col/o/n/o* ("colon"); *-rrhagia* ("discharge") | abnormal discharge from the colon |
| diabetes mellitus (dy-ah-BEET-ees meh-LY-tuhs) | from the Greek word *diabetes* ("siphon"); and the Latin word *mellitus* ("sweetened with honey") | a chronic metabolic disease characterized by the body's decreased ability to utilize carbohydrates and its enhanced ability to utilize proteins and lipids |
| duodenitis (doo-odd-eh-NY-tihs) | *duoden/o* ("duodenum"); *-itis* ("inflammation") | inflammation of the duodenum |
| enteralgia (en-teh-RAL-jee-uh); also enterodynia (en-teh-ro-DIN-ee-uh) | *enter/o* ("intestine"); *-algia* or *-dynia* ("pain") | abdominal pain |
| enteritis (ehn-teh-RY-tihs) | *enter/o* ("intestine"); *-itis* ("inflammation") | inflammation of the intestine |
| enterodynia (EN-teh-roh-DIHN-ee-uh) | *enter/o* ("intestine"); *-dynia* ("pain") | abdominal pain |
| enterogastritis (EN-teh-roh-gass-TRY-tihs) | *enter/o* ("intestine"); *gastr/o* ("stomach"); *-itis* ("inflammation") | inflammation of the intestine and stomach |
| enterohepatitis (EN-teh-roh-hep-ah-TY-tihs) | *enter/o* ("intestine"); *hepat/o* ("liver"); *-itis* ("inflammation") | inflammation of the intestine and liver |
| enteropathy (en-tehr-OP-ah-thee) | *enter/o* ("intestine"); *-pathy* ("disease") | any intestinal disease |
| enterorrhagia (en-teh-roh-RAY-jee-ah) | *enter/o* ("intestine"); *-rrhagia* ("discharge") | bleeding in the intestinal tract |
| enterospasm (EN-tehr-oh-spaz-uhm) | *enter/o* ("intestine"); *spasm* ("involuntary contraction") | painful peristalsis |
| enterostenosis (EN-tehr-oh-steh-NO-sihs) | *enter/o* ("intestine"); *stenosis* ("narrowing") | narrowing within the intestinal tract |
| gastritis (gas-TRY-tihs) | *gastr/o* ("stomach"); *-itis* ("inflammation") | inflammation of the stomach |
| gastrocele (GAS-troh-seel) | *gastr/o* ("stomach"); *-cele* ("hernia") | hernia of the stomach |
| gastrocolitis (GAS-troh-koh-LY-tihs) | *gastr/o* ("stomach"); *col/o/n/o* ("colon"); *-itis* ("inflammation") | inflammation of the stomach and colon |
| gastroduodenitis (GAS-troh-doo-oh-deh-NY-tihs) | *gastr/o* ("stomach"); *duoden/o* ("duodenum"); *-itis* ("inflammation") | inflammation of the stomach and duodenum |

## STUDY TABLE THE DIGESTIVE SYSTEM (continued)

| Term and Pronunciation | Analysis | Meaning |
|---|---|---|
| gastroenteritis (GAS-troh-en-teh-RY-tihs) | gastr/o ("stomach"); enter/o ("intestine"); -itis ("inflammation") | inflammation of the stomach and intestine |
| hepatitis (hep-ah-TY-tihs) | hepat/o ("liver"); -itis ("inflammation") | inflammation of the liver |
| hepatocele (HEH-pah-toh-seel) | hepat/o ("liver"); -cele ("protrusion") | protrusion of a part of the liver through an adjacent structure |
| hepatogenic (heh-pah-toh-JEN-ik) | hepat/o ("liver"); -genic ("origin") | originating in the liver |
| hepatopathy (heh-pah-TOP-ah-thee) | hepat/o ("liver"); -pathy ("disease") | any disease of the liver |
| hepatorrhexis (HEP-ah-toh-REK-sihs) | hepat/o ("liver"); -rrhexis ("rupture") | rupture of the liver |
| jejunitis (jeh-joo-NY-tihs) | jejun/o ("jejunum"); -itis ("inflammation") | inflammation of the jejunum |
| pancreatalgia (PAN-kree-ah-TAL-jee-ah) | pancreat/o ("pancreas"); -algia ("pain") | pain in the general area of the pancreas |
| pancreatitis (PAN-kree-ah-TY-tihs) | pancreat/o ("pancreas"); -itis ("inflammation") | inflammation of the pancreas |
| pancreatopathy (PAN-kree-ah-TOP-ah-thee) | pancreat/o ("pancreas"); -pathy ("disease") | any disease of the pancreas |
| sialoadenitis (SY-ah-loh-ah-deh-NY-tihs) | sialoaden/o ("salivary gland"); -itis ("inflammation") | inflammation of a salivary gland |
| sialoangiitis (SY-ah-loh-an-jee-EYE-tihs) | sialoangi/o ("salivary duct"); -itis ("inflammation") | inflammation of a salivary duct |
| sialorrhea (SY-ah-loh-REE-ah) | sial/o ("saliva or salivary glands and ducts"); -rrhea ("flow") | excessive production of saliva |
| sialostenosis (SY-ah-loh-steh-NO-sihs) | sial/o ("saliva or salivary glands and ducts"); -stenosis ("narrowing") | narrowing of a salivary duct |
| **DIAGNOSIS & TREATMENT** | | |
| colonoscope (ko-LAWN-uh-skope) | colon/o ("colon"); -scope ("device used in visual examination") | device used in colonoscopy |
| colonoscopy (ko-luh-NAW-skuh-pee) | colon/o ("colon"); -scope ("visual examination") | visual examination of the colon with a colonoscope |
| duodenoscopy (doo-oh-deh-NOS-kuh-pee) | duoden/o ("duodenum"); -scopy ("visual examination") | visual examination of the duodenum with the aid of an endoscope |
| enteroscope (en-TEHR-oh-skope) | enter/o ("intestine"); -scope ("visual examination") | device for visually examining the intestines |
| enteroscopy (en-tehr-OS-koh-pee) | enter/o ("intestine"); -scopy ("visual examination") | visual examination of the intestines |
| hepatoscopy (he-pah-TOSS-kuh-pee) | hepat/o ("liver"); -scopy ("visual examination") | examination of the liver |
| sialography (sy-ah-LOG-rah-fee) | sial/o ("saliva or salivary glands and ducts"); -graphy ("record") | radiography of salivary glands and ducts |

## STUDY TABLE THE DIGESTIVE SYSTEM (continued)

| Term and Pronunciation | Analysis | Meaning |
| --- | --- | --- |
| **PRACTICE & PRACTITIONERS** | | |
| enterology | *enter/o* ("intestine"); *-logy* ("study") | branch of medical science dealing with the structure and diseases of the intestinal tract |
| gastroenterologist (GAS-troh-en-tehr-OL-oh-jist) | *gastr/o* ("stomach"); *enter/o* ("intestine"); *-logist* ("practitioner") | a specialist in the diagnosis and treatment of digestive system disorders |
| gastroenterology (GAS-troh-en-tehr-OL-oh-jee) | *gastr/o* ("stomach"); *enter/o* ("intestine"); *-logy* ("study of") | the specialty concerned with the digestive system |
| **SURGICAL PROCEDURES** | | |
| cholecystectomy (KOH-lee-siss-TEK-toh-mee) | *cholecyst/o* ("gallbladder"); *-ectomy* ("excision") | excision of the gallbladder |
| cholecystotomy (KOH-lee-siss-TOT-oh-mee) | *cholecyst/o* ("gallbladder"); *-tomy* ("incision") | incision into the gallbladder |
| colectomy (ko-LEK-toh-mee) | *col/o/n/o* ("colon"); *-ectomy* ("excision") | excision of all or part of the colon |
| colopexy (KOH-loh-pehk-see) | *col/o/n/o* ("colon"); *-pexy* ("surgical fixation") | fixation of the colon |
| colostomy (koh-LOSS-tuh-mee) | *col/o/n/o* ("colon"); *-stomy* ("surgical opening") | surgical establishment of an opening into the colon |
| colotomy (ko-LOT-uh-mee) | *col/o/n/o* ("colon"); *-tomy* ("incision") | incision into the colon |
| duodenectomy (doo-oh-deh-NEK-toh-mee) | *duoden/o* ("duodenum"); *-ectomy* ("excision") | excision of the duodenum |
| duodenorrhaphy (doo-oh-deh-NOR-ah-fee) | *duoden/o* ("duodenum"); *-rrhaphy* ("suture") | suture of the duodenum |
| duodenostomy (doo-oh-deh-NOS-toh-mee) | *duoden/o* ("duodenum"); *-stomy* ("surgical opening") | surgical establishment of an opening in the duodenum |
| duodenotomy (doo-oh-deh-NOT-oh-mee) | *duoden/o* ("duodenum"); *-tomy* ("incision") | incision of the duodenum |
| enterectomy (en-teh-REK-toh-mee) | *enter/o* ("intestine"); *-ectomy* ("excision") | excision of part of the intestine |
| enteropexy (EN-teh-roh-pek-see) | *enter/o* ("intestine"); *-pexy* ("surgical fixation") | surgical fixation of part of the intestine |
| enterorrhaphy (en-tehr-OR-ah-fee | *enter/o* ("intestine"); *-rrhaphy* ("suture") | suturing of the intestine |
| gastrectomy (gas-TREK-toh-mee) | *gastr/o* ("stomach"); *-ectomy* ("excision") | excision of part of the stomach |
| hepatopexy (HEH-pah-to-pek-see) | *hepat/o* ("liver"); *-pexy* ("surgical fixation") | fixation of the liver |
| hepatorrhaphy (he-pah-TOR-ah-fee) | *hepat/o* ("liver"); *-rrhaphy* ("suture") | suturing of the liver |
| jejunectomy (jeh-joo-NEK-toh-mee) | *jejun/o* ("jejunum"); *-ectomy* ("excision") | excision of all or part of the jejunum |
| jejunoplasty (jeh-JOON-oh-plass-tee) | *jejun/o* ("jejunum"); *-plasty* ("surgical repair") | surgical repair of the jejunum |

## 📖 STUDY TABLE THE DIGESTIVE SYSTEM (*continued*)

| Term and Pronunciation | Analysis | Meaning |
|---|---|---|
| jejunotomy (jeh-joo-NOT-oh-mee) | *jejun/o* ("jejunum"); *-tomy* ("incision") | incision into the jejunum |
| pancreatotomy (PAN-kree-ah-TOT-ah-mee) | *pancreat/o* ("pancreas"); *-tomy* ("incision") | incision into the pancreas |
| sialoadenectomy (SY-al-oh-ah-deh-NEK-tah-mee) | *sialoaden/o* ("salivary gland"); *-ectomy* ("excision") | excision of a salivary gland |
| sialoadenotomy (SY-al-oh-ah-deh-NOT-ah-mee) | *sialoaden/o* ("salivary gland"); *-tomy* ("incision") | incision of a salivary gland |
| **ENHANCEMENT TERMS** | | |
| cirrhosis (sih-RO-sihs) | from the Greek word *kirrhos* ("yellow"); *-osis* ("condition") | a serious liver condition characterized by diffuse deterioration of hepatic cells |
| diverticulitis (DY-vur-tik-yu-LY-tihs) | from a Latin word *deverticulm* ("side road"); *-itis* ("inflammation") | inflammation of a diverticulum |
| diverticulosis (DY-vur-tik-yu-LOH-sihs | from a Latin word *deverticulm* ("side road"); *-osis* ("condition") | presence of diseased diverticula in the intestine |
| diverticulum (dy-vur-TIK-yu-lum); plural: *diverticula* | from a Latin word *deverticulm* ("side road") | a small pouch or sac leading off the main part of the intestine or bladder |
| ileostomy (ILL-ee-OS-to-mee) | *ile/o* ("ileum"); *-stomy* ("a surgical opening") | a surgical opening into the ileum |
| peristalsis | *peri-* ("around"); *stalsis* (Greek word for "constriction") | involuntary muscular contractions that propel contents forward through the digestive tract |

## ABBREVIATION TABLE

**COMMON ABBREVIATIONS:**
**The Digestive System**

| Abbreviation | Meaning |
|---|---|
| DM | diabetes mellitus |
| GB | gallbladder |
| GBS | gallbladder x-ray series |
| GERD | gastroesophageal reflux disorder |
| GI | gastrointestinal |
| NGT | nasogastric tube |
| S&D | stomach and duodenum |
| UGI | upper gastrointestinal |

# Exercises

## Exercise 11-1 Choosing the Correct Term

Fill in the blanks.

Digestion begins in the mouth and proceeds through the pharynx, 1)_____, 2)_____, 3)_____, and 4)_____. After swallowing (or deglutition), chewed (or masticated) food moves through the GI tract via involuntary muscle contractions, called 5)_____. In the stomach, food is converted to a liquid called 6)_____, as a result of the action of enzymes and acid. It then moves to the 7)_____, where 90% of nutrient absorption occurs, then to the 8)_____ or 9)_____, where the other 10% of absorption occurs and waste material is compacted for elimination.

Several diseases of the intestinal tract can cause inflammation of the colon, which is termed 10)_____. This inflammation can result in ulcerations that, in turn, cause bleeding from the intestinal tract or 11)_____. This condition is often accompanied by painful peristalsis or 12)_____. A specialist in this field, an 13)_____, would determine the extent and location of the disease by visual inspection, using a 14)_____. The disease may be treated medically or surgically, the second option requiring incision into the colon, called a 15)_____ or even removal of part of the colon, called a 16)_____.

# Exercises

## Exercise 11-2 Converting Nouns to Adjectives

Convert each of the following nouns to its adjective form using one of the following suffixes: *al, ic, ary, ive.*

| Noun | Adjective Form |
| --- | --- |
| 1. jejunum | _____ |
| 2. pancreas | _____ |
| 3. esophagus | _____ |
| 4. digestion | _____ |
| 5. enzyme | _____ |
| 6. bile | _____ |
| 7. antrum | _____ |
| 8. intestine | _____ |
| 9. duodenum | _____ |
| 10. saliva | _____ |
| 11. intestine | _____ |

12. diabetes          _____
13. choelcystis       _____
14. colon             _____
15. pancreas          _____

# Exercises

## Exercise 11-3 Matching Terms with Definitions

Match the numbers in Column 1 with the letters in Column 2 according to the corresponding terms and definitions they designate.

| Term | Definition |
|------|------------|
| 1. _____ fundus | A. branch of medicine concerned with the GI tract |
| 2. _____ cholecystis | B. secretion of the pancreas essential in digestion |
| 3. _____ duodenum | C. opening in the diaphragm through which the esophagus passes to get to the stomach |
| 4. _____ lipid | D. the digestive tract |
| 5. _____ alimentary canal | E. name given to the first 10 inches of the small intestine |
| 6. _____ ileum | F. one of the four parts making up the stomach |
| 7. _____ esophageal hiatus | G. the gallbladder |
| 8. _____ enterology | H. the final 12-foot-long segment of the small intestine |
| 9. _____ enzyme | I. to chew |
| 10. _____ masticate | J. a fat-soluble particle |
| 11. _____ hepatitis | K. incision into the jejunum |
| 12. _____ colonoscopy | L. excision of the gallbladder |
| 13. _____ enteralgia | M. inflammation of the liver |
| 14. _____ cholecystitis | N. inflammation of the stomach and intestine |
| 15. _____ cholecystectomy | O. painful peristalsis |
| 16. _____ gastroenteritis | P. surgical establishment of an opening into the colon |
| 17. _____ colostomy | Q. inflammation of the gallbladder |
| 18. _____ sialoangiitis | R. abdominal pain |
| 19. _____ jejunotomy | S. visual inspection of the colon |
| 20. _____ enterospasm | T. inflammation of a salivary duct |

# Exercises

## Exercise 11-4 Multiple Choice

Circle the term in the Choices column that correctly answers each of the following questions.

| Question | Choices |
| --- | --- |
| 1. What is the name of the area of the stomach between the fundus and its main body? | cardia; diaphragm; duodenal |
| 2. What part of the digestive tract is located between the pharynx and stomach? | esophagus; fundus; ileum |
| 3. What is the name of the chronic metabolic disease characterized by the body's decreased ability to utilize carbohydrates and its enhanced ability to utilize proteins and lipids? | cholecystitis; fundus; diabetes mellitus |
| 4. What is the name for a narrowing within the intestinal tract? | enterorrhagia; enterostenosis; enteropathy |
| 5. What is the term that means bleeding in the intestinal tract? | enterorrhagia; enterostenosis; enteropathy |
| 6. What generic term refers to an intestinal disease? | enterorrhagia; enterostenosis; enteropathy |
| 7. What term means hernia of the stomach? | gastritis; gastrocele; gastrocolitis |
| 8. What term means inflammation of the stomach and colon? | gastritis; gastrocele; gastrocolitis |
| 9. What term means inflammation of the stomach? | gastritis; gastrocele; gastrocolitis |
| 10. What term means inflammation of the stomach and intestine? | gastroduodentis; gastroenteritis; sialoangiitis |

# Exercises

## Exercise 11-5 True, False, and Correction

Read each statement, then indicate whether you think it is true or false. Write the correct answer in the "Correction, if False" column for any statements you identify as false.

| Statement | True | False | Correction, if False |
|---|---|---|---|
| 1. The part of the stomach near the entry to the duodenum is called the alimentary canal. | ____ | ____ | _____ |
| 2. Chyme is the term given to the liquefied food entering the duodenum. | ____ | ____ | _____ |
| 3. The word *deglutition*, from the Latin word "deglutio," simply means to swallow. | ____ | ____ | _____ |
| 4. The longest segment of the small intestine that leads into the large intestine is called the jejunum. | ____ | ____ | _____ |
| 5. The digestive organ composed of the fundus, cardia, body, and antrum is called the pancreas. | ____ | ____ | _____ |
| 6. *Colitis* is an abnormal discharge from the colon. | ____ | ____ | _____ |
| 7. The word element "*-itis*" in the word enterohepatitis (inflammation of the intestine and liver) means "liver." | ____ | ____ | _____ |
| 8. Visual examination of the intestines is accomplished with an enteroscope. | ____ | ____ | _____ |
| 9. Excision of part of the intestine is a duodenotomy. | ____ | ____ | _____ |
| 10. Excision of a salivary gland is a sialoadenectomy. | ____ | ____ | _____ |

# Exercises

## Exercise 11-6 Identifying the Parts of the Digestive System

Label the following parts on Figure 11-6.

+ esophagus
+ large intestine
+ small intestine
+ stomach

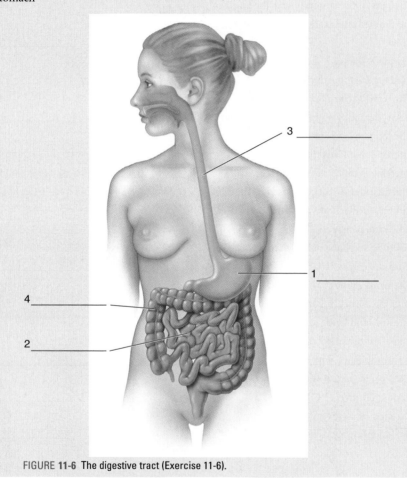

FIGURE **11-6**  The digestive tract (Exercise 11-6).

## ✓ Pre-Quiz Checklist

_____ Study the word roots specific to the digestive system in Table 11-1.
_____ Review the definitions and etymologies listed in the study table.
_____ Be sure you have checked your exercise responses with the answers in the Appendix. Consult the study table again to correct your errors before attempting the quiz.
_____ Review the spelling of the terms *ileum* and *ilium*. Remember that the ileum is part of the small intestine, and the ilium, which you learned in Chapter 6, is one of the three bones fused together to form the hip bone.

## ✓ Chapter Quiz

Write the answers to the following items in the spaces provided to the right.

1. What are the four main areas of the stomach?

1. _____

2. What are the endocrine and exocrine functions of the pancreas?

2. _____

   _____

   _____

   _____

3. Name the three pairs of salivary glands.

3. _____

   _____

   _____

4. What are the major jobs of the liver?

4. _____

   _____

   _____

   _____

   _____

5. Name the three parts of the small intestine.

5. _____

   _____

   _____

6. What does saliva consist of and what is its function?

6. _____

   _____

   _____

   _____

**☑ Chapter Quiz** *(continued)*

7. What is the main function of the gallbladder?

7. _____

_____

_____

_____

_____

8. Name the four segments of the large intestine.

8. _____

_____

_____

_____

9. Which portion of the small intestine empties the majority of nutrients into the bloodstream?

9. _____

_____

10. Describe the functions of the stomach.

10. _____

_____

_____

_____

_____

_____

11. Explain the job of an enterologist.

11. _____

_____

_____

12. What would hepatogenic cancer be referring to?

12. _____

13. Name the term for surgical repair of the jejunum.

13. _____

14. What is diabetes?

14. _____

_____

_____

_____

_____

15. What is enterorrhagia?

15. _____

_____

_____

_____

_____

16. What is the term for removal of all or part of the colon?

16. _____

17. What organ gets removed when one has a cholecystectomy?

17. _____

18. Define duodenotomy.

18. _____

19. What term means "hernia of the stomach"?

19. _____

20. What adjective would you use in naming a stomach ulcer? If the ulcer is in the duodenum, what adjective would you use?

20. _____; _____

Chapter **12**

# The Endocrine System

The cells in our bodies have not one but two ways of communicating with one another. The two communication systems are the *endocrine system* and the *nervous system,* and they work in similar ways. That is to say, both rely on chemicals for the messages they send. The endocrine system is a bit like e-mail or the telephone, while the nervous system is even faster, as you will learn in Chapter 16.

The endocrine system works so well that few people are even aware of it. If you are confronted by a sudden emergency, your brain relays messages to your adrenal glands from your senses, and adrenal secretions make it possible for you to react. However, sometimes the system doesn't work as it's supposed to, and that's why there are *endocrinologists,* practitioners of *endocrinology.*

## WORD ELEMENTS SPECIFIC TO THE ENDOCRINE SYSTEM

The roots and suffixes shown in Table 12-1 are often found in terms related to the endocrine system. You will recognize them in many of the terms you will learn in this chapter.

| TABLE 12-1 | COMMON ROOTS AND SUFFIXES RELATED TO THE ENDOCRINE SYSTEM |
|---|---|
| Root or Suffix | Refers to |
| aden/o | gland |
| adren/o; adrenal/o | adrenal glands |
| endocrin/o | endocrine |
| hypophys/o | pituitary gland |
| parathyr/o; parathyroid/o | parathyroid gland |
| ren/o | kidney |
| thyr/o; thyroid/o | thyroid gland |
| -ine | suffix used in the formation of names of chemical substances |
| -tropin (from the Greek word *trophe*) | suffix meaning "nourishment" or "stimulation" |

## HORMONES AND GLANDS

The endocrine system encompasses hormones and the glands that produce them. However, many endocrine secretions come from glands that belong to other systems. While these so-called "mixed-function" organs are mentioned in the following discussion, this chapter focuses mainly on the four glands that have endocrine functions only. Even among those four endocrine glands, however, two have dual status; they are the *pituitary* and *pineal* glands, both of which also belong to the nervous system. And the *hypothalamus,* another part of the nervous system, is one of the "mixed-function" organs mentioned above. (You will find terminology associated with mixed-function organs, which include the brain, heart, liver, stomach, pancreas, and others, in the chapters dealing with their particular systems.)

Chemically speaking, there are only three kinds of hormones: *amino acid derivatives, peptide hormones,* and *lipid derivatives,* but each can serve a wide variety of purposes. As you already know, the root *aden/o* can refer to any gland in the body. Thus, *adenectomy, adenitis,* and *adenotomy* might mean removal of, inflammation of, or incision of any gland. When referring to a particular gland, use a different root (or include a second one) to clarify which one. For example, use *adrenalitis* to mean inflammation of the adrenal glands and *adenohypophysitis* to mean inflammation of the pituitary gland.

## THE FOUR EXCLUSIVELY ENDOCRINE GLANDS

The glands that have endocrine secretions as their only job are the *pineal gland,* the *pituitary gland,* the *thyroid glands,* and the *adrenal glands.*

The adjective *endocrine* indicates that a particular gland's secretions are internal, rather than external; that is, secretions are not expelled through a duct. Glands that do expel their secretions through a duct are called *exocrine glands.* Perspiration is an example of an exocrine secretion, and *epinephrine,* also known as *adrenaline,* is an example of an endocrine secretion. Figure 12-1 shows the locations of the endocrine glands.

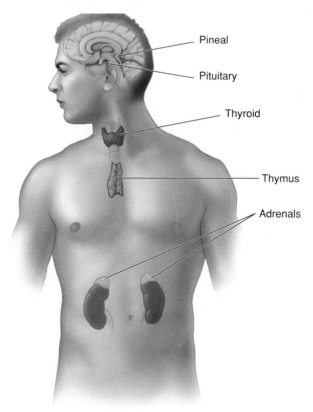

FIGURE **12-1** The endocrine glands.

## The Pineal Gland

The pineal gland (Figure 12-2) secretes the hormone *melatonin.* Studies using animals as subjects indicate that melatonin may have a regulatory effect on the reproductive system. It is also an antioxidant and as such is beneficial. But researchers also think it may be a factor in seasonal affective disorder (SAD), which affects people who live in areas with long, dark winters.

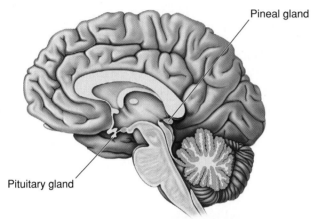

FIGURE **12-2** Location of the pineal and pituitary glands. *From:* Bear MF, Connors BW, Parasido MA. *Neuroscience: Exploring the Brain.* 2nd ed. Philadelphia: Lippincott Williams & Wilkins; 2001.

## The Pituitary Gland

The pituitary gland, also known as the *hypophysis,* is really two glands: the anterior pituitary and the posterior pituitary. The anterior pituitary, also known as the *adenohypophysis,* produces seven different hormones, as shown in Table 12-2.

| TABLE 12-2 ANTERIOR PITUITARY SECRETIONS | | |
|---|---|---|
| Term | Definition | Abbreviation |
| corticotropin | stimulates the adrenal glands | ACTH |
| gonadotropins | | |
|   1. follicle-stimulating hormone | stimulates estrogen production | FSH |
|   2. interstitial cell-stimulating hormone | stimulates testosterone production | ICSH |
|   3. leuteinizing hormone (lutropin) | stimulates ovulation | LH |
| melanocyte-stimulating hormone | stimulates melanin production | MSH |
| prolactin | stimulates milk production | PRL |
| somatotropin | stimulates growth | GH |
| thyrotropin | stimulates the thyroid | TSH |

Glands work together in complex ways. For example, *somatotropin* is secreted only after it receives a growth-releasing hormone from the hypothalamus, which is part of the brain. The somatotropin thus secreted by the anterior pituitary signals the liver to release *somatomedin,* which does the actual job of stimulating growth in the body's cells. In fact, the brain instructs all of the glands when to secrete hormones.

The posterior pituitary gland, or *neurohypophysis,* secretes two very important hormones: *antidiuretic hormone* (ADH) and *oxytocin* (OT). Antidiuretic hormone regulates the amount of electrolytes in extracellular fluid by preventing the kidneys from expelling too much water. Oxytocin helps the muscles in childbirth and in the new mother's milk production process.

### The Thyroid and Parathyroid Glands

The thyroid and parathyroid glands help regulate growth and metabolism (Figure 12-3). The thyroid secretes *thyroxine* ($T_4$) and *triiodothyronine* ($T_3$). Although the thyroid secretes more $T_4$ than $T_3$, it is the $T_3$ that does most of the work of regulating metabolism. Other organs and tissues can, and do, convert $T_4$ to $T_3$ as needed. The thyroid also secretes *calcitonin* (CT), a hormone secreted to prevent too much calcium from absorption into the bones. The parathyroid secretes *parathyroid hormone* (PTH), which also slows the constant calcium loss from bone tissue.

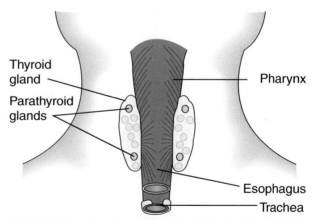

FIGURE **12-3** Location of the thyroid and parathyroid glands. *From: Cohen BJ, Taylor JJ, Memmler RL, eds. Memmler's The Structure and Function of the Human Body.* 8th ed. Baltimore, MD: Lippincott Williams & Wilkins; 2005.

### The Adrenal Glands

The adrenal glands, located at the top of each kidney (Figure 12-4), secrete *epinephrine* and *norepinephrine* whenever the brain indicates that immediate physical action is needed.

Epinephrine is a synonym for *adrenaline,* which is the common term. Norepinephrine is a synonym for *noradrenaline,* which is not as common as its synonym. As you may already know, these two hormones not only increase one's heart rate

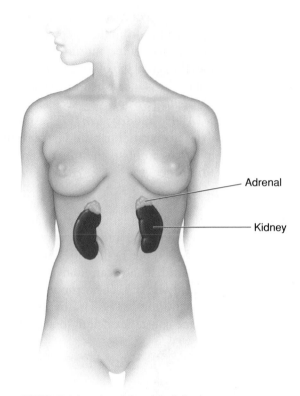

FIGURE 12-4 Location of the adrenal glands.

and blood pressure, they also increase blood sugar and release fats from the tissues. In short, these hormones give the body what it needs for quick action. The adrenal glands also secrete several dozen steroids. These hormones, known as *cortico-steroids,* are essential to life. One of them is called *aldosterone,* which helps the body retain the correct number of sodium ions.

An interesting fact about aldosterone is that its presence stimulates us to prefer salty foods, since salt is, of course, a sodium-based condiment. So the endocrine system not only tells our cells what to do; it also stimulates us to eat foods that contain what the cells need.

## COMMON ENDOCRINE SYSTEM DISORDERS AND PROCEDURES

### Adrenal Gland Disorders

The common disorders of the adrenal glands contain suffixes you have encountered many times in previous chapters and yield terms such as *adrenalectomy, adrenalopathy,* and *adrenalomegaly,* which you can probably define even before viewing Table 12-3.

## Pituitary Gland Disorders

As you learned in the previous chapter, another name for the pituitary gland is the hypophysis. Accordingly, the root *hypophys/o* is used to form terms associated with disorders of the pituitary gland, such as *hypophysectomy* and *hypophysitis.* Any pituitary dysfunction can be simply called *pituitarism. Hypopituitarism* names a condition that inhibits the secretion of pituitary hormones, and *hyperpituitarism* names a condition that leads to the excessive secretion of hormones.

Diabetes mellitus is caused by either the insufficient production of insulin in the pancreas (Type 1) or the failure of the body's cells to absorb glucose (Type 2). Although Type 1 was formerly called *juvenile diabetes* because it usually begins in childhood, it continues throughout life. Type 2 was formerly called *adult-onset diabetes* because it most often occurs in middle life. Both types have essentially the same symptoms, but Type 2 is approximately 10 times more common than Type 1. Often, the term *diabetes mellitus,* whether Type 1 or Type 2, is shortened to *diabetes.* There is another kind of diabetes, however, called *diabetes insipidus,* which results when the posterior pituitary does not produce enough ADH (antidiuretic hormone). However, apart from its connection with the endocrine system and one symptom (frequent urination), it has nothing to do with diabetes mellitus.

## Thyroid Disorders

The term for excision of the parathyroid gland is, as one might expect, *parathyroidectomy,* and *thyromegaly* is the term signifying an enlarged thyroid. Those and other common thyroid disorders are listed in Table 12-3.

| TABLE 12-3 | COMMON ENDOCRINE SYSTEM DISORDERS AND PROCEDURES |
|---|---|
| Term | Definition |
| adenectomy | excision of a gland |
| adenitis | inflammation of a gland |
| adenogenous | originating in a gland |
| adenohypophysitis | inflammation of the anterior pituitary gland |
| adenotomy | incision of a gland |
| adrenalectomy | surgical removal of one or both adrenal glands |
| adrenalitis | inflammation of the adrenal glands |
| adrenalopathy (sometimes also adrenopathy) | any disorder of the adrenal glands |
| adrenomegaly | enlarged adrenal glands |
| goiter | chronic enlargement of the thyroid gland caused by insufficient iodine in the diet |
| hyperglycemia | excessive sugar in the blood |
| hyperpituitarism | excessive hormone secretion by the pituitary gland |

| TABLE 12-3 | COMMON ENDOCRINE SYSTEM DISORDERS AND PROCEDURES *(continued)* |
| --- | --- |
| **Term** | **Definition** |
| hyperthyroidism | condition caused by an overactive thyroid; usually caused by an immune system disorder known as Grave's disease. |
| hypophysectomy | excision of the pituitary gland |
| hypophysitis | inflammation of the pituitary gland |
| hypopituitarism | a condition characterized by inadequate secretion of one or more of the anterior pituitary hormones |
| parathyroidectomy | excision of a parathyroid gland |
| pituitarism | any pituitary dysfunction |
| thyroaplasia | congenital condition characterized by insufficient thyroid secretion |
| thyroidectomy | excision of the thyroid gland |
| thyroiditis | inflammation of the thyroid gland |
| thyromegaly | enlargement of the thyroid gland |
| thyroparathyroidectomy | excision of the thyroid and parathyroid glands |
| thyrotomy | incision of the thyroid |

 **DECIPHERING MEDICAL DOCUMENTS**

**Read the following excerpt from a history and physical examination report, and answer the questions that follow:**

*This is a 78-year-old male with a history of diabetes, hypertension who was found lying on the floor by his wife and EMS was called. The patient was transported to the Emergency Room. On arrival he was confused and combative and had a blood sugar of higher than 600. The patient's initial vital signs were normal. The IV fluids and IV regular insulin were given as well as IV Haldol. The patient is being admitted in the hospital for further evaluation and management. The past medical history is unclear and from the medication list includes hypertension, hypercholesterolemia, Type 2 diabetes mellitus, and osteoarthritis.*

1. Since *hypercholesterolemia* has not been explained in the chapter, analyze the term.
2. What is Type 2 diabetes mellitus?
3. Analyze the term osteoarthritis.
4. What is another word for hypertension?

📖 **STUDY TABLE** THE ENDOCRINE SYSTEM

| Term and Pronunciation | Analysis | Meaning |
|---|---|---|
| **STRUCTURE & FUNCTION** | | |
| adenogenous (ad-eh-NAW-jeh-nuhs) | *aden/o* ("gland"); *-genous* ("producing") | originating in a gland |
| adenohypophysis (AD-eh-noh-hy-POFF-ih-sihs) | *aden/o* ("gland"); *hypophysis* from the Greek word for "undergrowth" (because of its location below the hypothalamus) | the anterior pituitary gland |
| adrenal glands (ah-DREE-nahl) | *ad-* ("near"); *ren/o* ("kidney"); *-al* (adjective suffix) | glands, located one at the top of each kidney |
| adrenaline (ah-DREN-ah-lihn) | *adrenal/o* ("adrenal gland"); *-ine* (suffix often used in the names of chemical substances) | synonym for epinephrine, a powerful stimulant capable of producing a range of effects, such as increases in muscular strength and endurance |
| aldosterone (al-DOSS-teh-rone) | chemical name with an uncertain history | one of the corticosteroids, hormones produced by the adrenal glands |
| amino acid derivatives (ah-MEEN-oh) | *amino-* (a prefix denoting a particular kind of chemical compound) | one of the three chemical classes of hormones |
| antidiuretic hormone (ADH) (AN-tee-dy-uh-RET-ik) | *anti-* ("against"); *di-* ("through"); *-uret* (from *uresis,* "urination"); *-ic* (adjective suffix) | hormone secreted by the posterior pituitary gland to prevent the kidneys from expelling too much water |
| calcitonin (CT) (kal-sih-TOH-nihn) | *calci-* ("calcium"); *-tonin* ("stretching") | hormone secreted by the thyroid to prevent too much calcium from absorption into the bones |
| corticosteroids (KOR-tih-ko-STEHR-oyds) | *cortico* ("cortex"); *steroid* (a particular group of chemical substances, including many hormones) | steroid produced by the cortices of the adrenal glands |
| corticotropin (ACTH) (KOR-tih-ko-TROH-pihn) | *cortico* ("cortex"); *tropin* ("nourishment" or "stimulation") | pituitary secretion that stimulates the adrenal glands |
| endocrine (EN-doh-krin) | *endo-* ("inside"); *crine* from the Greek word *krino* ("to separate") | adjective describing a gland that delivers its secretions directly into extracellular fluid |
| epinephrine (EP-ih-NEFF-rihn) | *epi-* ("around"); *nephr/o* ("kidney"); *-ine* (suffix often used in the names of chemical substances) | synonym for adrenaline, a powerful stimulant capable of producing a range of effects, such as increases in muscular strength and endurance |
| exocrine (EX-oh-krihn) | *exo-* ("outside"); *crine* from the Greek word *krino* ("to separate") | adjective describing a gland that delivers its secretions through a duct onto the skin or other epithelial surface |
| gonadotropin (FSH) (GO-nad-oh-TROH-pin) | *gonad/o* ("gonad"); *-tropin* ("nourishment" or "stimulation") | follicle-stimulating hormone; hormone promoting gonadal growth |

**STUDY TABLE** THE ENDOCRINE SYSTEM *(continued)*

| Term and Pronunciation | Analysis | Meaning |
|---|---|---|
| gonadotropin (ICSH) (GO-nad-oh-TROH-pin) | *gonad/o* ("gonad"); *-tropin* ("nourishment" or "stimulation") | interstitial cell–stimulating hormone; hormone promoting gonadal growth in the male |
| gonadotropin (LH) (GO-nad-oh-TROH-pin) | *gonad/o* ("gonad"); *-tropin* ("nourishment" or "stimulation") | luteinizing hormone; stimulates ovulation |
| hypophysis (hy-POFF-ih-sihs) | from a Greek word meaning "undergrowth" (because of its location below the hypothalamus) | synonym for pituitary gland |
| lipid derivatives (LIH-pihd) | *lipid* from the Greek word *lipos* ("fat") | one of the three chemical classes of hormones |
| melanocyte-stimulating hormone (MSH) (MEL-an-oh-syte) | *melan/o* ("dark color"); *-cyte* from the Greek word *kytos* (meaning "cell") | hormone secreted from the anterior pituitary gland |
| melatonin (mel-ah-TONE-ihn) | no helpful etymology | hormone secreted by the pineal gland |
| neurohypophysis (NUHR-oh-hy-POFF-ih-sihs) | *neur/o* ("nerve"); *hypophysis* (Greek for "undergrowth," because of its location below the hypothalamus) | synonym for posterior pituitary gland |
| noradrenaline (nor-ah-DREN-ah-lihn) | *nor-* (chemical prefix); *adrenal/o* ("adrenal gland"); *-ine* (suffix often used in the names of chemical substances) | synonym for norepinephrine; produced in smaller amounts than adrenaline; has strong vasoconstrictive effects |
| norepinephrine (NOR-ehp-ih-NEFF-rihn) | *nor-* (chemical prefix); *epi-* ("around"); *nephr/o* ("kidney"); *-ine* (suffix often used in the names of chemical substances) | synonym for noradrenaline; produced in smaller amounts than epinephrine; has strong vasoconstrictive effects |
| oxytocin (OT) (ox-ih-TOH-sihn) | from the Greek word *oxytokos* ("swift birth") | hormone secreted by the posterior pituitary gland |
| parathyroid gland (pahr-ah-THY-royd) | *para-* ("adjacent"); *thyr/o* ("shield"); *-oid* ("similar to") | secretes parathyroid hormone (PTH), which slows the loss of calcium from bone |
| parathyroid hormone (PTH) (pahr-ah-THY-royd) | *para-* ("adjacent"); *thyr/o* ("shield"); *-oid* ("similar to"); hormone (from the Greek verb *hormao*, "to set in motion") | a hormone that slows calcium loss from bones |
| peptide hormones (PEP-tyde) | peptide (chemical term derived from the Greek adjective *peptos*, meaning "digested") | one of the three chemical classes of hormones |
| pineal gland (PIHN-ee-ahl) | from the Latin word *pineus*, meaning "pine" ("shaped like a pine cone"); *-al* (adjective suffix) | gland that secretes melatonin, an antioxidant that is otherwise not well understood |
| pituitary gland (pih-TOO-ih-tahr-ee) | from the Latin word *pituita* ("phlegm") | synonym for hypophysis |
| prolactin (PRL) (pro-LAK-tihn) | *pro-* ("before"); *lactin* ("milk") | a secretion of the anterior pituitary gland |

📖 **STUDY TABLE** THE ENDOCRINE SYSTEM (*continued*)

| Term and Pronunciation | Analysis | Meaning |
|---|---|---|
| somatotropin (SO-mah-toh-TROH-pihn) | *somat/o* ("body"); *-tropin* ("nourishment" or "stimulation") | hormone secreted by the anterior pituitary gland to signal the liver to secrete somatomedin, which stimulates growth |
| suprarenal glands (SOO-prah-REEN-ahl) | *supra-* ("above"); *ren/o* ("kidney"); *-al* (adjective suffix) | another name for the adrenal glands |
| thyroid gland (THY-royd) | from the Greek word *thyreoeides* ("shield"); *-oid* ("similar to") | one of the four glands belonging solely to the endocrine system; located in the throat area |
| thyrotropin (TSH) (thy-ROT-roh-pihn) | *thyr/o* ("thyroid gland"); *-tropin* ("nourishment" or "stimulation") | thyroid-stimulating hormone |
| thyroxine ($T_4$) (thy-ROK-sihn) | *thyr/o* ("thyroid gland"); *-ine* (chemical suffix) | a secretion of the thyroid gland |
| triiodothyronine ($T_3$) (try-EYE-oh-doh-THY-roh-neen) | *tri-* ("three"); *iod/o* ("iodine;") *thyr/o* ("thyroid gland"); *-ine* (chemical suffix) | another secretion of the thyroid gland, which is often synthesized from thyroxine ($T_4$) by bodily organs |
| **COMMON DISORDERS** | | |
| adenitis (ad-eh-NY-tihs) | *aden/o* ("gland"); *-itis* ("inflammation") | inflammation of a gland |
| adenohypophysitis (AD-eh-noh-hy-poff-ih-SY-tihs) | *aden/o* ("gland"); *hypophysis* from the Greek word for "undergrowth" (because of its location below the hypothalamus); *-itis* ("inflammation") | inflammation of the hypophysis |
| adrenalitis (ah-dree-nah-LY-tiss) | *adrenal/o* ("adrenal gland"); *-itis* ("inflammation") | inflammation of an adrenal gland |
| adrenalopathy (ah-dree-nah-LOP-ah-thee); sometimes also adrenopathy (ah-dree-NOP-ah-thee) | *adrenal/o* ("adrenal gland"); *-pathy* ("disease") | any disease of the adrenal glands |
| adrenomegaly (ah-dree-noh-MEG-ah-lee) | *adren/o* ("adrenal gland"); *-megaly* ("enlargement") | enlargement of the adrenal glands |
| diabetes insipidus (DY-ah-BEET-ehs ihn-SIP-ih-duhs) | from the Greek word *diabetes* ("siphon"); from the Latin word *insipidus* ("tasteless") | condition brought about by the posterior pituitary's failure to produce enough ADH (antidiuretic hormone) |
| diabetes mellitus, Type 1 and Type 2 (DY-ah-BEET-ehs meh-LY-tuhs) | from the Greek word *diabetes* ("siphon"); from the Latin word *mellitus* ("honey") | condition brought about by insufficient production of insulin in the pancreas (Type 1) or the failure of the body's cells to absorb glucose (Type 2) |
| goiter (GOY-tuhr) | from the Latin word *guttur* ("throat") | chronic enlargement of the thyroid gland |
| hyperglycemia (hy-puhr-gly-SEEM-ee-ah) | *hyper-* ("greater or above"); *glyc/o* ("sugar"); *-emia* ("blood") | excessive sugar in the blood |

📖 **STUDY TABLE** THE ENDOCRINE SYSTEM *(continued)*

| Term and Pronunciation | Analysis | Meaning |
|---|---|---|
| hyperpituitarism (HY-puhr-pih-TOO-iht-ahr-izm) | *hyper-* ("greater or above"); *pituitary* from the Latin word *pituita* ("phlegm"); *-ism* ("condition") | excessive hormone secretion by the pituitary gland |
| hyperthyroidism (HY-puhr-THY-royd-izm) | *hyper-* ("greater or above"); *thyroid/o* ("thyroid gland"); *-ism* ("condition") | condition caused by an overactive thyroid; usually caused by an immune system disorder known as Graves disease |
| hypophysitis (hy-poh-fih-SY-tihs) | *hypophys/o* ("hypophysis"); *-itis* ("inflammation") | inflammation of the pituitary gland |
| hypopituitarism (hy-poh-pih-TOO-ih-tahr-izm) | *hypo-* ("less or below"); *pituitary* from the Latin word *pituita* ("phlegm"); *-ism* ("condition") | condition of diminished hormone secretion from the anterior pituitary gland |
| pituitarism (pih-TOO-iht-ahr-izm) | *pituitary* from the Latin word *pituita* ("phlegm"); *-ism* ("condition") | any pituitary dysfunction |
| thyroaplasia (THY-roh-a-PLAY-zee-ah) | *thyr/o* ("thyroid gland"); *-aplasia* ("deficiency") | congenital condition characterized by low thyroid output |
| thyroiditis (thy-roy-DY-tihs) | *thyroid/o* ("thyroid gland"); *-itis* ("inflammation") | inflammation of the thyroid gland |
| thyromegaly (thy-roh-MEG-ah lee) | *thyr/o* ("thyroid gland"); *-megaly* ("enlargement") | enlargement of the thyroid gland |
| **PRACTICE & PRACTITIONERS** | | |
| endocrinologist (en-do-krih-NOL-oh-jist) endocrinology | *endo-* ("inside;") *crin/o* from the Greek word *krino* ("to separate"); *-logist* ("practitioner") | medical specialist in endocrinology |
| endocrinology | *endo-* ("inside;") *crin/o* from the Greek word *krino* ("to separate"); *-logy* ("study") | medical specialty of the endocrine system |
| **SURGICAL PROCEDURES** | | |
| adenectomy (ad-eh-NEK-toh-mee) | *aden/o* ("gland"); *-ectomy* ("excision") | excision of a gland |
| adenotomy (ad-eh-NOT-oh-mee) | *aden/o* ("gland"); *-tomy* ("incision") | incision of a gland |
| adrenalectomy (ah-dree-nah-LEK-toh-mee) | *adrenal/o* ("adrenal gland"); *-ectomy* ("excision") | surgical removal of one or both adrenal glands |
| hypophysectomy (HY-poh-fih-SEK-toh-mee) | *hypophys/o* ("hypophysis"); *-ectomy* ("excision") | surgical removal of the hypophysis (pituitary gland) |
| parathyroidectomy (PAHR-ah-thy-royd-EK-toh-mee) | *parathyroid/o* ("parathyroid gland"); *-ectomy* ("excision") | surgical excision of the parathyroid gland |
| thyroidectomy (THY-royd-EK-toh-mee) | *thyroid/o* ("thyroid gland"); *-ectomy* ("excision") | excision of the thyroid gland |
| thyroparathyroidectomy (THY-roh-pehr-ah-THY-roy-DEK-toh-mee) | *thyr/o* ("thyroid gland"); *parathyroid/o* ("parathyroid gland"); *-ectomy* ("excision") | excision of the thyroid and parathyroid glands |
| thyrotomy (thy-ROT-oh-mee) | *thyr/o* ("thyroid gland"); *-tomy* ("incision") | surgery performed on the thyroid gland |

## STUDY TABLE THE ENDOCRINE SYSTEM (continued)

| Term and Pronunciation | Analysis | Meaning |
|---|---|---|
| **ENHANCEMENT TERMS** | | |
| Addison (or Addison's) disease | named for its discoverer, Thomas Addison, an English physician | a disorder characterized by a failure of the adrenal glands to produce hydrocortisone and, in some cases, aldosterone |
| Cushing (or Cushing's) syndrome | named for its discoverer, Harvey Cushing, an American physician | a hormonal disorder caused by too much hydrocortisone |
| Graves (or Graves') disease | named for its discoverer, Robert Graves, an Irish physician | a common form of hyperthyroidism resulting from overproduction of thyroxine; caused by a false immune system response |
| hydrocortisone (hy-droh-KOR-tih-sone) | *hydr/o* ("watery"); *cortisone* (chemical name) | an adrenal gland hormone secretion |

## ABBREVIATION TABLE

### COMMON ABBREVIATIONS:
**The Endocrine System**

| Abbreviation | Meaning |
|---|---|
| ACTH | corticotrophin |
| ADH | antidiuretic hormone |
| BS | blood sugar |
| DM | diabetes mellitus |
| FBS | fasting blood sugar |
| FSH | follicle-stimulating hormone |
| GH | growth hormone |
| ICSH | interstitial cell–stimulating hormone |
| IDDM | insulin-dependent diabetes mellitus (Type 1) |
| LH | leuteinizing hormone |
| MSH | melanocyte-stimulating hormone |
| NIDDM | non–insulin-dependent diabetes mellitus (Type 2) |
| PRL | prolactin |
| TSH | thyrotropin |

# ✏ Exercises

## Exercise 12-1 Choosing the Correct Term
Fill in the blanks.

The pineal gland secretes melatonin, which may be a factor in SAD, which stands for 1)_____ .
The pituitary gland, also called the 2)_____, is actually two glands: the 3)_____
pituitary, also known as the 4)_____, and the posterior pituitary or 5)_____ .
The thyroid and parathyroid glands help regulate growth and metabolism. The adrenal glands, also called the
6)_____ glands, are located at the top of each 7)_____ and
secrete 8)_____ and 9)_____ whenever the brain tells the body to get ready for
physical action. The adrenal glands also secrete several steroids.

Adenitis refers to 10)_____ of any 11)_____. However, if a particular gland is
meant, a different root is used to clarify which one. Inflammation of the pituitary gland is called 12)_____,
and inflammation of the adrenal glands, pituitary gland, and thyroid gland are as follows: 13)_____,
14)_____, and 15)_____ .

# Exercises

## Exercise 12-2 Converting Nouns to Adjectives
Convert each of the following nouns to its adjective form using one of the
following suffixes: *al, ic.*

| Noun | Adjective Form |
| --- | --- |
| 1. adrenaline | _____ |
| 2. hypothalamus | _____ |
| 3. hormone | _____ |
| 4. steroid | _____ |
| 5. diuresis | _____ |
| 6. gland | _____ |

# Exercises

## Exercise 12-3 Matching Terms with Definitions

Match the numbers in Column 1 with the letters in Column 2 according to the corresponding terms and definitions they designate.

|  | Term | Definition |
|---|---|---|
| 1. \_\_\_\_\_ gonadotropin (FSH) | | A. synonym for epinephrine, which is an adrenal hormone secreted when immediate physical action may be needed by the body |
| 2. \_\_\_\_\_ melatonin | | B. thyroid-stimulating hormone, secreted by the anterior pituitary |
| 3. \_\_\_\_\_ adenogenous | | C. one of the corticosteroids produced by the adrenal glands, which helps the body retain the correct amount of sodium ions |
| 4. \_\_\_\_\_ antidiuretic hormone | | D. an anterior pituitary hormone that stimulates estrogen production |
| 5. \_\_\_\_\_ adrenalin | | E. synonym for pituitary gland |
| 6. \_\_\_\_\_ hypophysis | | F. hormone secreted by the thyroid to prevent excessive calcium absorption into the bones |
| 7. \_\_\_\_\_ calcitonin | | G. originating in a gland |
| 8. \_\_\_\_\_ aldosterone | | H. pineal gland hormone, which is an antioxidant |
| 9. \_\_\_\_\_ parathyroid gland | | I. hormone secreted by the posterior pituitary to prevent the kidneys from expelling too much water |
| 10. \_\_\_\_\_ thyrotropin (TSH) | | J. secretes PTH (parathyroid hormone), which slows the loss of calcium from bone |
| 11. \_\_\_\_\_ thyromegaly | | K. disease of the adrenal glands |
| 12. \_\_\_\_\_ adenohypophysitis | | L. condition of diminished hormone secretion from the anterior pituitary gland |
| 13. \_\_\_\_\_ goiter | | M. originating in a gland |
| 14. \_\_\_\_\_ pituitarism | | N. inflammation of the anterior pituitary gland |
| 15. \_\_\_\_\_ thyroparathyroidectomy | | O. chronic enlargement of the thyroid, caused by insufficient iodine in the diet |
| 16. \_\_\_\_\_ adenogenous | | P. excessive pituitary secretion |
| 17. \_\_\_\_\_ adrenalopathy | | Q. enlargement of the thyroid gland |
| 18. \_\_\_\_\_ hypopituitarism | | R. excision of a gland |
| 19. \_\_\_\_\_ adenectomy | | S. any pituitary dysfunction |
| 20. \_\_\_\_\_ hyperpituitarism | | T. excision of the thyroid and parathyroid glands |

# Exercises

## Exercise 12-4 Identifying the Parts of the Endocrine System

Label the following endocrine glands on Figure 12-5.

* adrenal
* pineal
* pituitary
* thyroid

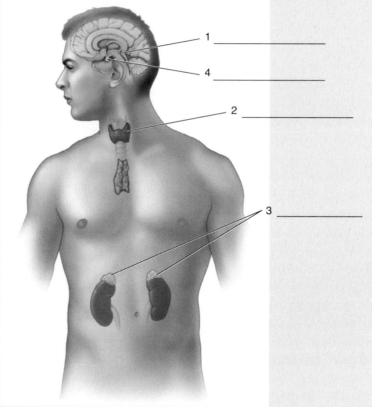

1 _____

4 _____

2 _____

3 _____

FIGURE **12-5** Identifying parts of the endocrine system (Exercise 12-4).

# Exercises

## Exercise 12-5 Abbreviations for the Pituitary Hormones

Write the abbreviation for each of the hormones below:

| Hormone | Function | Abbreviation |
|---|---|---|
| 1. somatotropin | stimulates growth | _____ |
| 2. thyrotropin | stimulates the thyroid | _____ |
| 3. corticotropin | stimulates the adrenal glands | _____ |
| 4. gonadotropin | stimulates estrogen production | _____ |
| 5. gonadotropin | stimulates testosterone production | _____ |
| 6. gonadotropin | stimulates ovulation | _____ |
| 7. prolactin | stimulates milk production | _____ |
| 8. melanocyte-stimulating hormone | stimulates melanin production | _____ |

# Exercises

## Exercise 12-6 Building Medical Terms

Build terms to satisfy the following definitions, and then analyze each term by identifying its word elements.

| Definition | Term | Analysis |
|---|---|---|
| 1. anterior pituitary gland | _____ | _____ |
| | | _____ |
| | | _____ |
| 2. inflammation of the hypophysis | _____ | _____ |
| | | _____ |
| | | _____ |
| 3. medical specialty of the endocrine system | _____ | _____ |
| | | _____ |
| | | _____ |
| 4. hormone secreted by the posterior pituitary gland to prevent the kidneys from expelling too much water | _____ | _____ |
| | | _____ |
| | | _____ |
| 5. synonym for adrenaline, a powerful stimulant capable of producing a range of effects, such as increases in muscular strength and endurance | _____ | _____ |
| | | _____ |
| | | _____ |

| Definition | Term | Analysis |
|---|---|---|
| 6. excessive hormone secretion by the pituitary gland | _____ | _____ _____ _____ |
| 7. surgical removal of one or both adrenal glands | _____ | _____ _____ _____ |
| 8. excision of the thyroid and parathyroid glands | _____ | _____ _____ _____ |
| 9. hormone secreted by the posterior pituitary gland | _____ | _____ _____ _____ |
| 10. congenital condition characterized by low thyroid output | _____ | _____ _____ _____ _____ |

# Exercises

## Exercise 12-7 Assembling and Defining Terms
Using the Term Analysis, assemble and define each term.

| Term Analysis | Term | Definition |
|---|---|---|
| 1. ad- (near); ren/o (kidney); -al (adjective suffix) | _____ | _____ _____ _____ |
| 2. cortico (cortex); steroid (a particular group of chemical substances, including many hormones | _____ | _____ _____ _____ |
| 3. gonad/o (gonad); -tropin (nourishment or stimulation) | _____ | _____ _____ |
| 4. adrenal/o (adrenal gland); -megaly (enlargement) | _____ | _____ _____ _____ |

| Term Analysis | Term | Definition |
|---|---|---|
| 5. hypo- (less or below); pituitary from the Latin word *pituita* (phlegm); -ism (condition) | _____ | _____ |
| 6. endo- (inside); crin/o from the Greek word *krino*, to separate; -logist (practitioner) | _____ | _____ |
| 7. tri- (three); iod/o (iodine); thry/o (thyroid gland); -ine (chemical suffix | _____ | _____ |
| 8. aden/o (gland); -ectomy (excision) | _____ | _____ |
| 9. thyr/o (thyroid gland); -megaly (enlargement) | _____ | _____ |
| 10. thyr/o (thyroid gland); -tomy | _____ | _____ |

## ✓ Pre-Quiz Checklist

_____  Study the word roots specific to the endocrine system (Table 12-1).
_____  Review the definitions and etymologies listed in the study table.
_____  Check the exercises with the answers in the Appendix and consult the review table again to correct your errors.
_____  Review the abbreviations table.

☑ **Chapter Quiz**

Write the answers to the following items in the spaces provided.

1. What are the human body's two "communication systems"?

   1. _____
   _____
   _____
   _____

2. Describe the difference between exocrine and endocrine glands.

   2. _____
   _____
   _____
   _____
   _____
   _____

3. Name the three types of hormones.

   3. _____
   _____
   _____

4. What are the four "exclusively" endocrine glands?

   4. _____
   _____
   _____

5. List the seven anterior pituitary hormones.

   5. _____
   _____
   _____
   _____
   _____
   _____
   _____

6. What hormones does the thyroid secrete and what are their functions?

   6. _____
   _____
   _____
   _____

7. Name one steroidal hormone secreted by the adrenal glands and describe its function.

   7. _____
   _____
   _____
   _____

8. Why are the adrenal glands sometimes called the suprarenal glands?

   8. _____
   _____

9. Which two important hormones does the pituitary gland secrete, and what are their functions?

   9. _____
   _____
   _____
   _____

## ✓ Chapter Quiz *(continued)*

10. What seasonal disease is thought to be associated with melatonin?

10. _____

11. List the terms that describe surgical removal of each of the following: a) any gland, b) the adrenal gland, c) the pituitary gland, d) the parathyroid gland, e) the thyroid gland, f) both the thyroid and parathyroid glands.

11. _____
_____
_____
_____
_____
_____

12. What is a goiter?

12. _____
_____
_____

13. What term is used to describe a disease process that is caused by a glandular dysfunction?.

13. _____

14. Name a medical specialist who treats glandular problems.

14. _____

15. Explain thyroaplasia.

15. _____
_____
_____

16. What is adrenomegaly?

16. _____

17. What term describes an excessive secretion of the pituitary gland?

17. _____

18. What is Graves disease?

18. _____
_____
_____

19. What is an incision into the thyroid gland called?

19. _____

20. What causes goiter?

20. _____
_____
_____

## Chapter 13

# The Immune System

## CHAPTER CONTENTS

The immune system enables the human body to ward off many kinds of assaults. If you fall off your skateboard and bruise your knee, the immune system sends whatever is needed to heal the wound and to prevent infection at the site. If you find yourself in a classroom or some other public place with a lot of people who are coughing and sneezing, your immune system will be alert for and react to the pathogens you breathe in.

The specialists who diagnose and treat immune system disorders are called *immunologists,* and the specialty itself is called *immunology.* The following paragraphs introduce terms that name parts of the immune system, along with those relating to common disorders, diagnosis, and treatment.

While studying this chapter, please keep in mind that all the cells named are kinds of white blood cells.

## WORD ROOTS SPECIFIC TO THE IMMUNE SYSTEM

The roots shown in Table 13-1 are often found in terms related to the Immune System. You will recognize them in many of the terms you will learn in this chapter.

| **TABLE 13-1** COMMON WORD ROOTS RELATED TO THE IMMUNE SYSTEM ||
|---|---|
| Root | Refers to |
| lymph/o; lymphat/o | lymph or lymphatic system |
| lymphangi/o | lymph vessels |
| immun/o | immune system |
| lymphaden/o | lymph nodes |
| splen/o | spleen |
| tonsill/o | lymph node, usually palatine tonsil |
| thym/o | thymus |

## PHAGOCYTES

*Phagocytes* are often the first immune system cells on the scene when injury occurs. They prevent infection by cleaning away pathogens and debris. Two types of phagocytes are *microphages* and *macrophages.* Microphages, which constantly circulate in the bloodstream, are more plentiful than macrophages but are short-lived. Macrophages live longer than microphages, and they reside in critical areas, such as the pleural and abdominal cavities, as first-response defenders.

## LYMPHOCYTES

When *leukocytes* (white blood cells) in the bloodstream are needed to fight infection, they leave the blood and enter the lymphatic system; they are then called *lymphocytes.* The average human body contains one trillion lymphocytes, which include three different types: *NK cells, T cells,* and *B cells.*

## NK Cells

*NK (natural killer) cells* travel throughout the body, constantly looking for cells with unusual components in their membranes. When NK cells find these "foreign" cells, they destroy them using proteins called *perforins.* Natural killer cells can combat viral infection and even destroy malignant cells.

## T Cells

T cells make up about 80% of the total number of lymphocytes. They are so named because they depend on the *thymus* for activation. They go to work only after being prompted by a specific *antigen,* a substance that induces sensitivity. Antigens also stimulate the immune system to generate *antibodies,* which can produce immunity from future attacks by the same type of antigen.

Although most antigens signal a disease-causing agent, some do not. For example, antigens in red blood cells (RBCs) determine each person's specific blood type. Individuals whose RBCs contain only the A antigen have Type A blood, while those with only the B antigen have Type B blood. Those with neither A nor B antigens have Type O blood, and those with both the A and B antigen have Type AB blood. As this example indicates, our individual immune systems discriminate between antigens that are normal to us ("good" antigens), and those that are not ("bad" antigens). It also shows why blood transfusions can be dangerous in certain circumstances. For instance, if a Type A patient receives blood from a Type B donor, the B antigens in the transfused blood will signal the Type A patient's immune system to attack.

Unlike NK cells, which roam the body looking for intruders, T cells attack only when they recognize a specific antigen, and then only after receiving instructions from special T cells that distinguish between good and bad antigens.

## B Cells

*B cells* are derived from bone marrow. Like NK cells, they roam the body looking for intruders. But unlike NK cells, they stop in lymph tissue to seek out foreign antigens. However, they do not attack until the special T cells instruct them to do so. Figure 13-1 shows each of the three types of cells in the immune system.

  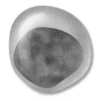

T lymphocyte    B lymphocyte    Natural killer
(T cell)    (B cell)    (NK cell)
FIGURE **13-1** The three types of lymphocytes, the first-response cells of the immune system.

## THE LYMPHATIC SYSTEM

The *lymphatic system* comprises the vessels through which lymphocytes travel, the lymph in which they travel, and the organs necessary to direct their functions.

### Lymph

Like blood plasma, *lymph* is a fluid that consists mostly of water. It also contains a low concentration of proteins in solution and, of course, lymphocytes. The word *lymph* is also used as an adjective in naming lymph vessels, lymph nodes, etc.

> A second adjective, *lymphatic*, is most often used when referring to the whole system and some specific parts of the system, such as the *right lymphatic duct.* Either adjective, however, is acceptable in any context.

### Lymph Vessels

*Lymph vessels* (Figure 13-2), also called *lymph ducts,* return cells back into the bloodstream. The largest of the lymph vessels, which correspond to the largest of the circulatory system veins, are the *thoracic duct* and the right lymphatic duct.

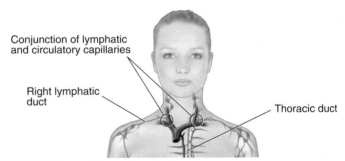

FIGURE **13-2** Lymphatic vessels and ducts.

Both NK cells and B cells originate in bone marrow. Some lymph cells find their way into the thymus, where they are eventually converted into T cells. The lymphatic capillaries are similar in some ways to the capillaries of the circulatory system. In fact, blood capillaries and lymphatic capillaries are physically joined together.

### The Thymus

The thymus gland, located behind the sternum (Figure 13-3), secretes hormones, known collectively as *thymosin,* which help T cells develop. The thymus is most active in children and gradually and continuously loses some of its function with maturation and further aging.

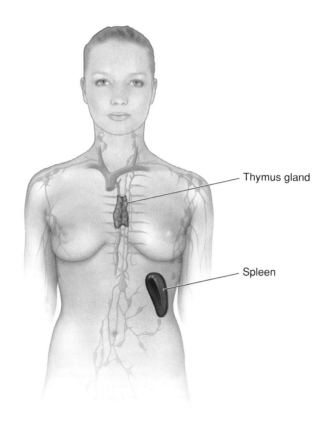

FIGURE **13-3** Location of the thymus and spleen.

## The Spleen

The spleen, which contains phagocytes, removes damaged red blood cells and recycles and stores reclaimed iron from others.

## Lymph Nodes

*Lymph nodes* are structures of variable size that contain macrophages that filter out disease-causing antigens and other debris as the lymph flows through. These antigens are then exposed to lymphocytes to start the immune response. Most lymph nodes are quite small, about 1/25th of an inch in diameter. The larger lymph nodes can be about an inch in diameter and are sometimes called *lymph glands.* Swollen glands are the result of large numbers of phagocytes and lymphocytes in the node; this condition may also reveal the presence of an infection or injury in the area of the swollen gland.

## Tonsils

Any collection of lymph tissue can be called a *tonsil.* Figure 13-4 shows the palatine, pharyngeal, and lingual tonsils, which are the ones we normally think of when we see or hear the word "tonsils."

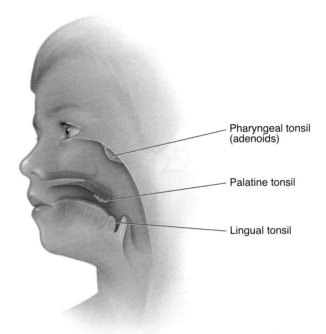

Pharyngeal tonsil
(adenoids)

Palatine tonsil

Lingual tonsil

FIGURE **13-4** Location of the tonsils.

## ABBREVIATION TABLE

**COMMON ABBREVIATIONS:**
**The Immune System**

| Abbreviation | Meaning |
| --- | --- |
| Ab | antibody |
| ADCC | antibody-dependent cell-mediated cytotoxicity |
| Ag | antigen |
| AIDS | acquired immune deficiency syndrome |
| APC | antigen-presenting cell |
| BCR | B cell (antigen) receptor (Ig) |
| BM | bone marrow |
| CBC | complete blood count |
| CD | celiac disease (allergy to gluten) |
| ELISA | enzyme-linked immunosorbent assay |
| ESR | erythrocyte sedimentation rate |
| HIV | human immunodeficiency virus |
| HLA | human leukocyte antigen (MHC) |
| Ig | immunoglobulin (antibody) |
| LFA | leukocyte functional antigen |
| LGL | large granular lymphocyte (NK cell) |
| NK | natural killer cell |
| RA | rheumatoid arthritis |

## ABBREVIATION TABLE *(continued)*

### COMMON ABBREVIATIONS:
The Immune System

| Abbreviation | Meaning |
|---|---|
| RIA | radioimmunoassay |
| SLE | systemic lupus erythematosus (usually shortened to lupus), an autoimmune disorder |
| TCR | T-cell (antigen) receptor |

## DECIPHERING MEDICAL DOCUMENTS.

**Read the following excerpt from a government report, and answer the questions that follow:**

*. . . The human immune and inflammatory systems protect us from a multitude of these and other agents in our environment, usually by one or more of the following four general types of immune reactions: Type I reactions are mediated by IgE antibodies and are the cause of most "allergic" reactions. Approximately 8% to 10% of the population have adverse symptoms due to Type I reactions to pollens, dust, mold, animal dander, or food. Type II (cytotoxic) reactions target molecules on the surface of cells and initiate processes leading to the death of that specific cell (hemolytic anemia). Type III reactions are "immune-complex" reactions in which a protective antibody attaches to an antigen and initiates an inflammatory reaction . . .*

1. What type of reactions cause most allergic reactions?
2. Given that certain kinds of immunoglobulins are designated by a third letter, what abbreviation in the excerpt indicates an immunoglobulin?
3. Analyze and define *hemolytic,* and then compare your definition with one from a medical dictionary.
4. Analyze and define *cytotoxic,* and then compare your definition with one from a medical dictionary.

## COMMON IMMUNE SYSTEM DISORDERS AND PROCEDURES

Some disorders are caused when the immune system targets a person's own cells. This condition is known as *autoimmunity.* Graves disease, which was introduced in Chapter 12, is an example of an autoimmune disease, which is organ-specific, affecting the thyroid gland. However, autoimmunity can affect nearly any part of the body.

### Lymphatic System Disorders

The general term for all the lymph vessel and node diseases is *lymphopathy.* These conditions range from *lymphatitis* (inflammation of nodes or vessels) to *lymphoma* (tumor of the lymph tissue). The root for lymph nodes is usually *lymphaden/o,* while the one for the vessels is *lymphang/i/o.*

### Thymus and Spleen Disorders

The roots for thymus and spleen are *thym/o* and *splen/o,* which yield terms such as *thymitis* and *splenomalacia.*

## Disorders of the Tonsils

A common disorder and procedure related to the tonsils is *tonsillitis* (inflammation of the tonsils) and *tonsillectomy* (excision of the tonsils), nearly always referring to the palatine tonsils in both instances. However, tonsillitis usually does not signal the need for a tonsillectomy.

Please refer to Table 13-2 for the names of more common disorders of the immune system.

| **TABLE 13-2** COMMON DISORDERS AND PROCEDURES ASSOCIATED WITH THE IMMUNE SYSTEM | |
| --- | --- |
| Term | Definition |
| autoimmunity | immune to oneself |
| lymphadenopathy | any disease of the lymph nodes; chronic or excessively swollen lymph nodes |
| lymphadenectomy | excision of lymph nodes |
| lymphadentitis | inflammation of a lymph node (or nodes) |
| lymphangiectomy | excision of a lymph vessel |
| lymphangitis; also sometimes lymphangiitis | inflammation of lymph vessels |
| lymphoma | tumor of lymph tissue |
| lymphangiography | radiography of the lymph vessels |
| lymphangioplasty | surgical repair of lymph vessels |
| lymphangiotomy | incision of lymph vessels |
| lymphatitis | inflammation of the lymph vessels or nodes |
| lymphopathy | any disease of the lymph vessels or nodes |
| immunodeficiency | impairment of the immune system |
| splenitis | inflammation of the spleen |
| splenectomy | excision of the spleen |
| splenomalacia | softening of the spleen |
| splenomegaly | enlargement of the spleen |
| splenopathy | any disease of the spleen |
| splenorrhagia | hemorrhage from a ruptured spleen |
| splenorrhaphy | suture of a ruptured spleen |
| splenotomy | incision of the spleen |
| tonsillitis | inflammation of a tonsil (commonly the palatine tonsil) |
| tonsillectomy | excision of a tonsil |
| tonsillotomy | incision of a tonsil |
| thymectomy | excision of the thymus |
| thymitis | inflammation of the thymus |

## STUDY TABLE  THE IMMUNE SYSTEM

| Term and Pronunciation | Analysis | Meaning |
|---|---|---|
| **STRUCTURE & FUNCTION** | | |
| antibody | *anti-* ("against"); *body* ("a foreign substance" and "antigen") | a molecule generated in specific opposition to an antigen |
| antigen (AN-tih-jehn) | *anti-* ("against"); *-gen* ("origin" or "production") | substance that induces sensitivity or an immune response in the form of antibodies |
| autoimmunity (aw-toh-ih-MYUN-iht-ee) | *auto-* ("self"); *immunity* from the Latin word *immunis* ("free from service") | literally, immune to oneself |
| B cell | B ("bone marrow") | lymphocytes that work with T cells to fight off infection |
| leukocyte (LUKE-oh-site) | *leuk/o* ("white"); *-cyte* ("cell") | white blood cell |
| lymph (limf) | from the Latin word *lympha* ("water") | fluid that flows through the lymphatic system; adjective synonymous with *lymphatic* |
| lymph duct (limf) | from the Latin word *lympha* ("water") | another term for lymph vessel |
| lymph gland (limf) | from the Latin word *lympha* ("water") | a large lymph node |
| lymph node (limf) | from the Latin word *lympha* ("water"); *node* from the Latin word *nodus* ("knot") | structures of variable size that contain macrophages that filter out disease-causing antigens and other debris as the lymph flows through |
| lymph vessel (limf) | from the Latin word *lympha* ("water") | vessel (or duct) within the lymphatic system |
| lymphatic system (lim-FAT-tik) | from the Latin word *lympha* ("water"); *-ic* (adjective suffix) | collectively, the vessels, nodes, and capillaries that carry the lymph and its disease-fighting cells to the areas in which they are needed |
| lymphocyte (LIHM-foh-syte) | *lymphat/o* ("lymphatic system"); *-cyte* ("cell") | white blood cell in the lymphatic system |
| macrophage (MAK-roh-fayj) | *macro-* ("large"); *phage* from the Greek word *phago* ("eat") | large phagocyte |
| microphage (MIKE-roh-fayj) | *micro-* ("small"); *phage* from the Greek word *phago* ("eat") | small phagocyte |
| NK cell | NK (*natural killer*) | type of lymphocyte; natural killer |
| perforin (PUR-for-ihn) | from the Latin word *perforo* ("to bore into") | protein that NK cells use to kill invading cells |
| phagocyte (FAG-oh-syte) | from the Greek word *phago* ("eat"); *-cyte* ("cell") | white blood cells that clear away pathogens and debris |
| right lymphatic duct (lim-FAT-ik) | *lymphat/o* ("lymphatic system") | large lymph vessel |
| spleen (SPLEEN) | from the Greek word *splen* ("spleen") | immune system organ that gets rid of damaged red blood cells and reclaims and stores iron |

## STUDY TABLE  THE IMMUNE SYSTEM (continued)

| Term and Pronunciation | Analysis | Meaning |
|---|---|---|
| T cell | T ("thymus") | cells that make up about 80% of lymphocytes; the T denotes their work with the thymus |
| thoracic duct (thoh-RASS-ik) | *thorac/o* ("thorax"); *-ic* (adjective suffix) | large lymph vessel located in the chest area |
| thymosin (THY-MOH-sihn) | from the Greek word *thymos* ("an abnormal growth") | hormone secreted by the thymus that helps create T cells |
| thymus (THY-muhs) | from the Greek word *thymos*, meaning an abnormal growth | immune system gland located behind the sternum |
| tonsil (TON-sihl) | from the Latin word *tonsilla* ("tonsil") | collection of lymph tissue; in common understanding, the lingual, pharyngeal, and (especially) the palatine tonsils |
| **COMMON DISORDERS** | | |
| immunodeficiency (IM-yu-noh-dee-FISH-ehn-see) | *immun/o* ("immune system"); *-deficiency* (common English word) | impairment of the immune system |
| lymphadenopathy (lim-fah-deh-NOP-ah-thee) | from the Latin word *lympha* ("water"); *aden/o* ("gland"); *-pathy* ("disease") | chronic or excessively swollen lymph nodes; any disease of the lymph nodes |
| lymphadenitis (LIM-FAD-eh-NY-tiss) | from the Latin word *lympha* ("water"); *aden/o* ("gland"); *-itis* ("inflammation") | inflammation of a lymph node (or nodes) |
| lymphangitis (lim-fan-JY-tihs); also sometimes lymphangiitis (lim-FAN-jee-EYE-tihs); see also lymphatitis | from the Latin word *lympha* ("water"); ang/i/o ("vessel"); -itis ("inflammation") | inflammation of lymph vessels |
| lymphatitis (lim-fah-TY-tihs) | *lymphat/o* ("lymphatic system"); *-itis* ("inflammation") | inflammation of the lymph vessels or nodes |
| lymphoma (lim-FOH-mah) | *lymph/o* ("lymphatic system"); *-oma* ("tumor") | tumor of lymph tissue |
| lymphopathy (lim-FOP-ah-thee) | *lymph/o* ("lymphatic system"); *-pathy* ("disease") | disease of the lymph vessels or nodes |
| splenitis (splee-NY-tihs) | *splen/o* ("spleen"); *-itis* ("inflammation") | inflammation of the spleen |
| splenomalacia (SPLEE-noh-mah-LAY-she-ah) | *splen/o* ("spleen"); *-malacia* ("softening") | softening of the spleen |
| splenomegaly (splee-noh-MEG-ah-lee) | *splen/o* ("spleen"); *-megaly* ("enlargement") | enlargement of the spleen |
| splenopathy (splee-NOP-ah-thee) | *splen/o* ("spleen"); *-pathy* ("disease") | any disease of the spleen |
| splenorrhagia (SPLEE-noh-RAY-jee-ah) | *splen/o* ("spleen"); *-rrhagia* ("hemorrhage") | hemorrhage from a ruptured spleen |
| thymitis (thy-MY-tihs) | *thym/o* ("thymus"); *-itis* ("inflammation") | inflammation of the thymus |
| tonsillitis (TAWN-sih-LY-tihs) | *tonsill/o* ("tonsil"); *-itis* ("inflammation") | inflammation of a tonsil (commonly the palatine tonsil) |

## STUDY TABLE  THE IMMUNE SYSTEM (continued)

| Term and Pronunciation | Analysis | Meaning |
|---|---|---|
| **DIAGNOSIS & TREATMENT** | | |
| lymphangiography (lim-FAN-jee-OG-rah-fee) | from the Latin word *lympha* ("water"); *ang/i/o* ("vessel"); *-graphy* ("x-ray") | radiography of the lymph vessels |
| **PRACTICE & PRACTITIONERS** | | |
| immunologist (im-yu-NOL-oh-jist) | from the Latin word *immunis* ("free from service"); *-logist* ("practitioner") | a medical practitioner specializing in the immune system |
| immunology (IM-yu-NOL-oh-jee) | from the Latin word *immunis* ("free from service"); *-logy* ("study") | the medical specialty dealing with the immune system |
| **SURGICAL PROCEDURES** | | |
| lymphadenectomy (lim-fah-deh-NEK-toh-mee) | from the Latin word *lympha* ("water"); *aden/o* ("gland"); *-ectomy* ("excision") | excision of lymph nodes |
| lymphangiectomy (lim-FAN-jee-EK-tah-mee) | from the Latin word *lympha* ("water"); *ang/i/o* ("vessel"); *-ectomy* ("excision") | excision of a lymph vessel |
| lymphangioplasty (lim-FAN-jee-oh-plass-tee) | from the Latin word *lympha* ("water"); *ang/i/o* ("vessel"); *-plasty* ("surgical repair") | surgical repair of lymph vessels |
| lymphangiotomy (lim-FAN-jee-OT-oh-mee) | from the Latin word *lympha* ("water"); *ang/i/o* ("vessel"); *-tomy* ("incision") | incision of lymph vessels |
| splenectomy (splee-NEK-toh-mee) | *splen/o* ("spleen"); *-ectomy* ("excision") | excision of the spleen |
| splenorrhaphy (splee-NOR-ah-fee) | *splen/o* ("spleen"); *-rrhaphy* ("suture") | suture of a ruptured spleen |
| splenotomy (splee-NOT-oh-mee) | *splen/o* ("spleen"); *-tomy* ("incision") | incision of the spleen |
| thymectomy (thy-MEK-toh-me) | *thym/o* ("thymus"); *-ectomy* ("excision") | excision of the thymus |
| tonsillectomy (TAWN-sih-LEK-toh-mee) | *tonsill/o* ("tonsil"); *-ectomy* ("excision") | excision of a tonsil |
| tonsillotomy (TAWN-sih-LOT-oh-mee) | *tonsill/o* ("tonsil"); *-tomy* ("incision") | incision of a tonsil |
| **ENHANCEMENT TERMS** | | |
| allergen (AL-ur-jehn) | from two Greek words: *allos* ("other") and *ergon* ("work") yielding *allergy*; *-gen* ("origin") | an allergy-producing substance |
| immunosuppressant (IM-yu-no-suh-PRESS-ant) | from the Latin word *immunis* ("free from service") and *suppressant* (common English word) | something that interferes with the immune system |
| inflammation (in-flah-MAAY-shun) | a common English word | redness and irritation caused by injury or abnormal stimulation by a physical, chemical, or biologic agent |
| pathogen (PATH-oh-jehn) | *path/o* ("disease"); *-gen* ("origin") | substance that produces disease |

📖 **STUDY TABLE** THE IMMUNE SYSTEM (*continued*)

| Term and Pronunciation | Analysis | Meaning |
|---|---|---|
| phagocytosis (FAG-oh-sy-TOE-sihs) | from the Greek word *phago* ("eat"); *-cyte* ("cell"); *osis* ("condition") | process of white blood cells clearing away pathogens and debris |
| reaction (ree-AK-shun) | common English word | an action of an antibody on a specific antigen; also, in reference to immune responses, an abnormal or unwanted reaction |
| toxin (TOX-sihn) | from the Greek word *toxikon* ("poison") | a poisonous substance |

# 🖎 Exercises

## Exercise 13-1 Choosing the Correct Term

Fill in the blanks.

The word *leukocyte* is a synonym for 1)_____ in the blood system. When leukocytes are needed to fight infection, they leave the blood and enter the 2)_____ system, after which entry they are called 3)_____. The three different types of lymphocytes are NK cells, T cells, and B cells. The "NK" in NK cells stands for 4)_____, and it kills "foreign" cells using proteins called 5)_____. The "T" in T cells refers to the 6)_____ because they depend on the thymus for activation. The T cells must be sensitized by a specific 7)_____ in order to start working. The "B" in B cells stands for bone, as they originate in bone marrow. The B cells stop at 8)_____ to attack foreign antigens, but not until they get "permission" from 9)_____. When injury occurs to a body part, the 10)_____ system sends what is needed to heal the wound.

## Exercises

## Exercise 13-2 Converting Nouns to Adjectives

Convert each of the following nouns to its adjective form using one of the following suffixes: *-oid,- al, -ar, -ic, -ine.*

| Noun | Adjective Form |
|---|---|
| 1. pharynx | _____ |
| 2. lymph | _____ |
| 3. lymphocyte | _____ |
| 4. phagocyte | _____ |

| Noun | Adjective Form |
|------|----------------|
| 5. leukocyte | _____ |
| 6. lymph | _____ |
| 7. sternum | _____ |
| 8. palate | _____ |
| 9. tonsil | _____ |
| 10. pathogen | _____ |
| 11. spleen | _____ |
| 12. cell | _____ |
| 14. thorax | _____ |
| 14 inflammation | _____ |
| 15. allergen | _____ |

# Exercises

## Exercise 13-3 Matching Terms with Definitions

Match the numbers in Column 1 with the letters in Column 2 according to the corresponding terms and definitions they designate.

| Term | Definition |
|------|------------|
| 1. _____ thymus | A. protein that NK cells use to kill invading cells |
| 2. _____ tonsil | B. substance that induces sensitivity or an immune response |
| 3. _____ lymph node | C. cells that make up about 80% of lymphocytes, the "T" denoting their work with the thymus |
| 4. _____ perforin | D. immune system gland, located behind the sternum |
| 5. _____ spleen | E. fluid that flows through the lymphatic system |
| 6. _____ T cell | F. type of lymphocyte; "natural killer" cell |
| 7. _____ lymph | G. structures of variable size that contain macrophages, which filter out disease-causing antigens and other debris as the lymph flows through |
| 8. _____ antigen | H. collection of lymph tissue (in common understanding, the lingual, pharyngeal and the palatine) |
| 9. _____ B cell | I. lymphocytes that work with T cells to fight off infection |
| 10. _____ NK cell | J. immune system organ that gets rid of damaged red blood cells and reclaims and stores iron |

| Term | Definition |
|---|---|
| 11. _____ lymphoma | K. hemorrhage from a ruptured spleen |
| 12. _____ splenomegaly | L. impairment of the immune system |
| 13. _____ thymitis | M. tumor of lymph tissue |
| 14. _____ lymphadenopathy | N. inflammation of a tonsil (commonly the palatine) |
| 15. _____ immunodeficiency | O. radiography of the lymph vessels |
| 16. _____ splenorrhagia | P. inflammation of lymph vessels |
| 17. _____ lymphangiography | Q. chronic or excessively swollen lymph nodes or any disease of the lymph nodes |
| 18. _____ tonsillitis | R. any disease of the spleen |
| 19. _____ splenopathy | S. inflammation of the thymus |
| 20. _____ lymphangitis | T. enlargement of the spleen |

# Exercises

## Exercise 13-4 Locating the Lymphatic Organs and Vessels

Label the following lymphatic organs and vessels on Figure 13-5:
* conjunction of lymphatic and circulatory capillaries
* right lymphatic duct
* thoracic duct

2 _____

_____

3 _____

1 _____

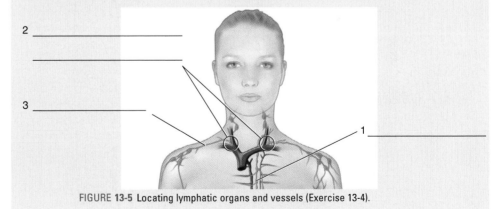

FIGURE 13-5 Locating lymphatic organs and vessels (Exercise 13-4).

# Exercises

## Exercise 13-5 Locating the Tonsils

Label the following on Figure 13-6:

* lingual tonsils
* palatine tonsils
* pharyngeal tonsils

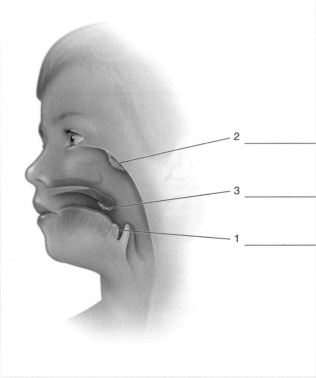

FIGURE **13-6** Locating the tonsils (Exercise 13-5).

# Exercises

## Exercise 13-6 Building Medical Terms

Build terms to satisfy the following definitions, and then analyze each term by identifying its word elements.

| Definition | Term | Analysis |
|---|---|---|
| 1. molecule generated in specific opposition to an antigen | _____ | _____ _____ |
| 2. white blood cell | _____ | _____ _____ _____ |
| 3. white blood cell in the lymphatic system | _____ | _____ _____ |
| 4. impairment of the immune system | _____ | _____ _____ |
| 5. inflammation of the spleen | _____ | _____ _____ _____ |
| 6. softening of the spleen | _____ | _____ _____ _____ |
| 7. any disease of the spleen | _____ | _____ _____ _____ |
| 8. inflammation of the thymus | _____ | _____ _____ _____ |
| 9. medical practitioner specializing in the immune system | _____ | _____ _____ _____ |
| 10. incision of a tonsil | _____ | _____ _____ _____ |

# Exercises

## Exercise 13-7 Multiple Choice

Circle the term in the Choices column that correctly answers each of the following questions.

| Question | Choices |
| --- | --- |
| 1. What is the substance that induces sensitivity or an immune response in the form of antibodies? | antigen; autoimmunity; immunology |
| 2. What is the term that means literally, "immune to oneself"? | immunology; autoimmunity; antigen |
| 3. What is the name for the medical specialty that deals with the immune system? | antigen; autoimmunity; immunology |
| 4. Name the immune system organ that gets rid of damaged red blood cells and reclaims and stores iron. | lymphadentitis; lymphangitis; spleen |
| 5. What is the term that describes the inflammation of a lymph node (or nodes)? | lymphadentitis; lymphangitis; spleen |
| 6. What is the term that describes the inflammation of the lymph vessels? | lymphadentitis; lymphangitis; spleen |
| 7. What term would you use to request an x-ray of a patient's lymph vessels? | lymphangiectomy; lymphangiography; lymphangioplasty |
| 8. What is the word that means "excision of a lymph vessel"? | lymphangiectomy; lymphangiography; lymphangioplasty |
| 9. What is the term for a surgical repair of a lymph vessel (or vessels)? | lymphangiectomy; splenotomy; lymphangioplasty |
| 10. What term means "incision of the spleen"? | lymphangiectomy; splenotomy; lymphangioplasty |

## ✔ Pre-Quiz Checklist

_____  Study the word roots specific to the immune system (Table 13-1).
_____  Review the term analysis column in the study table to make sure you understand all the word elements.
_____  Check the exercises with the answers in the Appendix and consult the review table again to correct your errors before attempting the quiz.

## ✔ Chapter Quiz

Write the answers to the following items in the spaces provided.

1. Of what does lymph mostly consist?

1. _____
_____
_____
_____
_____

2. Name the three types of lymphocytes.

2. _____
_____

3. Describe the job of a phagocyte. Name the two types.

3. _____
_____
_____
_____
_____
_____
_____

4. Name the two largest lymph vessels.

4. _____
_____

5. Describe the spleen's functions.

5. _____
_____
_____
_____
_____
_____

6. What is the job of the thymus?

6. _____
_____
_____

☑ **Chapter Quiz** *(continued)*

7. What are lymph nodes? Describe their function.

7. _____
_____
_____
_____
_____
_____

8. Why do lymph nodes often become "swollen" when an infection is present in the body?

8. _____
_____
_____
_____

9. Name the three tonsils that are most commonly referred to.

9. _____
_____

10. Where is the thymus located?

10. _____
_____

11. What is the difference between lymphadenitis and lymphangitis?

11. _____
_____
_____
_____
_____
_____

12. What would excision of each of the following be called? a) lymph node(s), b) lymph vessel, c) spleen, d) tonsils, e) thymus

12. _____
_____
_____
_____
_____
_____

13. What gland and organ are responsible for controlling immune responses?

13. _____
_____

14. Give an example of a type of antigen that is not a disease-causing agent.

14. _____

15. Explain how blood types are named.

15. _____
_____
_____
_____

16. What would happen if a person with Type A blood were to receive blood from a Type B donor?

16. _____
_____
_____
_____

## ✓ Chapter Quiz (continued)

17. What do chronically swollen lymph nodes signal?

17. _____

18. What does the Latin word *lympha* mean?
    Why has *lymph* become the common root
    for terms about the lymphatic system?

18. _____
    _____
    _____

19. What tonsils does the common form of
    tonsillitis refer to?

19. _____

20. What term covers all instances of an impaired
    immune system?

20. _____

# Chapter 14

# The Urinary System

CHAPTER CONTENTS

The urinary system removes wastes and toxins from the body. It also regulates the amount of water in the body and the amount and kinds of *electrolytes* (compounds in solution that conduct electricity) that it contains. Urinary system malfunctions can occur at any time throughout the lifespan, but their likelihood increases with age because of decreased general muscle tone and the kidneys' reduced capacity to function. This chapter outlines the normal structures and functions of the urinary system and introduces the terms that describe many abnormal conditions, as well as commonly used treatments and procedures.

## WORD ELEMENTS SPECIFIC TO THE URINARY SYSTEM

The word elements shown in Table 14-1 are found in terms related to the urinary system. You will recognize them in many of the terms you will learn in this chapter.

| TABLE 14-1 WORD ELEMENTS RELATED TO THE URINARY SYSTEM | |
|---|---|
| Word Elements | Refers to |
| cyst/o | bladder |
| lith/o | stone |
| nephr/o, ren/o | kidney |
| olig/o | little, few |
| pyel/o | pelvis |
| py/o | pus |
| ureter/o | ureter |
| urethr/o | urethra |
| urin/o | urine |
| poly- | prefix meaning "much" or "many" |
| -iasis | suffix meaning "condition" or "state" |

## AN OVERVIEW OF THE URINARY SYSTEM

The urinary system is composed of the *kidneys, urinary bladder, ureters,* and *urethra.* Figure 14-1 shows the locations of each of these, which are discussed below.

### Kidneys

As vital organs, the kidneys share some physical characteristics with the heart. For example, each kidney has layers. A thin covering called the *renal capsule* encloses and gives shape to the kidney. A thicker layer of fatty tissue, called the *perirenal fat,* surrounds the renal capsule. Finally, a thin layer of connective tissue, called the *renal fascia,* forms each kidney's protective outer covering. The *hilum* is the indented, or narrowest, part of the kidney, where blood vessels and nerves enter. Figure 14-2 shows the structure of the kidneys.

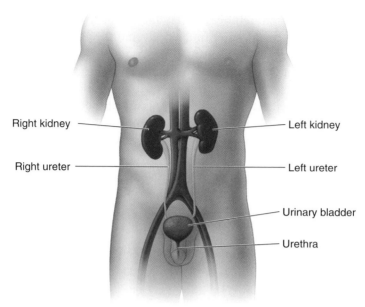

FIGURE **14-1** Location of urinary system components. *From:* Cohen BJ, Taylor JJ, Memmler RL, eds. *Memmler's The Structure and Function of the Human Body.* 8th ed. Baltimore, MD: Lippincott Williams & Wilkins; 2005.

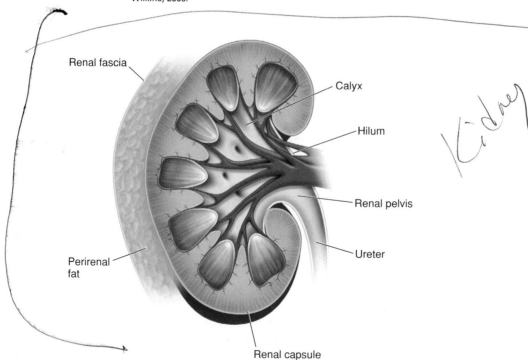

FIGURE **14-2** The kidneys. *From:* Cohen BJ, Taylor JJ, Memmler RL, eds. *Memmler's The Structure and Function of the Human Body.* 8th ed. Baltimore, MD: Lippincott Williams & Wilkins; 2005.

The kidneys produce *urine,* which is water that contains other substances in solution. In producing urine, the kidneys remove two natural products of metabolism, *urea* and *uric acid,* along with other waste products from the blood. The kidneys also filter, reabsorb, and secrete non-waste products back into the system.

The kidneys contain about 2.5 million *nephrons,* tiny structures in which the urine-making process begins. The capillary network found inside each nephron is called a *glomerulus,* which assists in filtration.

The root *nephr/o* is often used in naming kidney disorders, but *ren/o* may also be used at times. Applying some of the standard suffixes yields *nephritis, nephralgia, nephrectomy, nephrology, nephromegaly* (or *renomegaly*), *nephropathy* (or *renopathy*), *nephrorrhaphy,* and *nephrotomy.* However, the adjective *renal* is used more often than its counterpart, *nephric.*

The English word *calculus* (plural: *calculi*) is also a Latin word meaning "small stone or pebble." A calculus in a kidney is commonly called a kidney stone and in the gallbladder a gallstone. However, *renal calculus,* rather than *kidney stone,* is the medical phrase one would likely find in a medical report.

In forming medical terms having to do with *calculi* in the kidneys and gallbladder, the Greek root *lith/o* is often used in preference to the roots based on the Latin word *calculus.* Thus, a *nephrolithotomy* would be an incision into a kidney to remove a renal calculus (refer again to Table 14-1).

## Ureters

After urine is produced and processed in the kidneys, it is transported by two tubes, called *ureters,* one extending from each kidney to either side of the urinary bladder. Peristalsis, or involuntary muscle contractions (see Chapter 11), moves the urine through the ureters and into the urinary bladder.

## Urinary Bladder

The *urinary bladder* (Figure 14-3) collects urine so that it can be expelled in significant quantities at intervals. The process of urine expulsion, called *urination* or *micturition,* begins when a circular muscle called the *internal sphincter* relaxes, thus permitting urine to enter the opening of the urethra. This first section of the urethra extends only a few inches and is met at the other end by another circular muscle called the *external urethral sphincter.*

The root *cyst/o* is used in the construction of terms having to do with the urinary bladder. Unfortunately, the same terms are often used to mean the gallbladder. *Cystalgia* and *cystopexy* can mean, respectively, pain and surgical fixation of the urinary bladder or the gallbladder. *Cystectomy,* likewise, can refer to either bladder. But since the word *cyst* refers to an abnormal growth, cystectomy can also simply mean excision of a cyst.

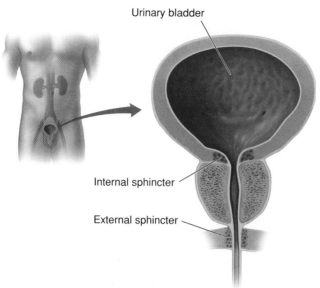

FIGURE **14-3** Location of the urinary bladder, internal sphincter, and external sphincter. *From:* Cohen BJ, Taylor JJ,  Memmler RL, eds. *Memmler's The Structure and Function of the Human Body.* 8th ed. Baltimore, MD: Lippincott Williams & Wilkins; 2005.

## Urethra

The *urethra*, the tube that carries urine out of the body, is connected to the bottom of the bladder. The *micturition reflex* sends a signal that it is time to open the external urethral sphincter and permit the urine to enter the urethra proper so that it can be expelled.

## ABBREVIATION TABLE

**COMMON ABBREVIATIONS:**
**The Urinary System**

| Abbreviation | Meaning |
| --- | --- |
| Abdo | abdomen |
| Abdo E&S | abdomen erect and supine (lying face upwards) |
| AXR | abdominal x-ray |
| BPH | benign prostatic hypertrophy |
| GFR | glomerular filtration rate |
| IVP | intravenous pyelogram (same as IVU): contrast is injected into a vein and is excreted by the kidney to show the urinary system |
| IVU | intravenous urogram (same as IVP) |

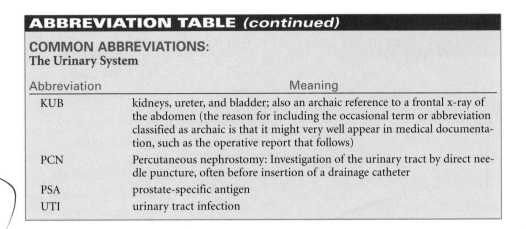

## ABBREVIATION TABLE *(continued)*

### COMMON ABBREVIATIONS:
### The Urinary System

| Abbreviation | Meaning |
|---|---|
| KUB | kidneys, ureter, and bladder; also an archaic reference to a frontal x-ray of the abdomen (the reason for including the occasional term or abbreviation classified as archaic is that it might very well appear in medical documentation, such as the operative report that follows) |
| PCN | Percutaneous nephrostomy: Investigation of the urinary tract by direct needle puncture, often before insertion of a drainage catheter |
| PSA | prostate-specific antigen |
| UTI | urinary tract infection |

 **DECIPHERING MEDICAL DOCUMENTS**

**Read the following excerpt from an operative report, and answer the questions that follow.**

*Operation: Cystoscopy, removal of left ureteral stent, and left retrograde pyelogram. The patient was placed in the lithotomy position, and a KUB was obtained. The genitalia were prepped and draped in a sterile fashion. Cystoscopy was performed with a #22 French cystoscope. The stent was identified coming from the left ureteral orifice, and the end was grasped with forceps and removed through the cystoscope.*

1. What is cystoscopy?
2. What is a KUB?
3. Analyze the term *ureteral*.

## COMMON URINARY SYSTEM DISORDERS AND PROCEDURES

Table 14-2 provides a quick reference for the meanings of the terms naming disorders and procedures associated with the urinary system.

| TABLE 14-2 | DISORDERS AND PROCEDURES ASSOCIATED WITH THE URINARY SYSTEM |
|---|---|
| **Term** | **Definition** |
| cystalgia | pain in a bladder, most often used to signify the urinary bladder |
| cystectomy | excision of either the urinary bladder or the gallbladder; (excision of the gallbladder is properly, and most often, called a *cholecystectomy*; since *cyst* also means "cyst," a *cystectomy* can also refer to the surgical removal of a cyst) |
| cystopexy | surgical fixation of either the gallbladder or the urinary bladder; this term is included because it is typical of the dual use of *cysto* |

| TABLE 14-2 | DISORDERS AND PROCEDURES ASSOCIATED WITH THE URINARY SYSTEM (continued) |
|---|---|

| Term | Definition |
|---|---|
| nephralgia | pain in the kidneys |
| nephrectomy | removal of a kidney |
| nephritis | inflammation of the kidneys |
| nephrolithotomy | incision into the kidney to remove a calculus (kidney stone) |
| nephromegaly | enlargement of one or both kidneys; renomegaly |
| nephropathy | any disease of the kidney |
| nephrorrhaphy | suture of the kidney |
| nephrotomy | incision into a kidney |
| renal calculus | a kidney stone |
| renal hypoplasia | an abnormally small kidney |
| renomegaly | enlargement of one or both kidneys; nephromegaly |
| renopathy | any disease of the kidney; the preferred term is *nephropathy* |
| ureteralgia | pain in a ureter |
| ureterectomy | excision of part or all of a ureter |
| ureteritis | inflammation of a ureter |
| ureterography | radiography of the ureter |
| ureterolithotomy | incision into the ureter to remove a calculus (stone) |
| ureteroplasty | surgical repair of a ureter |
| ureterorrhaphy | suture of a ureter |
| urethralgia | pain in the urethra (sometimes also called *urethrodynia*) |
| urethrectomy | excision of all or part of the urethra |
| urethritis | inflammation of the urethra |
| urethrostenosis | narrowing of the urethra |
| urinalysis | analysis of urine |

## STUDY TABLE THE URINARY SYSTEM

| Term and Pronunciation | Analysis | Meaning |
|---|---|---|
| **STRUCTURE & FUNCTION** | | |
| calculus (KAL-kyu-luhs); plural: calculi (KAL-kyu-lye) | a Latin word meaning "a small stone or pebble" | a kidney stone (in the context of this body system) |
| electrolyte (ee-LEK-troh-lyte) | *electr/o* ("electricity"); *-lyte* from the Greek word *lytos* ("soluble") | electricity-conducting compound in solution |
| external sphincter (SFINK-tehr) | sphincter is from a Greek word meaning "band" | muscle that controls the release of urine from the first section of the urethra for subsequent expulsion |
| glomerulus (gloh-MER-yu-luhs) | from the Latin word *glomus* ("ball-shaped mass") | capillary network found inside each nephron |

## STUDY TABLE THE URINARY SYSTEM *(continued)*

| Term and Pronunciation | Analysis | Meaning |
|---|---|---|
| hilum (HY-luhm) | Latin word for "trifle" | narrow part of the kidney where blood vessels and nerves enter |
| internal sphincter muscle (SFINK-tehr) | from a Greek word meaning "band" | muscle that controls the release of urine from the bladder into the first section of the urethra |
| kidneys (KID-neez) | origin unknown; may be from two Anglo-Saxon words *cwith* and *neere* ("womb" and "belly," respectively) | pair of organs that excrete urine |
| micturition (mihk-chu-RISH-uhn) | from the Latin verb *micturire* ("to desire to make water") | urination |
| micturition reflex (mihk-chu-RISH-uhn) | from the Latin verb *micturire* ("to desire to make water") | reflex that signals the external sphincter to open |
| nephron (NEFF-ron) | from the Greek word *nephros* ("kidney") | tiny structure within the kidney in which the urine-production process begins |
| perirenal fat (PEHR-ih-REE-nahl) | *peri-* ("around"); *ren/o* ("kidney"); *-al* (adjective suffix) | fatty tissue surrounding the renal capsule |
| renal capsule (REE-nahl) | *ren/o* ("kidney"); *-al* (adjective suffix) | thin inner covering enclosing the kidney |
| renal fascia (REE-nahl FASH-ee-ah) | *ren/o* ("kidney"); *-al* (adjective suffix); *fascia* (Latin word for "band") | protective outer covering of the kidney |
| urea (yu-REE-ah) | from the Greek word *ouron* ("urine") | natural waste product of metabolism that is excreted in urine |
| ureters (yu-REE-tehrs; also YUR-eh-tehrs) | from the Greek word *oureter* ("urinary canal") | two tubes that transfer urine from the kidneys to the urinary bladder |
| urethra (yu-REE-thrah) | from the Greek word *ourethra* | tube that conducts urine away from the bladder for expulsion |
| uric acid (YUR-ik) | from the Greek word *ouron* ("urine") and *-ic* (adjective suffix) | natural waste product of metabolism that is excreted in urine |
| urinary bladder (YUR-ihn-ayr-ee BLAD-dehr) | from the Greek word *ouron* ("urine") and the Old English word *blaedre* | temporary storage receptacle for urine |
| urine (YUR-ihn) | from the Greek word *ouron* ("urine") | water and soluble substances excreted by the kidneys |
| **COMMON DISORDERS** | | |
| cystalgia (sihs-TAL-jee-ah) | *cyst/o* ("bladder"); *-algia* ("pain") | pain in a bladder, most often used to signify the urinary bladder |
| nephralgia (neh-FRAL-jee-ah) | *nephr/o* ("kidney"); *-algia* ("pain") | pain in the kidneys |
| nephritis (neh-FRY-tihs) | *nephr/o* ("kidney"); *-itis* ("inflammation") | inflammation of the kidneys |
| nephromegaly (neh-fro-MEG-ah-lee) | *nephro* ("kidney"); *megaly* ("enlargement") | enlargement of one or both kidneys; renomegaly |
| nephropathy (neh-FROP-ah-thee) | *nephr/o* ("kidney"); *-pathy* ("disease") | any disease of the kidney |

## STUDY TABLE THE URINARY SYSTEM *(continued)*

| Term and Pronunciation | Analysis | Meaning |
|---|---|---|
| renal calculus (REE-nahl KAL-ku-luhs) | *ren/o* ("kidney"); *-al* (adjective suffix); *calculus* ("stone") | a kidney stone |
| renal hypoplasia (REE-nahl HY-poh-PLAYZ-ee-ah) | *ren/o* ("kidney"); *hypo-* ("under"); *-plasia* ("form") | an underdeveloped kidney |
| renomegaly (REE-noh-MEG-ah-lee) | *ren/o* ("kidney"); *-megaly* ("enlargement") | enlargement of one or both kidneys; nephromegaly |
| renopathy (reh-NOP-ah-thee) | *ren/o* ("kidney"); *-pathy* ("disease") | any disease of the kidney; the preferred term is *nephropathy* |
| ureteralgia (yu-ree-teh-RAL-jee-aj) | *ureter/o* ("ureter"); *-algia* ("pain") | pain in a ureter |
| ureteritis (yu-ree-teh-RY-tihs) | *ureter/o* ("ureter"); *-itis* ("inflammation") | inflammation of a ureter |
| urethralgia (yu-ree-THRAL-jee-ah) | *urethr/o* ("urethra"); *algia* ("pain") | pain in the urethra (sometimes also called *urethrodynia*) |
| urethritis (yu-ree-THRY-tihs) | *urethr/o* ("urethra"); *-itis* ("inflammation") | inflammation of the urethra |
| urethrostenosis (yu-REE-throh-steh-NO-sihs) | *urethr/o* ("urethra"); *-stenosis* ("narrowing") | narrowing of the urethra |

### DIAGNOSIS & TREATMENT

| Term and Pronunciation | Analysis | Meaning |
|---|---|---|
| ureterography (yu-REE-teh-ROG-rah-fee) | *ureter/o* ("ureter"); *-graphy* ("x-ray") | radiography of the ureter |
| urinalysis (yur-ih-NAL-ih-sihs) | *urin/o* ("urine"); *analysis* (common English word) | analysis of urine |

### PRACTICE & PRACTITIONERS

| Term and Pronunciation | Analysis | Meaning |
|---|---|---|
| nephrologist (neh-FROL-oh-jist) | *nephr/o* ("kidney"); *-logist* ("practitioner") | a medical specialist who diagnoses and treats disorders of the kidneys |
| nephrology (neh-FROL-oh-jee) | *nephr/o* ("kidney"); *-logy* ("study") | medical specialty dealing with the kidneys |
| urologist (yu-ROL-oh-jist) | from the Greek word *ouron* ("urine"); *-logist* ("practitioner") | a medical specialist who diagnoses and treats disorders of the urinary system |
| urology (yu-ROL-oh-jee) | from the Greek word *ouron* ("urine"); *-logy* ("study") | the medical specialty dealing with the urinary system |

### SURGICAL PROCEDURES

| Term and Pronunciation | Analysis | Meaning |
|---|---|---|
| cystectomy (sihs-TEK-toh-mee) | *cyst/o* ("bladder"); *-ectomy* ("excision") | excision of either the urinary bladder or the gallbladder; excision of the gallbladder is properly, and most often, called a *cholecystectomy*; since *cyst* also means *cyst*, a *cystectomy* can also mean "surgical removal of a cyst" |
| cystopexy (SIHS-toh-pek-see) | *cyst/o* ("bladder"); *-pexy* ("surgical fixation") | surgical fixation of either the gallbladder or the urinary bladder; this term is included because it is typical of the dual use of *cysto* |

## STUDY TABLE THE URINARY SYSTEM *(continued)*

| Term and Pronunciation | Analysis | Meaning |
|---|---|---|
| nephrectomy (neh-FREK-toh-mee) | *nephr/o* ("kidney"); *-ectomy* ("excision") | removal of a kidney |
| nephrolithotomy (NEH-froh-lih-THOT-oh-mee) | *nephr/o* ("kidney"); *lith/o* ("stone"); *-tomy* (incision) | incision into the kidney to remove a calculus (kidney stone) |
| nephrorrhaphy (neh-FROR-ah-fee) | *nephr/o* ("kidney"); *-rrhaphy* ("suture") | suture of the kidney |
| nephrotomy (neh-FROT-oh-mee) | *nephr/o* ("kidney"); *-tomy* ("incision") | incision into a kidney |
| ureterectomy (yu-ree-teh-REK-toh-mee) | *ureter/o* ("ureter"); *-ectomy* ("excision") | excision of part or all of a ureter |
| ureterolithotomy (yu-REE-tehr-oh-lih-THOT-oh-mee) | *ureter/o* ("ureter"); *lith/o* ("stone") *-tomy* ("incision") | incision into the ureter to remove a stone |
| ureteroplasty (yu-REE-tehr-oh-plass-tee) | *ureter/o* ("ureter"); *-plasty* ("surgical repair") | surgical repair of a ureter |
| ureterorrhaphy (yu-ree-tehr-OR-rah-fee) | *ureter/o* ("ureter"); *-rrhaphy* ("suture") | suture of a ureter |
| urethrectomy (yur-ee-THEK-toh-mee) | *urethr/o* ("urethra"); *-ectomy* ("excision") | excision of all or part of the urethra |
| **ENHANCEMENT TERMS** | | |
| albuminuria (al-byu-mihn-YUR-ee-ah) | from the Latin word *albumen* ("white of an egg") | presence of protein in urine |
| anuria (an-YUR-ee-ah) | *a-* ("not"); *ur/o* ("urine"); *-ia* ("condition") | absence of urine formation |
| cystocele (SIHS-toh-seel) | *cyst/o* ("bladder"); *-cele* ("hernia') | hernia of the bladder |
| cystoscopy (sihs-TOS-ko-pee) | *cyst/o* ("bladder"); *-scopy* ("visual inspection") | visual inspection of the bladder by means of a cystoscope |
| dialysis (dy-AL-ih-sihs) | from the Greek verb *dialyo* ("separate") | filtration to remove colloidal particles from a fluid |
| diuretic (dy-yu-REHT-ik) | From the Latin word *diureticus* | promoting the excretion of urine |
| dysuria (dihs-YUR-ee-ah) | *dys-* ("difficult"); *ur/o* ("urine"); *-ia* (condition) | difficult or painful urination |
| glomerulonephritis (glom-MER-yu-lo-neh-FRY-tihs) | from the Latin verb *glomerare* ("to form into a ball"); *nephr/o* ("kidney"); *-itis* ("inflammation") | renal disease characterized by inflammation of glomeruli (not the result of kidney infection) |
| glycosuria (gly-kohs-YUR-ee-ah) | *glyc/o* ("sugar"); *-urea* ("urine") | urinary excretion of carbohydrates |
| hematuria (he-mat-YUR-ee-ah) | *hemat/o* ("blood"); *ur/o* ("urine"); *-ia* ("condition") | urinary excretion of blood |
| lithotripsy (LITH-oh-trip-see) | *lith/o* ("stone"); *tripsy* from a Greek word *tripsis* ("rubbing") | treatment in which a stone in the kidney, urethra, or bladder is broken up into small particles |
| nephrolithiasis (NEFF-ro-lih-THY-ah-sihs) | *nephr/o* ("kidney"); *lith/o* ("stone"); *-iasis* ("condition") | the presence of renal calculi |
| nephroureterocystectomy (NEH-fro-yu-REH-teh-roh-sihs-TEK-toh-mee) (Note: This term is included | *nephr/o* ("kidney"); *ureter/o* ("ureter"); *cyst/o* ("bladder"); | excision of a kidney, ureter, and at least part of the urinary bladder |

📖 **STUDY TABLE** THE URINARY SYSTEM (continued)

| Term and Pronunciation | Analysis | Meaning |
|---|---|---|
| to show how roots are sometimes strung together to simplify an otherwise wordy description of a procedure) | -ectomy ("excision") | |
| oliguria (oh-lih-GUR-ee-ah) | olig/o ("little or few"); ur/o ("urine");-ia ("condition") | diminished urine production |
| polyuria (pol-ee-YUR-ee-ah) | poly- ("much or many"); ur/o ("urine"); -ia ("condition') | excessive urine production |
| pyelography (PY-eh-LOG-rah-fee) | pyel/o ("pelvis"); -graphy ("x-ray") | radiography of the pelvic area: kidney, ureters, and urinary bladder |
| pyuria (pu-YOUR-ee-ah) | py/o ("pus"); ur/o ("urine"); -ia ("condition") | pus in the urine |
| uremia (yu-REE-mee-ah) | ur/o ("urine"); -emia ("blood") | an excess of urea in the blood |
| urinogenous (yur-ih-NOJ-eh-nuhs) | urin/o ("urine"); gen/o ("origin"); -ous (adjective suffix) | adjective denoting urine production |
| urinometry (yur-ih-NOM-ih-tree) | urin/o ("urine"); -metry ("measurement") | test of urine for specific gravity |

📝 **Exercises**

**Exercise 14-1 Choosing the Correct Term**
Fill in the blanks.

When urine passes from the 1) _Kidneys_ it is transported by two tubes called 2) _ureters_, one extending from each kidney to either side of the 3) _urinary bladder_. Urine moves through the ureters to the urinary bladder by means of 4) _peristalsis_. The urinary bladder collects 5) _urine_, so that it can be expelled in large quantities. The tube that empties the urine from the urinary bladder and expels it from the body is called the 6) _urethra_. Urine is expelled into the first portion of the urethra, when a muscle called the 7) _urethral internal sphincter_ relaxes. When the 8) _micturition urethra sphincter_ reflex sends a signal that it is time to open and expel urine from the body, another circular muscle, called the 9) _external urethra sphincter_, allows urine to pass from the first section of the 10) _urethra_.

A kidney stone, properly called a 11) _renal calculus_, is formed in the kidney and, subsequently, passes through that kidney's ureter, where it causes acute pain 12) _ureteralgia_ and inflammation 13) _ureteritis_. A specialist in the urinary system, called a 14) _urologist_, would diagnose this problem, using x-ray technology in the process of 15) _ureterography_. If the calculus is unable to pass through the ureter, it may cause blockage in the flow of urine from that kidney and possibly require removal by means of a surgical procedure called a 16) _ureterolithotomy_. If the calculus does pass through the ureter, it enters the urinary bladder and, subsequently, the urethra. When it is in the urethra, the calculus may again cause pain 17) _urethralgia_ and inflammation 18) _urethritis_.

# Exercises

## Exercise 14-2 Matching Terms with Definitions

Match the numbers in Column 1 with the letters in Column 2 according to the corresponding terms and definitions they designate.

| Term | Definition |
|---|---|
| 1. _G_ nephron | A. capillary network found inside each nephron |
| 2. _D_ urethra | B. urination |
| 3. _I_ external sphincter | C. muscle that controls the release of urine from the bladder into the first section of the urethra |
| 4. _A_ glomerulus | D. tube that conducts urine away from the bladder for expulsion |
| 5. _B_ micturition | E. electricity-producing compound in solution |
| 6. _J_ uric acid | F. narrow part of the kidney where blood vessels and nerves enter |
| 7. _H_ ureters | G. tiny structure within the kidney in which the urine-production process begins |
| 8. _F_ hilum | H. two tubes that transfer urine from the kidneys to the urinary bladder |
| 9. _E_ electrolyte | I. muscle that controls the release of urine from the first section of the urethra for subsequent expulsion |
| 10. _C_ internal sphincter | J. natural waste product of metabolism excreted in the urine |
| 11. _P_ nephralgia | K. a kidney stone |
| 12. _R_ urinometry | L. excision of a kidney, ureter, and at least part of the urinary bladder |
| 13. _N_ urethrostenosis | M. adjective denoting urine production |
| 14. _T_ cystalgia | N. narrowing of the urethra |
| 15. _L_ nephro-ureterocystectomy | O. any disease of the kidney |
| 16. _S_ ureterography | P. pain in the kidneys |
| 17. _K_ renal calculus | Q. incision into the kidney to remove a calculus (kidney stone) |
| 18. _M_ urinogenous | R. test of urine for specific gravity |
| 19. _Q_ nephrolithotomy | S. radiography of the ureter |
| 20. _O_ nephropathy | T. pain in the bladder (most often used to signify the urinary bladder) |

# Exercises

## Exercise 14-3 Identifying the Parts of the Urinary System

Label the following parts of the urinary system in Figure 14-4.

- left kidney
- left ureter
- right kidney
- right ureter
- urethra
- urinary bladder

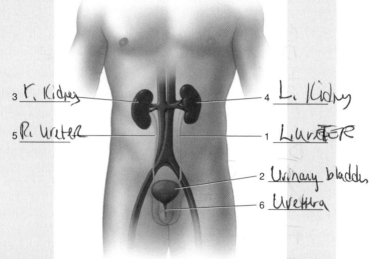

3 R. Kidney

5 R. ureter

4 L. Kidney

1 L ureter

2 Urinary bladder

6 Urethra

FIGURE 14-4 Parts of the urinary system (Exercise 14-3).

# Exercises

## Exercise 14-4 Building Medical Terms

Build terms to satisfy the following definitions, and then analyze each term by identifying its word elements.

| Definition | Term | Analysis |
|---|---|---|
| 1. electricity-conducting compound in a solution | Electrolyte | electro Electric.. |
| 2. narrow part of the kidney where blood vessels and nerves enter | hilum | tripple |
| 3. pain in a bladder, most often used to signify the urinary bladder | Cystalgia | Cyst/o Algia |
| 4. pain in a ureter | uteralgia | uete Algis |
| 5. analysis of urine | Urinalysis | Urine |
| 6. medical specialty dealing with the urinary system | urology | Urine |

7. surgical fixation of either
   the gallbladder or the
   urinary bladder
   *Cystopexy    Cept/Pexy*

8. incision into a kidney
   *Nephrotomy    Kidney/Incision*

9. thin inner covering enclosing
   the kidney
   *Renal Capsule    Kidney*

10. excision of all or part of
    the urethra
    *Urethrectomy    Excision of all of.*

## Exercises

### Exercise 14-5 Assembling and Defining Terms

Using the Term Analysis, assemble and define each term.

| Term Analysis | Term | Definition |
|---|---|---|
| 1. olig/o (little or few); ur/o (urine); -ia (condition) | *Obligarie* | *diminished with produ Lotsa of Urine* |
| 2. poly- (much or many); ur/o (urine); -ia (condition) | *Polyuria* | *Reflux Signal Sphincter* |
| 3. noun from the Latin verb *micturire* (to desire to make water) | *micturition Reflex* ~~Renal Calculus~~ | ~~Softening of Renal gland~~ |
| 4. ren/o (kidney); -al (adjective suffix; fascia (Latin word for band) | *Renal Fascia* | *Outer covering of Kidney* |
| 5. ren/o (kidney); -al (adjective suffix); calculus (stone) | *Renal Fascis* | *Softening of Renal* |
| 6. ren/o (kidney); hypo (under); -plasia (form) | *Renal Hypoplasia* | *Undeveloped Kidney* |
| 7. ren/o (kidney); -megaly (enlargement) | *Renal-Enlargment -megaly* | *Enlargment* |
| 8. ureter/o (ureter); graphy (x-ray) | *Ureterography* | *Xray* |
| 9. nephr/o (kidney); -logy (study) | *Nephrology* | *Study of Kidney* |
| 10. ren/o (kidney); -pathy (disease) | *Renopathy* | *Disease* |

# Exercises

## Exercise 14-6 Multiple Choice

Circle the term in the Choices column that correctly answers each of the following questions.

| Question | Choices |
|---|---|
| 1. What term means an excess of urea in the blood? | hematuria; uremia; glomerular |
| 2. What is the name of the capillary network found inside each nephron? | globular; glomerulus; glomerular |
| 3. What is the name of the pair of organs that excrete urine? | internal sphincters; kidneys; nephrons |
| 4. What are the tiny structures within the kidneys in which the urine-production process begins? | internal sphincters; kidneys; nephrons |
| 5. What is the term for an enlargement of one or both kidneys? | nephropathy; nephromegaly; nephrolithotomy |
| 6. What is the term for any disease of the kidney? | nephropathy; nephromegaly; nephrolithotomy |
| 7. What is the term for the tube that conducts urine away from the bladder for expulsion? | ureter; urethra; urethalgia |
| 8. What is the term for pain in the urethra? | urethritis; urethra; urethalgia |
| 9. What is the term for excision of part or all of a ureter? | ureterorrhaphy; urethra; ureterectomy |
| 10. What is the term for suture of a ureter? | ureterorrhaphy; urethra; ureterectomy |

# Exercises

## Exercise 14-7 True, False, and Correction

Put an X in the True or False column next to each statement. Write the correct answer in the "Correction, if False" column for any statements you identify as false.

| Statement | True | False | Correction, if False |
|---|---|---|---|
| 1. Testing urine for specific gravity is urinometry. | ✓ | | |
| 2. Renal fascia is the fatty tissue surrounding the renal capsule. | | ✓ | Perirenal Fat |
| 3. The two tubes that transfer urine from the kidneys to the urinary bladder are the urethritis. | | ✓ | Ureters |
| 4. A natural waste product of metabolism that is excreted in urine is called urea. | | ✓ | Uric Acid |
| 5. The urinary bladder serves as temporary storage receptacle for urine. | ✓ | | |
| 6. Narrowing of the urethra is referred to as urethrostenosis. | ✓ | | |
| 7. The word element -logist in urologist means study. | | ✓ | Practitioner |
| 8. An incision into the kidney to remove a kidney stone is called a nephrectomy. | | ✓ | Nephrolithotomy |
| 9. An incision into the ureter to remove a stone is called a ureteroplasty. | ✓ | | |
| 10. Inflammation of the urethra is called ureteralgia. | | ✓ | Ureitis |

---

### ✓ Pre-Quiz Checklist

_____ Study the word elements specific to the urinary system (Table 14-1).

_____ Review the definitions and etymologies in the study table.

_____ Check your answers to all the exercises with the answers in the Appendix and consult the study table again to correct any errors before attempting the quiz.

## ✓ Chapter Quiz

Write the answers to the following items in the spaces provided.

1. What is the hilum?

    1. _____
       _____
       _____
       _____

2. Name the three layers of the kidney, from innermost to outermost.

    2. _____
       _____
       _____

3. Name two natural products of metabolism that the kidneys remove.

    3. _____
       _____

4. What reflex sends a signal indicating that it is time to open the external sphincter to permit urination?

    4. _____
       _____

5. Which sphincter muscle allows urine into the first section of the urethra?

    5. _____
       _____

6. What is the capillary network found inside each nephron called, and what does it do?

    6. _____

7. What are ureters, and what is their job?

    7. _____
       _____
       _____
       _____
       _____
       _____

8. By what action does urine travel through the ureters?

    8. _____

9. What is the urethra, and what is its function?

    9. _____
       _____

10. Give the name of the medical specialty dealing with the kidneys.

    10. _____

11. What term denotes surgical removal of the urinary bladder?

    11. _____

12. What is the term for an underdeveloped kidney?

    12. _____

13. Give the terms for pain in the following areas: a) urinary bladder, b) kidney, c) ureter, and d) urethra.

    13. _____

14. Name two of the many tests that can be performed on the urine.

    14. _____

15. Cystectomy can have two meanings other than removal of the urinary bladder. What are they?

    15. _____
        _____
        _____

## ✓ **Chapter Quiz** *(continued)*

16. Define nephrectomy.                                          16. _____

17. What organs are removed when a                              17. _____
    nephroureterocystectomy is performed?

18. What is the synonym for nephromegaly?                       18. _____

19. Nephropathy means any disease of                           19. _____
    the kidney. What is its synonym?

20. In Question 19 above, which of the two terms is preferred? 20. _____

# Chapter 15

# The Reproductive System

CHAPTER CONTENTS

The reproduction process begins with *fertilization, which* occurs when a male *gamete* (also called a *sperm* or *spermatozoon*; plural: *spermatozoa*) fertilizes a female gamete (also called an *ovum*; plural: *ova*). The collective name for any female or male organ that produces a gamete is *gonad*. The single cell formed at fertilization is called a *zygote,* which contains a full complement of *chromosomes* carrying the DNA of a unique new person. The period of *gestation* is the time lapse between the formation of the zygote and birth.

In the paragraphs, illustrations, and tables that follow, you will encounter key terms used in describing the reproduction process, along with a few terms associated with genetics, one of several related specialties.

## WORD ROOTS SPECIFIC TO THE REPRODUCTIVE SYSTEM

The roots shown in Table 15-1 are often found in terms related to the reproductive system. You will recognize them in many of the terms you will learn in this chapter.

| TABLE 15-1 | COMMON ROOTS RELATED TO THE REPRODUCTIVE SYSTEM |
|---|---|
| Root | Refers to |
| cervic/o; trachel/o | cervix |
| colp/o; vagin/o | vagina |
| men/o | menses |
| oo | egg |
| oophor/o | ovary (also egg) |
| orch/i/o; orchid/o | testes |
| ovari/o | ovary |
| salping/o | tube (sometimes a reference to the uterine tube) |
| spermat/o | sperm |
| uter/o; hyster/o; metr/o | uterus |

## THE MALE REPRODUCTIVE CYCLE

The male reproductive cycle comprises the production of the male gametes. This process, called *spermatogenesis,* involves a cell-division process known as *meiosis,* which produces *haploid cells* having only the chromosomes of the potential male parent.

Male gamete production occurs in the *testes* (singular: *testis*), and the dynamics of the process rely on the secretion of *androgens,* which are male sex hormones. The most significant of these is *testosterone.* After spermatogenesis is complete, the *spermatozoa* (singular: *spermatozoon*) travel to the *epididymis,* an organ adjacent to the testes, where they become functional.

In summary, the testes produce and store the spermatozoa; the epididymis stores and develops them into a functional state; and the *prostate gland* produces,

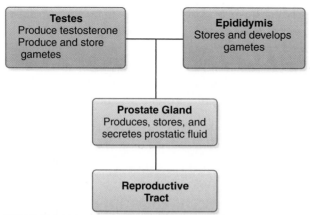

FIGURE 15-1 Male reproductive functions (diagram).

stores, and secretes a fluid medium called *prostatic fluid.* The combination of the gametes and their associated glandular secretions, along with the prostatic fluid, is called *semen* (Figure 15-1).

Leaving the epididymis, spermatozoa enter the *ductus deferens,* also called the *vas deferens,* and eventually find their way into the *urethra,* which is part of both the male urinary and male reproductive systems. As you discovered in Chapter 14, the urethra attaches to the bottom of the urinary bladder. It is also surrounded by and connected to the prostate gland (Figure 15-2).

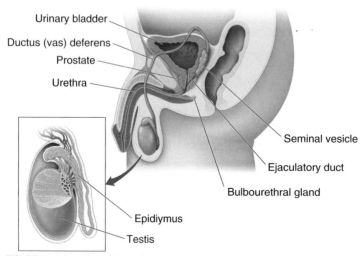

FIGURE 15-2 Location of the male reproductive system. *From:* Cohen BJ, Taylor JJ, Memmler RL, eds. *Memmler's The Structure and Function of the Human Body.* 8th ed. Baltimore, MD: Lippincott Williams & Wilkins; 2005.

# THE FEMALE REPRODUCTIVE CYCLE

## The Fertilization Stage

Like the male reproductive cycle, the female reproductive cycle provides gametes for fertilization. But it does a great deal more by also providing an environment suitable for development of the zygote.

The female counterpart to spermatogenesis is *oogenesis,* which occurs in the *ovaries* (singular: *ovary*). Stimulated by follicle-stimulating hormone (FSH; see Chapter 12), the ovaries begin the process of oogenesis, which continues with the secretion of other required hormones, called *progestins,* the principal one of which is *progesterone.* As a result, the ovaries produce *oocytes,* which are haploid cells that eventually become the gametes.

Hormonal activity controls all phases of the reproduction cycles in both men and women, but in women, it also controls something called the *uterine cycle* or *menstrual cycle,* which has three phases: *secretory* (secretion of hormones), *proliferative* (proliferation of the ovum), and *menses* (the end of one cycle and the beginning of another). If male spermatozoa are present during *ovulation,* which occurs during the proliferative phase, the possibility of fertilization exists.

 Oogenesis and ovulation are not the same thing. *Oogenesis* is the formation of the ovum, and *ovulation* refers to its release from the ovary.

The *uterine tubes,* also known as *fallopian tubes,* connect the ovaries to the *uterus,* which is the reproductive organ in which the fertilized oocyte is implanted and in which the child develops. The *uterine cervix,* usually called simply the *cervix,* is located at the lower end of the uterus (Figure 15-3).

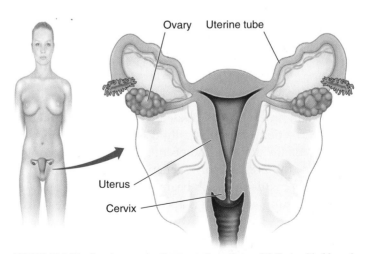

FIGURE **15-3** The female reproductive tract. *From:* Cohen BJ, Taylor JJ,  Memmler RL, eds. *Memmler's The Structure and Function of the Human Body.* 8th ed. Baltimore, MD: Lippincott Williams & Wilkins; 2005.

## The Gestation Stage

*Gestation,* a synonym for pregnancy, comes from the Latin verb *gesto,* meaning "to bear." When the single-cell zygote divides the first time, it is called an *embryo.* This term is used until approximately the eighth week of gestation. Between the eighth week and birth, which under normal circumstances occurs between weeks 38 to 40, the term *fetus* is used.

This process of cell division is called *mitosis.* Like meiosis, mitosis is a process of cell division, but each cell produced contains a full complement of both maternal and paternal chromosomes and is thus called a *diploid* cell. Mitosis occurs many billions of times during gestation (Figure 15-4).

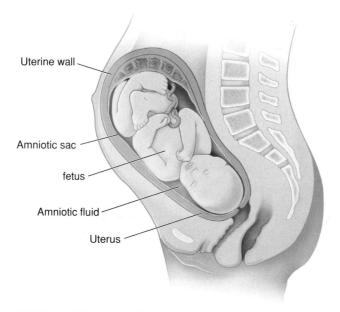

Uterine wall

Amniotic sac

fetus

Amniotic fluid

Uterus

FIGURE **15-4** Midsagittal section of a pregnant uterus with fetus. *From:* Cohen BJ, Taylor JJ, Memmler RL, eds. *Memmler's The Structure and Function of the Human Body.* 8th ed. Baltimore, MD: Lippincott Williams & Wilkins; 2005.

Diagnostic tests and procedures associated with pregnancy include *amniocentesis,* involving the extraction of amniotic fluid from the *amniotic sac,* which surrounds the fetus inside the uterus. Amniocentesis is most commonly employed to discover, or rule out, the presence of a genetic disorder, but it can also help in determining fetal lung maturity, which bears on the safety of an early delivery, or whether the mother's immune system is adversely affecting the fetus.

The medical term used in reference to a pregnant woman is *gravida,* which is usually followed by a number (most often a Roman numeral, e.g., I, II, etc.) that indicates the number of times she has been pregnant. Therefore, *gravida I* refers to a woman who is pregnant for the first time. Another way of designating the number of the pregnancy is by using Latin prefixes: *primigravida, secundigravida,* etc. Gravida comes from the Latin adjective *gravis,* which medical dictionaries list as meaning "heavy." However, other meanings of *gravis* include "profound" and "important." The medical term for a woman who has delivered a baby is *para,* and it is also followed by a number. Thus, a woman who has born her first child (or children in the case of a multiple birth) would be called a *gravida I, para I.* A woman who has carried and born a second child would be known as a *gravida II, para II,* etc. Para comes from the Latin verb *pario,* which means "to bring forth, produce, or create."

 **DECIPHERING MEDICAL DOCUMENTS**

**Read the following excerpt from a hospital report, and answer the questions that follow.**

*A 27-year-old gravida 2, para 1 woman without significant medical history. Bloodwork was normal before delivery of a stillborn 1 pound, 11 ounce infant during week 21. Although ultrasound studies during week 14 and amniocentesis during week 15 were unremarkable, intrauterine fetal demise had occurred during week 18.*

1. What does gravida 2, para 1 signify?
2. What is amniocentesis?
3. In the final sentence, both "fetal demise" and "stillborn" are self-evident terms. Using your knowledge of word elements, define intrauterine.

## REPRODUCTIVE SYSTEM DISORDERS AND PROCEDURES

The *Pap test,* which consists of the microscopic examination of cells from a mucosal surface, especially the uterine cervix, is widely used in diagnostic screening, as is *mammography,* examination of the breast by means of an imaging technique, such as radiography. Table 15-2 lists these and other common disorders and procedures associated with both the male and female reproductive systems and some of the procedures used in their diagnosis and treatment.

**TABLE 15-2**  COMMON DISORDERS AND PROCEDURES ASSOCIATED WITH THE REPRODUCTIVE SYSTEM

| Term | Definition |
|---|---|
| amniocentesis | extraction and diagnostic examination of amniotic fluid from the amniotic sac |
| cervicectomy; also, rarely, trachelectomy | excision of the uterine cervix |
| cervicitis; also trachelitis | inflammation of the uterine cervix |
| cervicoplasty | surgical repair of the uterine cervix OR the neck |
| cervicotomy; also trachelotomy | incision of the uterine cervix; *tracheotomy* is the term used to denote an incision into the neck (trachea), but *trachelotomy* refers to the uterine cervix and is synonymous with *cervicotomy* |

| TABLE 15-2 | COMMON DISORDERS AND PROCEDURES ASSOCIATED WITH THE REPRODUCTIVE SYSTEM *(continued)* |
|---|---|
| **Term** | **Definition** |
| hysteralgia; also hysterodynia | pain in the uterus |
| hysterectomy | surgical removal of the uterus |
| hysteropathy | any disease of the uterus |
| hysteropexy | surgical fixation of the uterus |
| hysteroplasty | surgical repair of the uterus |
| hysterotomy | incision of the uterus |
| mammography | examination of the breast by means of an imaging technique, such as radiography |
| oophorectomy | ovariectomy |
| oophoritis | inflammation of an ovary |
| oophoroplasty | surgical repair of an ovary |
| oophorotomy | incision into an ovary |
| orchialgia | pain in the testes |
| orchiectomy | removal of one or both testes (less commonly orchidectomy) |
| orchiopathy | any disease of the testes |
| orchioplasty | surgical repair of a testis |
| orchiotomy | incision into a testis |
| orchitis | inflammation of a testis |
| ovarialgia | pain in an ovary |
| ovariectomy | excision of one or both ovaries |
| ovariotomy | incision of an ovary |
| ovaritis | inflammation of an ovary (see also oophoritis) |
| Pap test | microscopic examination of cells from a mucosal surface, especially the uterine cervix |
| uteropexy | surgical fixation of the uterus (see also hysteropexy) |
| uteroplasty | surgical repair of the uterus (see also hysteroplasty) |
| uterotomy | incision of the uterus (see also hysterotomy) |

## STUDY TABLE   THE REPRODUCTIVE SYSTEM

| Term and Pronunciation | Analysis | Meaning |
|---|---|---|
| **STRUCTURE & FUNCTION** | | |
| amniotic sac (am-nee-OT-ic) | from the Greek word *amnios* ("lamb") | fluid-filled sac that surrounds the fetus inside the uterus |
| androgens (AN-droh-jehns) | from the Greek *andros* ("man"); *-gen* ("origin") | hormones that promote the production of male gametes |
| cervix (SURV-ihks) | Latin word for "neck" | common term for the uterine cervix |
| chromosome (KROM-oh-som) | from the Greek words *chroma* ("color") and *soma* ("body") | a gene-bearing bundle of DNA found in the nucleus of all cells |

## 📖 STUDY TABLE THE REPRODUCTIVE SYSTEM *(continued)*

| Term and Pronunciation | Analysis | Meaning |
|---|---|---|
| diploid cell (DIHP-loyd) | *dipl/o* ("double"); *-oid* ("similar") | cell containing both the maternal and paternal chromosomes |
| ductus deferens (DUK-tuhs DEHF-eh-rehnz) | ductus from the Latin word *ducto* ("to lead"); deferens from the Latin word *defero* ("to carry away") | duct leading out of the epididymis (also called the *vas deferens*) |
| embryo (EHM-bree-oh) | from the Greek word *embryon* ("young one") | name change from *zygote* after the first cell division and until the eighth week of pregnancy |
| epididymis (ehp-ih-DIHD-ih-muhs) | *epi-* ("on"); *didymus* from the Greek word *didumos* ("testes") | organ in which the male sperm become functional |
| fallopian (fah-LOHP-ee-ahn) tubes; also called uterine (YU-teh-rihn) tubes | from Gabriele Fallopio, 16th-century Italian priest, physician, and anatomist | tubes between the ovaries and the uterus |
| fertilization (FUR-tih-ly-ZAY-shun) | common English word | the joining of the male and female gametes (in the context of the human reproductive system) |
| fetus (FEE-tuhs) | Latin word for "offspring" | name change from *embryo* after the eighth week of pregnancy to birth |
| gamete (GAH-meet) | from the Greek words *gamete* ("wife") and *gametes* ("husband") | term given to both the female ovum and the male spermatozoon |
| gestation (jehs-TAY-shun) | from the Latin word *gesto* ("to bear") | development that occurs between the formation of the zygote and birth of the child |
| gonad (GOH-nad) | from the Greek word *goneos* ("generation") | gamete-generating organ (ovary or testis) |
| gravida (GRA-vee-dah) | from the Latin adjective *gravis* ("heavy, profound, or important") | a pregnant woman |
| haploid cell (HAP-loyd) | from the Greek word *haplous* ("single"); *-oid* ("similar") | cell containing only one set of chromosomes, those of either the potential father or the potential mother |
| meiosis (my-OH-sihs) | Greek word for "reduction" | cell division that produces cells with only one set of chromosomes, those of either the potential father or the potential mother |
| menses (MEN-seez) | plural form of the Latin word *mensis* ("month") | end of one uterine cycle and the beginning of another |
| menstrual cycle; also called the uterine cycle | adjectival form of *menses*, Latin for "months" | part of the reproductive system process in women, comprising three phases: secretory, proliferative, and menses |

## STUDY TABLE THE REPRODUCTIVE SYSTEM (continued)

| Term and Pronunciation | Analysis | Meaning |
|---|---|---|
| mitosis (my-TOH-sihs) | from the Greek word *mitos* ("thread") | process of cell division by which one cell becomes two, both of which contain the maternal and paternal chromosomes |
| oocytes (OO-sites) | *oo* ("egg"); *-cyte* ("cell") | the product of oogenesis that become the female gametes |
| oogenesis (oo-JEN-ih-sihs) | *oo* ("egg"); *-genesis* ("origin") | production of oocytes |
| ovulation (OH-vyu-LAY-shun) | from the Latin word *ovum* ("egg") | release of the female gamete that occurs during the proliferative stage of the uterine cycle |
| ovum (OH-vuhm); plural: ova (OH-vah) | Latin for "egg" | the female gamete; ovum is singular; ova is plural |
| para (PAR-ah) | from the Latin verb *pario* ("to bring forth, produce, or create") | a woman who has given birth |
| progesterone (pro-JESS-teh-rone) | *pro-* (common English prefix meaning "foreshadow" or "promote"); *ge-* (short form of *genesis*, meaning "origin"); *sterone* (from *sterol*, referring to a class of complex alcohols) | hormone produced in the ovaries |
| progestins (pro-JESS-tihns) | *pro-* (common English prefix meaning "foreshadow" or "promote"); *ge-* (short form of *genesis*, meaning "origin"); *stins* (from *sterol*, a class of complex alcohols) | female hormones generated in the ovaries and required for oogenesis |
| proliferative (pro-LIFF-ehr-ah-tihv) | from the Latin word *prolifer* ("bearing offspring") | adjectival form of *proliferation*; term signifying one part of the uterine cycle |
| prostate gland (PRAH-stayt) | from the Greek word *prostates* ("one who stands before") | male gland that produces and stores prostatic fluid, a fluid medium that is part of semen |
| prostatic fluid (prah-STAT-ik) | *-ic* (adjective suffix added to prostate); *fluid* (common English word) | product of the prostate gland |
| reproductive tract | both common English words | in the male reproductive system, the ductwork leading from the epididymus to the outside of the body |
| secretory (seh-KREET-ehr-ee) | from the French verb *sécréter* ("to secrete") | adjectival form of *secrete*; part of the uterine cycle |
| semen (SEE-mehn) | Latin word for "seed" | combination of male gametes, their associated glandular secretions, and prostatic fluid |

## STUDY TABLE  THE REPRODUCTIVE SYSTEM (continued)

| Term and Pronunciation | Analysis | Meaning |
|---|---|---|
| sperm (spurm); spermatozoon (SPUR-mah-tah-ZOH-on); spermatozoa (SPUR-mah-tah-ZOH-ah) | from the Greek word *sperma* ("seed") | the male gamete; sperm is singular or plural; spermatozoon is singular; spermatozoa is plural |
| spermatogenesis (SPUR-mah-toh-JEHN-ih-sihs) | *spermat/o* ("sperm"); *-genesis* ("origin") | production of sperm |
| testes (TEHS-teez); singular: testis (TEHS-tihs) | from the Latin word *testiculus*, which also gives us the synonym *testicles* | the organs that produce and store the male gametes |
| testosterone (tehs-TOSS-teh-rohn) | from the Latin word *testiculus* ("testes") and *sterol* (class of complex alcohols) | androgen prominent in male gamete production |
| urethra (yu-REETH-rah) | from the Greek word *ourethra* | male ductwork that acts as a part of both the male urinary and male reproductive systems |
| uterine cervix (YU-teh-rihn) | *uter/o* ("uterus"); *-ine* (adjective suffix); *cervix* (Latin word for "neck") | the "neck" located at the lower end of the uterus |
| uterine cycle; also called the menstrual cycle | *uter/o* ("uterus"); *-ine* (adjective suffix); *cycle* (common English word) | part of the reproduction system process in women, comprising three phases: secretory, proliferative, and menses |
| uterine tubes (YU-teh-rihn); also called fallopian (fah-LOHP-ee-ahn) tubes | *uter/o* ("uterus"); *-ine* (adjective suffix); *tubes* (common English word) | tubes between the ovaries and the uterus |
| uterus (YU-teh-ruhs) | Latin word for "womb" | reproductive organ in which the fertilized oocyte is implanted and in which the child develops |
| vas deferens (vas-DEHF-eh rehnz) | *vas/o* ("vessel"); *deferens* (from the Latin word *defero*, "to carry away") | duct leading out of the epididymis (also called the *ductus deferens*) |
| **COMMON DISORDERS** | | |
| cervicitis (sur-vih-SY-tihs); also trachelitis (trak-ih-LY-tihs) | *cervic/o* ("cervix"); *-itis* ("inflammation") | inflammation of the uterine cervix |
| hysteralgia (hiss-teh-RAL-jee-ah); also hysterodynia (HIHS-toh-roh-DIHN-ee-ah) | *hyster/o* ("uterus"); *-algia* ("pain") | pain in the uterus |
| hysteropathy (hiss-toh-ROP-ah-thee) | *hyster/o* ("uterus"); *-pathy* ("disease") | any disease of the uterus |
| oophoritis (oo-foh-RY-tihs) | *oophor/o* ("ovary"); *-itis* ("inflammation") | inflammation of an ovary |
| orchialgia (or-kee-AL-jee-ah) | *orch/i/o* ("testes"); *-algia* ("pain") | pain in the testes |
| orchiopathy (or-kee-OP-ah-thee) | *orch/i/o* ("testes"); *-pathy* ("disease") | any disease of the testes |

## STUDY TABLE THE REPRODUCTIVE SYSTEM (continued)

| Term and Pronunciation | Analysis | Meaning |
|---|---|---|
| orchitis (or-KY-tihs) | *orch/i/o* ("testes"); *-itis* ("inflammation") | inflammation of a testis |
| ovarialgia (oh-vahr-ee-AL-jee-ah) | *ovar/i/o* ("ovary"); *-algia* ("pain") | pain in an ovary |
| ovaritis (ohv-ah-RY-tihs) | *ovar/i/o* ("ovary"); *-itis* ("inflammation") | inflammation of an ovary (see also *oophoritis*) |
| **PRACTICE & PRACTITIONERS** | | |
| obstetrician (OB-steh-trish-uhn) | from the Latin word *obstetrix* ("midwife"); *-ian* ("practitioner") | a physician who specializes in the medical care of women during pregnancy and childbirth |
| obstetrics (ob-STET-rihks) | from the Latin word *obstetrix* ("midwife") | medical specialty concerned with the medical care of women during pregnancy and childbirth |
| **DIAGNOSIS & TREATMENT** | | |
| amniocentesis (am-nee-oh-sen-TEE-sihs) | from the Greek words *amnios* ("lamb"); and *kentesis* ("puncture") | extraction and diagnostic examination of amniotic fluid from the amniotic sac |
| mammography (mam-OG-rah-fee) | *mamm/o* ("breast"); *-graphy* ("x-ray") | examination of the breast by means of an imaging technique, such as radiography |
| Pap test | named for the stain (*Papanicolaou*) used in microscopic examination | microscopic examination of cells from a mucosal surface, especially the uterine cervix |
| **SURGICAL PROCEDURES** | | |
| cervicectomy (surv-ih-SEK-toh-mee); also, rarely, trachelectomy (trak-eh-LEK-toh-mee) | *cervic/o* ("cervix"); *-ectomy* ("excision") | excision of the uterine cervix |
| cervicoplasty (SURV-ih-ko-plass-tee) | *cervic/o* ("cervix"); *-plasty* ("repair") | surgical repair of the uterine cervix OR the neck |
| cervicotomy (surv-ih-KOT-oh-mee); also trachelotomy (trak-eh-LOT-oh-mee) | *cervic/o* ("cervix"); *-tomy* ("incision") | incision of the uterine cervix; *tracheotomy* is the term used to denote an incision into the neck (trachea); but *trachelotomy* refers to the uterine cervix and is synonymous with *cervicotomy* |
| hysterectomy (hiss-toh-REK-toh-mee) | *hyster/o* ("uterus"); *-ectomy* ("excision") | surgical removal of the uterus |
| hysteropexy (HISS-teh-roh-pek-see) | *hyster/o* ("uterus"); *-pexy* ("fixation") | surgical fixation of the uterus |
| hysteroplasty (HISS-teh-roh-plass-tee) | *hyster/o* ("uterus"); *-plasty* ("surgical repair") | surgical repair of the uterus |
| hysterotomy (hiss-teh-ROT-oh-mee) | *hyster/o* ("uterus"); *-tomy* ("incision") | incision of the uterus |
| oophorectomy (oo-foh-REK-toh-mee) | *oophor/o* ("ovary"); *-ectomy* ("excision") | excision of an ovary; ovariectomy |
| oophoroplasty (OO-foh-roh-plass-tee) | *oophor/o* ("ovary"); *-plasty* ("surgical repair") | surgical repair of an ovary |

## STUDY TABLE THE REPRODUCTIVE SYSTEM *(continued)*

| Term and Pronunciation | Analysis | Meaning |
|---|---|---|
| oophorotomy (oo-foh-ROT-oh-mee) | *oophor/o* ("ovary"); *-tomy* ("incision") | incision into an ovary |
| orchiectomy (or-kee-EK-toh-mee) | *orch/i/o* ("testes"); *-ectomy* ("excision") | removal of one or both testes (less commonly, *orchidectomy*) |
| orchioplasty (ORK-ee-oh-plass-tee) | *orch/i/o* ("testes"); *-plasty* ("surgical repair") | surgical repair of a testis |
| orchiotomy (or-kee-OT-ah-mee) | *orch/i/o* ("testes"); *-tomy* ("incision") | incision into a testis |
| ovariectomy (oh-vahr-ee-EK-toh-mee) | *ovar/i/o* ("ovary"); *-ectomy* ("excision") | excision of one or both ovaries |
| ovariotomy (oh-vahr-ee-OT-oh-mee) | *ovar/i/o* ("ovary"); *-tomy* ("incision") | incision of an ovary |
| uteropexy (YU-teh-roh-pek-see) | *uter/o* ("uterus"); *-pexy* ("surgical fixation") | surgical fixation of the uterus (see also *hysteropexy*) |
| uteroplasty (YU-teh-roh-plass-tee) | *uter/o* ("uterus"); *-plasty* ("surgical repair") | surgical repair of the uterus (see also *hysteroplasty*) |
| uterotomy (yu-the-ROT-oh-mee) | *uter/o* ("uterus"); *-tomy* ("incision") | incision of the uterus (see also *hysterotomy*) |

### ENHANCEMENT TERMS

| | | |
|---|---|---|
| amenorrhea (a-men-oh-REE-ah) | *a-* ("not"); *men/o* ("menses"); *-rrhea* ("flow") of menses | absence or abnormal cessation |
| Cesarean section (seh-SAYR-ee-ahn); other spellings are Caesarean and Caesarian | from the Latin word *Caesarianus* (after Julius Caesar, who authorities say was born in this way) | surgical operation through the abdominal wall and uterus for delivery of the baby |
| colposcopy (kole-POSS-koh-pee) | *colp/o* ("vagina"); *-scopy* ("visual examination") | examination of the vagina and cervix using an endoscopic instrument |
| dysmenorrhea (diss-men-oh-REE-ah) | *dys-* ("difficult"); *men/o* ("menses"); *-rrhea* ("flow") | difficult or painful menses |
| ectopic pregnancy (ek-TOP-ik) | *ec-* ("outside"); *-top* (from the Greek word *topos,* "place"); *-ic* (adjective suffix) | development of an impregnated ovum outside the uterus |
| endometriosis (EN-do-mee-tree-OH-sihs) | *endo-* ("inside"); *metr/o* ("uterus"); *-osis* ("condition") | tissue outside the uterus that resembles the inner lining of the uterus |
| hypermenorrhea (HY-pur-men-oh-REE-ah) | *hyper-* ("excessive"); *men/o* ("menses"); *-rrhea* ("flow") | prolonged or excessive menorrhea; also sometimes called *menorrhagia* |
| lactation (lak-TAY-shun) | from the Latin word *lactatio* ("suckle") | the production of milk |
| menopause (MEN-oh-paws) | *men/o* ("menses"); the Greek word *pausis* ("cessation") | permanent cessation of menses |
| menorrhagia (men-oh-RAJ-ee-ah) | *men/o* ("menses"); *-rrhagia* ("excessive discharge") | See *hypermenorrhea* |
| salpingitis (sal-pin-JY-tiss) | *salping/o* ("tube"); *-itis* ("inflammation") | inflammation of the uterine tube (see also Chapter 18 Study Table) |

## ABBREVIATION TABLE

### COMMON ABBREVIATIONS:
### The Reproductive System

| Abbreviation | Meaning |
| --- | --- |
| BPH | benign prostatic hyperplasia (hypertrophy) |
| CS | Cesarean section |
| D&C | dilation and curettage |
| DNA | deoxyribonucleic acid (the genetic code) |
| DUB | dysfunctional uterine bleeding |
| HSG | hysterosalpingogram |
| IVF | in vitro fertilization |
| OB | obstetrics |
| PID | pelvic inflammatory disease |
| PSA | prostate-specific antigen |
| TURP | transurethral resection of the prostate |

# Exercises

## Exercise 15-1 Choosing the Correct Term

Fill in the blanks.

Male gamete production occurs in the 1)_____. This process relies on the secretion of 2)_____ and most significantly 3)_____. After the production of sperm (or 4)_____) is complete, they travel to the 5)_____, an organ adjacent to the 6)_____, where they become functional. On leaving the epididymis, spermatozoa enter the 7)_____ and then travel to the 8)_____. The prostate gland, which surrounds and is connected to the urethra, produces 9)_____. This fluid, together with the combination of gametes and their glandular secretions, constitutes 10)_____.

11)_____ activity controls all of the phases of the reproduction cycles in both men and women, but in a woman, it also controls something called the 12)_____ or 13)_____ cycle. The ovaries secrete the required hormones, called 14)_____, the principal one of which is 15)_____. These hormones stimulate the ovaries to produce 16)_____, which become the 17)_____ for fertilization. The ovaries are connected to the uterus by the two 18)_____ or 19)_____ tubes.

# Exercises

## Exercise 15-2 Converting Nouns to Adjectives

Convert each of the following nouns to its adjective form using one of the following suffixes: *al, ar, ic, ous, ory, ine, ian.*

| Noun | Adjective Form |
|------|----------------|
| 1. testicle | _____ |
| 2. chromosome | _____ |
| 3. androgen | _____ |
| 4. epididymis | _____ |
| 5. prostate | _____ |
| 6. urethra | _____ |
| 7. spermatogenesis | _____ |
| 8. oogenesis | _____ |
| 9. uterus | _____ |
| 10. ovulation | _____ |
| 11. cervix | _____ |
| 12. ovary | _____ |
| 13. gestation | _____ |
| 14. fetus | _____ |
| 15. embryo | _____ |

# Exercises

## Exercise 15-3 Matching Terms with Definitions

Match the numbers in Column 1 with the letters in Column 2 according to the corresponding terms and definitions they designate.

| Term | Definition |
|------|------------|
| 1. _____ ductus deferens | A. combination of male gametes, their associated secretions, and prostatic fluid |
| 2. _____ prostate gland | B. removal of one or both testes |
| 3. _____ spermatogenesis | C. organs that produce and store male gametes |
| 4. _____ epididymis | D. duct leading out of the epididymis (also called the vas deferens) |
| 5. _____ orchiectomy | E. production of sperm |
| 6. _____ haploid cell | F. male gland that produces and stores prostatic fluid, a fluid medium that is part of semen |

| Term | Definition |
|------|-----------|
| 7. \_\_\_\_ semen | G. pain in the testes |
| 8. \_\_\_\_ testosterone | H. cell containing only one set of chromosomes (those of either the potential mother or potential father) |
| 9. \_\_\_\_ orchalgia | I. organ in which the male sperm become functional |
| 10. \_\_\_\_ testes | J. androgen prominent in male gamete production |
| 11. \_\_\_\_ hysterectomy and bilateral oophorectomy | K. inflammation of an ovary |
| 12. \_\_\_\_ salpingectomy | L. excision of the uterine cervix |
| 13. \_\_\_\_ ovarialgia | M. surgical fixation of the uterus |
| 14. \_\_\_\_ uteropexy or hysteropexy | N. release of the female gamete that occurs during the proliferative stage of the uterine cycle |
| 15. \_\_\_\_ period of gestation | O. surgical removal of a fallopian tube |
| 16. \_\_\_\_ cervicectomy or trachelectomy | P. the female gamete |
| 17. \_\_\_\_ ovaritis or oophoritis | Q. surgical removal of the uterus and right and left ovaries |
| 18. \_\_\_\_ uterine cervix | R. pain in the ovary |
| 19. \_\_\_\_ ovum | S. the "neck" located at the lower end of the uterus |
| 20. \_\_\_\_ ovulation | T. time lapse between zygote formation and birth |

# Exercises

## Exercise 15-4 Identifying the Parts of the Male Reproductive System

Label the following parts on Figure 15-5.

- ductus deferens
- epididymis
- testes
- urethra

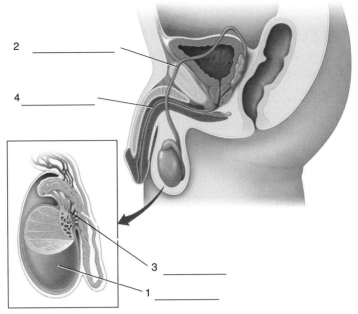

2 _____

4 _____

3 _____

1 _____

FIGURE **15-5** Identifying the parts of the male reproductive system (Exercise 15-4).

# Exercises

## Exercise 15-5 Locating Major Parts of the Female Reproductive System

Label the following parts on Figure 15-6.

- ◆ cervix
- ◆ ovaries
- ◆ uterine tubes
- ◆ uterus

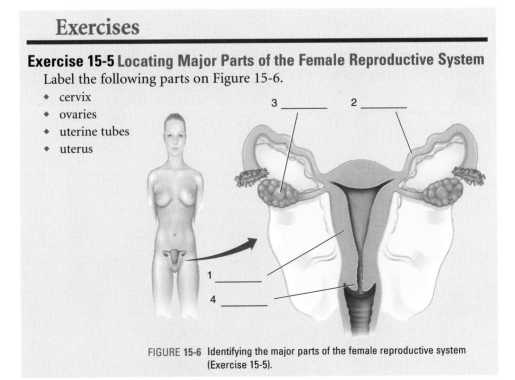

3 _____   2 _____

1 _____

4 _____

FIGURE **15-6** Identifying the major parts of the female reproductive system (Exercise 15-5).

# Exercises

## Exercise 15-6 Building Medical Terms

Build terms to satisfy the following definitions, and then analyze each term by identifying its word elements.

| Definition | Term | Analysis |
|---|---|---|
| 1. hormones that promote the production of male gametes | _____ | _____ _____ |
| 2. organ in which the male sperm become functional | _____ | _____ _____ |
| 3. gamete-generating organ, male or female | _____ | _____ _____ |
| 4. the product of oogenesis that becomes the female gamete | _____ | _____ _____ |
| 5. product of the prostate gland | _____ | _____ _____ _____ |
| 6. reproductive organ in which the fertilized oocyte is implanted and in which the child develops | _____ | _____ _____ _____ |
| 7. surgical repair of the uterine cervix | _____ | _____ _____ |
| 8. incision into an ovary | _____ | _____ _____ |
| 9. androgen prominent in male gamete production | _____ | _____ _____ |
| 10. absence of or abnormal cessation of menses | _____ | _____ _____ |

# Exercises

## Exercise 15-7 True, False, and Correction

Put an X in the True or False column next to each statement. Write the correct answer in the "Correction, if False" column for any statements you identify as false.

| Statement | True | False | Correction, if False |
|---|---|---|---|
| 1. Fertilization is the development that occurs between the formation of the zygote and birth of the child. | ____ | ____ | _____ |
| 2. The tubes between the ovaries and the uterus are called the fallopian tubes. | ____ | ____ | _____ |
| 3. The joining of the male and female gametes is called ovulation. | ____ | ____ | _____ |
| 4. The process of cell division by which one cell becomes two is known as oogenesis. | ____ | ____ | _____ |
| 5. The term for release of the female gamete that occurs during the proliferative stage of the uterine cycle is proliferation. | ____ | ____ | _____ |
| 6. The male ductwork that acts as a part of both the male urinary and male reproductive systems is called the urethra. | ____ | ____ | _____ |
| 7. Hysteralgia is pain in the uterus. | ____ | ____ | _____ |
| 8. Obstetrician is the medical specialty concerned with the medical care of women during the pregnancy and childbirth. | ____ | ____ | _____ |
| 9. Endometriosis is a difficult or painful menses. | ____ | ____ | _____ |
| 10. Mammography is the microscopic examination of cells from a mucosal surface, especially the uterine cervix. | ____ | ____ | _____ |

---

✓ **Pre-Quiz Checklist**

_____ Study the word roots given in Table 15-1.
_____ Using the study table, review the analyses and definitions.
_____ Review the exercises, and check your answers with the answers in the Appendix.
Consult the study table again to correct any errors before attempting the quiz.

---

✓ **Chapter Quiz**

Write the answers to the following items in the spaces provided.

1. Give two other names for a male gamete.

2. Explain the difference between meiosis and mitosis.

3. What is a gonad?

4. What does semen consist of?

5. Give another name for a female gamete.

6. Although gamete production occurs in the testes, what stimulus does the process require?

7. What is a zygote?

8. Explain the difference between a haploid and a diploid cell.

1. _____
_____
2. _____
_____
_____
_____
_____ ;
_____
_____
_____
3. _____
_____
4. _____
_____
_____
_____
5. _____
6. _____
_____
_____
_____
7. _____
_____
_____
_____
8. _____
_____
_____ ;
_____
_____
_____

## ✓ Chapter Quiz  *(continued)*

9. What dual purpose does a male urethra have?

9. _____
_____
_____
_____
_____

10. What parts of the male are considered part of the male reproductive "tract"?

10. _____
_____
_____
_____

11. Name the three phases of the uterine/menstrual cycle.

11. _____
_____
_____
_____
_____
_____
_____

12. In which phase of menstruation does ovulation occur?

12. _____

13. What tubes connect the ovaries to the uterus?

13. _____

14. When does a single-cell zygote become an embryo?

14. _____
_____

15. When is an embryo considered a fetus?

15. _____
_____

16. In which phase of the menstrual cycle is fertilization possible?

16. _____
_____

17. Where is the uterine cervix located?

17. _____
_____

18. What is the female counterpart of spermatogenesis?

18. _____

19. What stimulus is required for the ovaries to produce oocytes?

19. _____
_____
_____

20. What do oocytes eventually become?

20. _____

# Chapter 16

# The Nervous System

lthough the nervous system is more sophisticated than even the most complex computer, at least one parallel with the computer is useful in understanding how the nervous system works as a whole. The brain functions in much the same way as a computer's central processor, since information to be processed in the brain must pass between it and other parts of the body through the spinal cord. The brain and spinal cord are together known as the *central nervous system,* abbreviated CNS. The parts of the nervous system found throughout the rest of the body make up the *peripheral nervous system* (PNS), which is somewhat like a computer's operating system. This chapter introduces terms related to the CNS and PNS, along with terms naming nervous system disorders and procedures.

## WORD ELEMENTS SPECIFIC TO THE NERVOUS SYSTEM

The word elements shown in Table 16-1 are often found in terms related to the nervous system. You will recognize them in many of the terms you will learn in this chapter.

| TABLE 16-1 | COMMON WORD ELEMENTS OF THE NERVOUS SYSTEM |
|---|---|
| Word Element | Refers to |
| cephal/o; encephal/o | brain |
| cerebell/o | the cerebellum |
| cerebr/o | the cerebrum; also, the brain in general |
| cortic/o | outer layer or covering |
| gangli/o; ganglion/o | ganglia (singular: ganglion) |
| gli/o | glue |
| hydr/o | water |
| megal/o | large |
| mening/i/o | a membrane |
| myel/o | in connection with the nervous system, refers to the spinal cord and medulla oblongata |
| neur/o | a nerve cell; nervous system |
| phren/o | mind |
| psych/o | the mind |
| spin/o | the spinal cord |
| -mania | suffix meaning "morbid attraction to" or "impulse toward" |
| -phobia | suffix meaning "morbid or unreasonable fear" |

## THE PRACTICE AND THE PRACTITIONERS

Coupling the root *neur/o* with the suffix *-logy* yields the term *neurology,* which is the name of the medical specialty dealing with the nervous system. Specialists who treat nervous system disorders are called *neurologists, neurosurgeons, psychiatrists,* and *psychologists.*

## ANATOMY OF THE NERVOUS SYSTEM

Nerve tissue, along with its associated connective tissue and blood vessels, makes up both the CNS and PNS. Nerve tissue is composed of fundamental units called *neurons,* which are separated, supported, and protected by *neuroglia.* The three principal parts of a neuron cell are the *cell body,* the *dendrites,* and the *axon* (Figure 16-1). Axons are protected by the *myelin sheath,* an envelope of glial cells providing protection and electrical insulation to neurons.

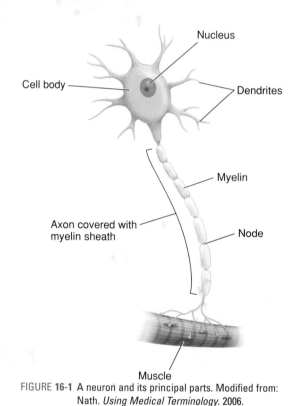

FIGURE **16-1** A neuron and its principal parts. Modified from: Nath. *Using Medical Terminology.* 2006.

## PHYSIOLOGY OF THE NERVOUS SYSTEM

*Dendrites,* which project outward from the cell body, act as antennae that receive and transmit messages between the neuron and muscles, skin, or other neurons. The cell body passes these messages to the axon, which is a tail-like "process," so called because it conducts electrical impulses away from the cell body. The connecting points for these message transfers are called *synapses.* Synaptic connections can occur between a neuron and a neuron or between a neuron and another cell. Within the connection, the cell that sends the message is called a *presynaptic cell,* and the cell receiving the message is the *postsynaptic cell.* The postsynaptic cell releases a chemical called a *neurotransmitter.* Hormones (see Chapter 12) are typical neurotransmitters.

When groups of neuron cell bodies occur within the CNS, each one is called a *nucleus* (plural: nuclei). However, when groups of neuron cell bodies occur within the PNS, each one is called a *ganglion* (plural: *ganglia*). Groupings of axons are called *nerves,* wherever they occur in the body. Neurons are grouped because they work together to carry out the highly complex sensing and processing actions required for everything we do.

As shown in Figure 16-2, information travels in two directions through the nervous system: sensory information passes either from or through the spinal cord to the brain; and command information passes from the brain to or through the spinal cord to effect an action. We can know which kind of information (sensory or command) and the direction the information is traveling (to or from the brain) by referring to the last word element in the term naming the path along which it flows. For example, the information traveling along the *spinothalamic* pathway (or tract) carries sensory information from the spinal cord *(spino)* to the thalamus, which is part of the brain. If the adjective denoting the pathway ended with *spinal* instead, as in the *corticospinal* pathway, we would know that the message moving along that pathway is command information because it is going from the brain to the spinal cord.

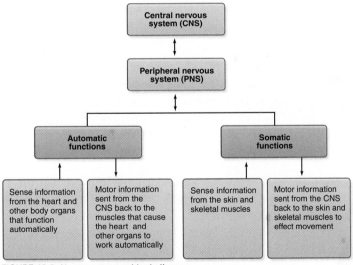

FIGURE **16-2** Nervous system block diagram.

## THE CENTRAL NERVOUS SYSTEM

### The Brain

As the the body's "central processor," the brain contains 98% of the body's *neural (nerve) tissue.*

From the outside, the brain is separable into four lobes: the *frontal, parietal, occipital,* and *temporal.* As shown in Figure 16-3, the brain is divisible into the following major parts: *cerebrum, cerebellum, diencephalon,* and *brain stem.*

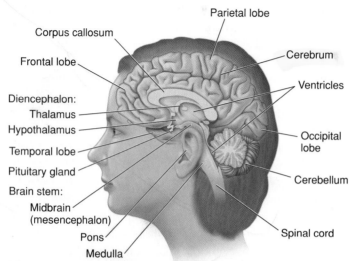

FIGURE **16-3** The brain. *Modified from:* Cohen BJ, Taylor JJ, Memmler RL, eds. *Memmler's The Structure and Function of the Human Body.* 8th ed. Baltimore, MD: Lippincott Williams & Wilkins; 2005.

## Cerebrum

The *cerebrum,* the largest part of the brain, is where memories and conscious thoughts are stored. It also directs some of our bodily movements. An outer layer of gray matter called the *cerebral cortex* protects the cerebrum, which is divided into two hemispheres. The term *basal ganglia* is commonly used when referring to the *basal nuclei* situated in the white matter of the cerebrum.

## Cerebellum

The *cerebellum,* like the larger cerebrum situated above it, also has two hemispheres. The cerebellum helps us perform learned body movements smoothly and maintain our equilibrium.

## Diencephalon

The *diencephalon* contains both the *thalamus* and the *hypothalamus.* The thalamus processes sensory information, and the hypothalamus, which is the hormone and emotion center of the brain, controls autonomic functions.

## Brain Stem

The *brain stem* contains the *mesencephalon* (or *midbrain*), the *pons,* and the *medulla oblongata.* The mesencephalon processes visual and audible sensory information.

Both consciousness and some *psychomotor* responses also occur within the mesencephalon. The pons (Latin for "bridge") passes information to the cerebellum and the thalamus to regulate subconscious somatic activities. The medulla oblongata sends sensory information to the thalamus to direct the autonomic functions of the heart, lungs, and other organs of the body. The cavities between the brain stem and the cerebrum are called *ventricles.*

### The Spinal Cord

The spinal cord and the brain communicate continuously with one another. The messages that flow back and forth bring about all the actions and functions that make life pleasurable, painful, and even possible. In the average-size adult, the spinal cord is about a foot and a half long and a half-inch wide. It is surrounded by membranes called spinal *meninges,* which absorb physical shocks that could damage the neural tissue. The outer layer of the spinal cord consists of *dura mater,* a dense collection of collagen fibers located along its length. The spinal cord is further protected by ligaments, tendons, and muscles. The structure of the spinal cord nerves is shown in Figure 16-4.

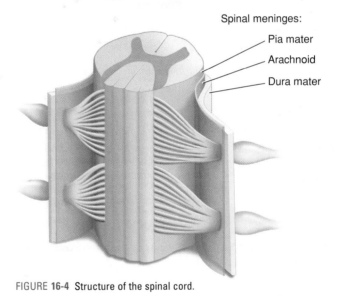

Spinal meninges:
Pia mater
Arachnoid
Dura mater

FIGURE **16-4** Structure of the spinal cord.

## THE PERIPHERAL NERVOUS SYSTEM

The PNS may be further divided into two subsystems: the *autonomic nervous system* and the *somatic nervous system.* Since some organs, such as the heart and lungs, work on their own, their performance is said to be *autonomic.* The word *autonomy,* which you may already know, is a common English word that means "self-sufficient." Conscious and habitual actions, on the other hand, are called *somatic,* which comes from a Greek word meaning "body."

Like the CNS, the PNS contains neurons, neuroglia, and associated tissue. The PNS also consists of the *cranial nerves* and *spinal nerves* emanating from the CNS, along with *receptors* and *effectors.* Receptors, which reside in all parts of the body, sense stimuli and transmit them to the CNS. Effectors respond to motor impulses from the CNS.

For example, many nerves, including the optic nerve, function together with the brain to create the sensation of sight. This process requires that a string of electrical messages, called *nerve impulses,* be exchanged between the PNS and CNS. These messages travel back and forth to the CNS from receptors and effectors by means of synapses and along axons.

The cranial nerves are connected directly to the brain, but they are nevertheless part of the PNS. The 12 pairs of cranial nerves, shown in Figure 16-5, are the *olfactory, optic, oculomotor, trochlear, trigeminal, abducent, facial, vestibulocochlear, glossopharyngeal, vagus, accessory,* and *hypoglossal.* As part of the PNS, these nerves are associated with bodily movements and functions within other systems.

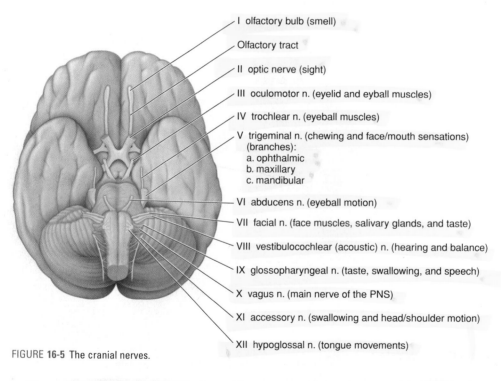

I olfactory bulb (smell)

Olfactory tract

II optic nerve (sight)

III oculomotor n. (eyelid and eyeball muscles)

IV trochlear n. (eyeball muscles)

V trigeminal n. (chewing and face/mouth sensations)
(branches):
a. ophthalmic
b. maxillary
c. mandibular

VI abducens n. (eyeball motion)

VII facial n. (face muscles, salivary glands, and taste)

VIII vestibulocochlear (acoustic) n. (hearing and balance)

IX glossopharyngeal n. (taste, swallowing, and speech)

X vagus n. (main nerve of the PNS)

XI accessory n. (swallowing and head/shoulder motion)

XII hypoglossal n. (tongue movements)

FIGURE **16-5** The cranial nerves.

Figure 16-6 shows the distribution of the 31 pairs of spinal nerves located along the regions of the spinal column.

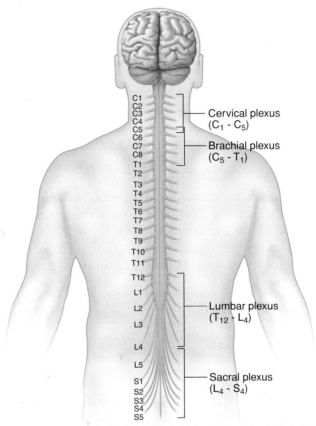

FIGURE **16-6** The spinal nerves. *Modified from:* Nath. *Using Medical Terminology.* 2006.

## ABBREVIATION TABLE

### COMMON ABBREVIATIONS:
**The Nervous System**

| Abbreviation | Meaning |
|---|---|
| ADHD | attention deficit hyperactivity disorder |
| EEG | electroencephalography |
| IQ | intelligence quotient |
| LP | lumbar puncture |
| MA | mental age |
| OBS | organic brain syndrome |
| OCD | obsessive-compulsive disorder |
| PERRLA | pupils equal, round, and reactive to light and accommodation |
| SAD | seasonal affective disorder |
| TENS | transcutaneous electrical nerve stimulation |
| WAIS | Wechsler Adult Intelligence Scale |
| WISC | Wechsler Intelligence Scale for Children |

## NERVOUS SYSTEM DISORDERS AND PROCEDURES

A *neurosis* is a fear of something that is not a hazard, at least not from a statistical point of view. Neuroses usually represent only a skewed perspective of reality, and although they can be debilitating, most people can overcome the anxiety such fears engender. Neuroses are often named by combining the suffix *-phobia* ("fear of something") with a root or prefix identifying the object feared, such as *pan-* ("all"). Thus, *panophobia* means "fear of everything" (Table 16-2).

A *psychosis,* on the other hand, represents a marked distortion of or sharp break from reality and is a serious personality disorder. *Schizophrenia,* a psychosis, involves delusions, such as believing that someone or something is controlling your thoughts. Another of its manifestations is hallucinations, most often "hearing" voices or other sounds. *Paranoia,* another personality disorder, is characterized by unreasonable suspicion or jealousy, along with a tendency to interpret everything others do as hostile. Some psychoses are indicated by the suffix *-mania.* Examples are *megalomania* (delusions of grandeur) and *kleptomania* (uncontrollable impulse to steal).

| TABLE 16-2 COMMON PHOBIAS | |
|---|---|
| Term | Definition |
| acrophobia | fear of heights |
| agoraphobia | fear of being outside your own house |
| arachnophobia | fear of spiders |
| claustrophobia | fear of being in a closed airless space |
| xenophobia | fear of foreigners |
| ankylophobia | fear of immobility of a joint (root in Chapter 6) |
| hemophobia | fear of blood (root in Chapter 9) |
| panophobia | fear of everything (prefix in Chapter 3) |
| xenoglossophobia | fear of foreign languages (second root in Chapter 11) |

Table 16-3 lists common nervous system disorders, along with some of the procedures used in their diagnosis and treatment.

| TABLE 16-3 | DISORDERS AND PROCEDURES COMMON TO THE NERVOUS SYSTEM |
|---|---|
| **Term** | **Definition** |
| agnosia | loss of sensory input recognition |
| Alzheimer disease; also Alzheimer's disease | a disease that may begin in late middle life; characterized by progressive mental deterioration that includes loss of memory and visual and spatial orientation |
| aphasia | loss of speech |
| cerebral thrombosis | blood clot in the brain |
| cerebral stroke | an acute clinical event, related to impairment of cerebral circulation, lasting more than 24 hours |
| cerebrovascular accident (CVA) | synonym for a cerebral stroke; an acute clinical event, related to impairment of cerebral circulation, lasting more than 24 hours |
| cerebrovascular disease | brain disorder involving a blood vessel |
| craniectomy | excision of part of the skull |
| craniotomy | incision into the skull |
| delirium | impaired consciousness |
| dementia | impaired intellectual function |
| dysphasia | impaired speech |
| encephalitis | inflammation of the brain |
| epilepsy | CNS disorder often characterized by seizures |
| glioblastoma | a cerebral tumor occurring most frequently in adults |
| glioma | tumor of glial tissue |
| hemiparesis | partial paralysis of one side of the body |
| hemiplegia | paralysis of one side of the body |
| Huntington disease (also Huntington's disease) | hereditary disorder of the CNS characterized by involuntary muscle movements and dementia |
| hydrocephalus | excessive cerebrospinal fluid in the brain |
| hyperesthesia | abnormal sensitivity to touch |
| meningioma | benign tumor of meninges |
| meningitis | inflamed meninges |
| multiple sclerosis | disease of the CNS; characterized by the formation of plaques in the brain and spinal cord |
| myelitis | inflamed spinal cord |
| myelography | radiography of the spinal cord and nerve roots |
| neuralgia | pain in a nerve |
| neuropathy | any disorder of the nervous system |
| neuroplasty | surgery to repair a nerve |
| paralysis | loss of motor control |
| paraplegia | paralysis of the lower extremities and, often, the lower trunk of the body |
| paresthesia | numbness |

| TABLE 16-3 | DISORDERS AND PROCEDURES COMMON TO THE NERVOUS SYSTEM *(continued)* |
|---|---|
| Term | Definition |
| Parkinson disease (also Parkinson's disease) | a neurologic condition characterized by difficulty in controlling muscles |
| plegia | paralysis |
| poliomyelitis | inflamed gray matter in the spinal cord |
| psychosis | general term covering severe mental or emotional disorders |
| quadriplegia | paralysis of all four limbs |
| sciatica | pain in the sciatic nerve, located in the lower back and extending down the thigh |
| seizure | sudden disturbance in brain function, sometimes producing a convulsion |
| syncope | fainting |

## 📖 STUDY TABLE  THE NERVOUS SYSTEM

| Term and Pronunciation | Analysis | Meaning |
|---|---|---|
| **STRUCTURE & FUNCTION** | | |
| autonomic nervous system (aw-to-NOM-ik) | *auto-* ("self"); *nom-* ("name"); *-ic* (adjective suffix) | the parts of the PNS that carry messages between the CNS and organs that function autonomously |
| axon (AX-ohn) | *axon* (Greek for "axis") | the part of a neuron that conducts electrical impulses |
| basal nuclei (BAY-suhl NEW-klee-eye); also often referred to as basal ganglia (BAY-suhl GAN-glee-ah) | *basal* (English adjective: "at or near the base of"); *nuclei* (plural of *nucleus*; common English word and Latin for "kernel") | nuclei within the white matter of the cerebrum |
| brain stem (brayn) | brain from *braegen* (Anglo-Saxon from Dutch, Low German, and in antiquity a Greek word meaning "upper part of the head") | the part of the brain that controls functions including heart rate, breathing, and body temperature |
| cell body | two common English words | one of the three parts of a neuron cell, the other two being the axon and dendrites |
| central nervous system | three common English words | the subdivision of the nervous system that includes the brain and spinal cord |
| cerebellum (SERR-uh-bell-uhm) | diminutive form of *cerebrum* (Latin for "brain") | the part of the brain that controls the skeletal muscles |
| cerebral cortex (seh-REE-bruhl KOR-tex) | *cerebr/o* ("brain"); *-al* (adjective suffix); *cortex* (Latin for "bark" as on a tree and "rind" as on a lemon) | the gray matter surrounding the cerebrum |
| cerebrum (seh-REE-bruhm) | Latin ("brain") | the largest part of the brain; controls conscious thought and stores memories |

## 📖 STUDY TABLE  THE NERVOUS SYSTEM  (continued)

| Term and Pronunciation | Analysis | Meaning |
|---|---|---|
| cranial nerves (KRAY-nee-uhl nerves) | *crani/o* ("skull"); *-al* (adjective suffix) | pairs of nerves entering and exiting the cranium: olfactory, optic, oculomotor, trochlear, abducent, trigeminal, vestibulocochlear, glossopharyngeal, vagal, accessory, hypoglossal |
| dendrite (DEN-dryte) | *dendrites* (Greek, "relating to a tree") | one of two processes extending from a neuron cell body, the other being the axon |
| diencephalon (dy-en-SEFF-uh-lohn) | *di-* ("through"); *encephal/o* ("brain") | the part of the brain containing both the thalamus and the hypothalamus |
| dura mater (DOO-ruh MAY-tuhr) | from *durus* (Latin for "hard") and *mater* (Latin for "mother") | the fibrous membrane protecting the CNS |
| effector (ee-FEK-tor) | that which produces an effect (from the Latin verb *efficere*, "to bring about") | cell that responds to nerve impulses by contraction (muscle), secretion (gland), etc. |
| frontal lobe (FRUN-tahl) | *frontal* (adjectival form of the English word *front*); *lobos* (Greek word for "lobe") | the front part of the brain from which voluntary muscle movements and other sensory and motor tasks are directed |
| ganglion (GANG-lee-ohn); plural: ganglia | *ganglion* (Greek word for "knot") | a group of neuron cell bodies grouped together in the PNS |
| hypothalamus (HY-po-thal-uh-muhs) | *hyp/o* ("below"); *thalamos* (Greek word for "bed") | the hormone and emotion center of the brain that controls autonomic functions |
| medulla oblongata (meh-DUH-luh ohb-lohng-GAH-tuh) | *medius* (Latin for "middle"); *oblongus* (Latin for "long") | the part of the brain stem that sends sensory information to the thalamus to direct the autonomic functions of the heart, lungs, and other viscera |
| meninges (meh-NIHN-jees) | the plural form of *meninx* (Greek for "membrane") | one of the dura mater layers surrounding both the brain and the spinal cord |
| mesencephalon (mez-ehn-SEFF-ah-lon) | *mes/o* ("middle"); *encephal/o* ("brain") | the middle part of the brain between the diencephalon and the pons |
| myelin sheath (MY-eh-lin) | *myel/o* ("bone marrow") | an envelope of glial cells providing protection and electrical insulation to neurons |
| nerve | a common English word with a specialized meaning when used as a medical term | a whitish, cordlike structure composed of one or more bundles of nerve fibers outside the CNS, together with their connective tissues and nourishing blood vessels |
| neural (NUHR-uhl) | *neur/o* ("nerve"); *-al* (adjective suffix) | an adjective to modify any noun having to do with neurology |

## STUDY TABLE  THE NERVOUS SYSTEM *(continued)*

| Term and Pronunciation | Analysis | Meaning |
|---|---|---|
| neural tissue (NUHR-uhl) | *neur/o* ("nerve"); *-al* (adjective suffix); *tissu* (French for "woven") | nerve tissue |
| neuroglia (nuhr-o-GLEE-uh) | *neur/o* ("nerve"); *gli/o* ("glue") | cells within both the CNS and PNS, which, although they are external to neurons, form an essential part of nerve tissue |
| neuron (NUHR-ohn) | *neur/o* ("nerve") | a nerve cell, including the cell body and its axon |
| neurotransmitter (NOO-roh-TRANS-mitt-ehr) | *neur/o* ("nerve"); *trans-* ("across"); *mitter* (from the Latin verb *mitto*, "to send") | chemical released by the postsynaptic cell to effect an action |
| nucleus (NEW-klee-uhs); plural: nuclei (NEW-klee-eye) | *nucleus* (Latin for "kernel") | a group of neuron cell bodies grouped together in the CNS |
| occipital lobe (AWK-sihp-ih-tuhl lobe) | adjectival form of *occiput* ("back of the head"); *lobos* (Greek word for "lobe") | the part of the brain that processes information from the sense of sight and other sensory and motor tasks |
| parietal lobe (pah-RY-uh-tuhl) | from the Latin word *paries* ("wall"); and the Greek word *lobos* ("lobe") | the part of the brain that processes information from the sense of touch and other sensory and motor tasks |
| peripheral nervous system (PNS) (puh-RIFF-uh-ruhl) | from the Latin word *peripheria* ("boundary" or "surrounding area") | made up of neurons, neuroglia, and associated tissue, including the cranial and spinal nerves and the sensory and motor nerves that extend throughout the body |
| pons (POHNS) | *pons* (Latin word for "bridge") | the part of the brain stem that passes information to the cerebellum and the thalamus to regulate subconscious somatic activities |
| postsynaptic cell (post-sy-NAP-tik) | *post-* ("after"); Greek word *synapsis* ("junction") | cell within the synaptic connection that receives an action message and releases a neurotransmitter |
| presynaptic cell (pree-sy-NAP-tik) | *pre-* ("before"); Greek word *synapsis* ("junction") | cell within a synaptic connection that sends a message to perform an action |
| psychomotor (SY-ko-mo-tuhr) | *psych/o* ("mind"); *motor* (from Latin *moveo*, "mover") | an adjective used to indicate the relation between psychic activity and muscular movement |
| receptor (ree-SEPP-tor) | from *recipio* (Latin for "to receive") | a sensory nerve ending |
| somatic nervous system (so-MAT-ik) | *soma* (Greek word for "body"); *-ic* (adjective suffix) | the parts of the PNS that carry impulses for conscious rather than habitual activity |
| spinal nerves (SPY-nahl) | *spin/o* ("spine"); *-al* (adjective suffix) | the 31 pairs of nerves located along the spinal column |

## 📖 STUDY TABLE  THE NERVOUS SYSTEM  *(continued)*

| Term and Pronunciation | Analysis | Meaning |
|---|---|---|
| spinothalamic (spyn-oh-thah-LAM-ik) | *spin/o* ("spine"); *thalamos* (Greek word for "thalamus"); *-ic* (adjective suffix) | adjective used to name a nerve pathway from the spine to the thalamus |
| synapse (SIH-naps) | *syn* (Greek for "together") and *hapto* (Greek for "clasp") | the connecting point between nerve cells or between a nerve cell and a receptor or effector cell |
| temporal lobe (TEM-puh-ruhl lobe) | from *temporalis* (Latin for "time"); *lobos* (Greek for "lobe") | the part of the brain that processes information from the senses of hearing, smell, and taste, and other sensory and motor tasks |
| thalamus (THAL-uh-muhs) | from *thalamos* (Greek word for "bed") | part of the brain that processes sensory information |
| ventricles (VEN-trik-uhls) | from *ventriculus* (Latin word for "belly") | cavities between the cerebrum and brain stem |
| **COMMON DISORDERS** | | |
| agnosia (ag-NO-seeya) | *a-* ("without"); *-gnosis* ("knowledge"); *-ia* ("condition") | loss of sensory input recognition |
| Alzheimer disease (ALZ-hy-mur); also Alzheimer's disease | an eponym | a disease that may begin in late middle life, characterized by progressive mental deterioration that includes loss of memory and visual and spatial orientation |
| aphasia (uh-FAY-jhah) | *a-* ("without"); *phasis* (Greek for "speech"); *-ia* ("condition") | loss of speech |
| cerebral stroke (she-REE-bruhl) | *cerebr/o* ("brain"); *-al* (adjective suffix); *stroke* (common English word) | an acute clinical event, related to impairment of cerebral circulation, lasting more than 24 hours |
| cerebral thrombosis (seh-REE-bruhl throm-BO-sihs) | *cerebr/o* ("brain"); *-al* (adjective suffix); *thrombosis* (Greek for "clot") | blood clot in the brain |
| cerebrovascular accident (CVA) (suh-ree-bro-VAS-ku-lahr) | *cerebr/o* ("brain"); *vascul/o* ("vessel"); *-ar* (adjective suffix) | a synonym for *cerebral stroke*, an acute clinical event, related to impairment of cerebral circulation, lasting more than 24 hours |
| cerebrovascular disease (suh-ree-bro-VAS-ku-lahr) | *cerebr/o* ("brain"); *vascul/o* ("vessel"); *-ar* (adjective suffix) | brain disorder involving a blood vessel |
| delirium (duh-LEER-ee-uhm) | from the Latin word *deliro* ("to become crazy") | impaired consciousness |
| dementia (duh-MEN-shah) | Latin word meaning "madness" or "folly" | impaired intellectual function |
| dysphasia (DISS-fay-jhah) | *dys-* ("difficult"); *phasis* ("speech"); *-ia* ("condition") | impaired speech |

## STUDY TABLE THE NERVOUS SYSTEM *(continued)*

| Term and Pronunciation | Analysis | Meaning |
|---|---|---|
| encephalitis (en-seff-uh-LY-tiss) | *encephal/o* ("brain"); *-itis* ("inflammation") | inflammation of the brain |
| epilepsy (EPP-ih-lepp-see) | *epilepsia* (Greek word for "seizure") | CNS disorder often characterized by seizures |
| glioblastoma (GLY-oh-blass-TOH-mah) | *gli/o* ("glue"); *blastos* (Greek word for "germ"); *-oma* ("tumor") | a cerebral tumor occurring most frequently in adults |
| glioma (gly-OH-muh) | *gli/o* ("glue"); *-oma* ("tumor") | tumor of glial tissue |
| hemiparesis (heh-mee-puh-REE-suhs) | *hemi-* ("half"); *paresis* ("weakness") | partial paralysis of one side of the body |
| hemiplegia (hehm-ee-PLEE-jee-ah) | *hemi-* ("half"); *plege* (Greek word for "stroke"); *-ia* ("condition") | paralysis of one side of the body |
| Huntington disease (HUN-ting-tuhn); also Huntington's disease | an eponym | hereditary disorder of the CNS |
| hydrocephalus (hy-dro-SEFF-uh-lehs) | *hydr/o* ("water"); *cephal/o* ("brain") | excessive cerebrospinal fluid in the brain |
| hyperesthesia (hy-per-ess-THEE-zyuh) | *hyper-* ("above"); Greek word *aisthesis* ("sensation"); *-ia* ("condition") | abnormal sensitivity to touch |
| kleptomania (klep-toh-MAY-knee-yah) | from the Greek verb *klepto* ("to steal"); *-mania* ("a morbid attraction to or impulse toward") | uncontrollable impulse to steal |
| megalomania (MEG-ah-loh-MAYN-ee-ah) | *megal/o* ("large"); *-mania* ("a morbid attraction to or impulse toward") | delusions of grandeur |
| meningioma (meh-nihn-jee-OH-muh) | *mening/i/o* ("membrane"); *-oma* ("tumor") | benign tumor of the meninges |
| meningitis (meh-nihn-JY-tiss) | *mening/i/o* ("membrane"); *-itis* ("inflammation") | inflamed meninges |
| multiple sclerosis (skleh-RO-sihs) | *multiple* (common English word); *scleros* (Greek word for "hard"); *-osis* ("condition") | disease of the CNS characterized by the formation of plaques in the brain and spinal cord |
| myelitis (my-eh-LY-tiss) | *myel/o* ("bone marrow" [of the spinal cord in nervous system terminology]); *-itis* ("inflammation") | inflammation of the spinal cord |
| neuralgia (nuh-RALL-jah) | *neur/o* ("nerve"); *-algia* ("pain") | pain in a nerve |
| neuropathy (nuh-ROP-ah-thee) | *neur/o* ("nerve"); *-pathy* ("disease") | any disorder of the nervous system |
| paralysis (pah-RALL-ih-sihs) | *para-* ("abnormal"); *-lysis* ("loosening") | loss of one or more muscle functions |
| paranoia (pahr-ah-NOY-ya) | Greek word for "madness" | a serious mental disorder characterized by unreasonable suspicion or jealousy, along with a tendency to interpret everything others do as hostile |
| paraplegia (pahr-ah-PLEE-jee-ah) | *para-* ("abnormal"); from *plege* (Greek word for "stroke"); *-ia* ("condition") | paralysis of the lower extremities and, often, the lower trunk of the body |

## 📖 STUDY TABLE THE NERVOUS SYSTEM (continued)

| Term and Pronunciation | Analysis | Meaning |
|---|---|---|
| paresthesia (per-ess-THEE-zyuh) | *para-* ("abnormal"); Greek word *aisthesis* ("sensation"); *-ia* ("condition") | numbness |
| Parkinson disease (PAR-kin-suhn); also Parkinson's disease | an eponym | disease of the nerves in the brain |
| phobia (FOH-bee-ah) | from the Greek word *phobos* ("fear") | a fear of something that is not a hazard from a statistical point of view |
| plegia (PLEE-jee-uh) | from *plege* (Greek word for "stroke"); *-ia* ("condition") | paralysis |
| poliomyelitis (pohl-ee-oh-MY-eh-LY-tiss) | *polio-* ("gray matter"); *myel/o* ("the marrow of the spinal cord"); *-itis* ("inflammation") | inflamed gray matter of the spinal cord |
| psychosis (sy-KO-sihs) | *psych/o* ("mind"); *-osis* ("condition") | a serious disorder involving a marked distortion of, or sharp break from, reality; general term covering severe mental or emotional disorders |
| quadriplegia (kwad-rih-PLEE-jee-ah) | *quadri-* ("four"); from *plege* (Greek word for "stroke"); *-ia* ("condition") | paralysis of all four limbs |
| schizophrenia (skits-oh-FREN-ee-ah) | from the Greek word *schizo* ("split"); *phren/o* ("mind"); *-ia* ("condition") | personality disorder involving delusions and/or hallucinations |
| sciatica (sy-AT-ih-kuh) | from *sciaticus* (Latin for "hip") | pain in the sciatic nerve; loosely, any back pain |
| seizure (SEE-zhur) | from *saisir* (French verb meaning "to grasp") | sudden disturbance in brain function sometimes producing a convulsion |
| syncope (SIN-kuh-pee) | Greek word for "swoon" | fainting |
| **PRACTICE & PRACTITIONERS** | | |
| neurologist (nuhr-AWL-ih-gihst) | *neur/o* ("nerve"); *-logist* ("practitioner") | a medical specialist who treats nervous system disorders |
| neurology (nuhr-AWL-uh-jee) | *neur/o* ("nerve"); *-logy* ("practice or study") | medical specialty dealing with the nervous system |
| neurosurgeon (NOO-roh-sur-juhn) | *neur/o* ("nerve"); *surgeon* from two Greek words, *cheir* ("hand") and *ergon* ("work") | surgeon who specializes in operations on the nervous system |
| psychiatrist (sy-KY-ah-trist) | *psych/o* ("mind"); *-iatrist* ("practitioner") | a medical doctor who specializes in the diagnosis and treatment of psychologic disorders |
| psychologist (sy-KOL-oh-jist) | *psych/o* ("mind"); *-logist* ("practitioner") | a doctor of psychology who specializes in the diagnosis and treatment of psychologic disorders |
| **DIAGNOSIS & TREATMENT** | | |
| myelography (my-eh-LOG-rah-fee) | *myel/o* ("marrow"); *-graphy* ("x-ray") | radiography of the spinal cord and nerve roots |

## STUDY TABLE THE NERVOUS SYSTEM *(continued)*

| Term and Pronunciation | Analysis | Meaning |
|---|---|---|
| **SURGICAL PROCEDURES** | | |
| craniectomy (KRAY-nee-ek-tuh-mee) | *crani/o* ("skull"); *-ectomy* ("excision") | excision of part of the skull |
| craniotomy (KRAY-nee-aw-tuh-mee) | *crani/o* ("skull"); *-tomy* ("incision") | incision into the skull |
| lobotomy (lo-BAWT-uh-mee) | from *lobos* (Greek for "lobe," a part of an organ); *-tomy* ("incision") | incision into a lobe |
| neuroplasty (NURR-oh-plass-tee) | *neur/o* ("nerve"); *-plasty* ("surgical repair") | surgery to repair a nerve |
| **ENHANCEMENT TERMS** | | |
| aneurysm (AN-yur-izm) | *angi/o* ("blood vessel"); *eurys* (Greek for "wide") | dilated blood vessel |
| ataxia (ah-TAK-see-ah) | *a-* ("not"); *taxis* (Greek word meaning "order") | lack of muscular coordination |
| cerebrospinal fluid (suh-REE-bro-SPY-nuhl) | *cerebr/o* ("brain"); *spin/o* ("spine"); *-al* (adjective suffix) | the fluid in and around the brain and spinal cord |

## DECIPHERING MEDICAL DOCUMENTS

**Read the following excerpt from a History and Physical Examination, and answer the questions that follow.**

CHIEF COMPLAINT: *Weakness, ataxia, confusion.*

HISTORY OF PRESENT ILLNESS: *Patient is an 86-year-old female with weakness, difficulty walking or standing, and pain in her right foot and leg that has been progressive for the last several weeks. Also, she has been having increasing confusion, especially over the last 3–4 days. No other modifying factors or associated signs or symptoms.*

REVIEW OF NEUROLOGIC SYSTEM: *Profound weakness with difficulty walking and ataxia.*

REVIEW OF HEENT: *Head is normal cephalic and atraumatic. Eyes PERRLA. Extraocular movements intact. Tympanic membranes patent. Posterior pharynx and oral mucosa moist and clear.*

ASSESSMENT: *Confusion, probable OBS of Alzheimer's type.*

1. What does ataxia mean? *LACK OF MUSCULAR COORDINATION*
2. What does the abbreviation PERRLA stand for? *Pupils, Equal round reactive to light & Accomodat*
3. What does the abbreviation OBS stand for? *Organic Brain Syndrome*

# 🪨 Exercises

## Exercise 16-1 Inserting the Correct Term

Fill in the blanks.

The 1) *Cerebrum* , the largest part of the brain, is where memories and thoughts are stored. It also directs some of our bodily movements. It's protected by an outer layer of gray matter called the 2) *Cerebral Cortex* and is divided into two hemispheres. The 3) *Cerebellum* also has two hemispheres. It helps us perform learned body movements smoothly and maintain our equilibrium.

The 4) *Thalamus* processes sensory information, and the 5) *HypoTHAlamus*, which is the hormone and emotion center of the brain, controls autonomic functions. They are both contained in the 6) *diencephalon*

The brain stem contains three "processors." The first is the 7) *Mesencephalon* which processes visual and audible sense information. Second is the 8) *Pons* , which passes information to the cerebellum and thalamus (to regulate subconscious somatic activities). The third is the 9) *Medulla Oblongata* which sends sensory information to the thalamus to direct the autonomic functions of the heart, lungs, and other organs of the body.

The 10) *Spinal Cord* and the brain communicate continuously with one another and bring about all the actions and functions that make life pleasurable and possible. The spinal cord is surrounded by membranes called spinal 11) *Meninges* to absorb physical shocks. The spinal cord is further protected by ligaments, tendons, and muscles. The outer layer of the spinal cord consists of 12) *dura Mater* , a dense collection of collagen fibers.

# Exercises

## Exercise 16-2 Defining Terms

Write a brief definition in the space next to each term.

| Term | Definition |
| --- | --- |
| 1. agnosia | Loss OF Sensory input |
| 2. aneurysm | dialated blood vessel |
| 3. cerebrovascular disease | Cebreal Stroke |
| 4. craniectomy | Excision OF Part OF Skull |
| 5. delirium | Impaired Consciouness |
| 6. dysphasia | Impaired Speech |
| 7. encephalitis | INFlamation OF Brain |
| 8. glioma | Tumor OF Glial tissue |
| 9. hemiparesis | Paralasis OF one Side |
| 10. meningioma | Benign tumor OF Meneqis |
| 11. multiple sclerosis | Disease OF CNS |
| 12. neuralgia | Nerve Pain |

| Term | Definition |
|---|---|
| 13. Parkinson disease (Parkinson's disease) | CNS / Difficulti Controlling Nervous System. |
| 14. poliomyelitis | Inflamed grey matter / Spinal Cord |
| 15. seizure | Sudden disturbance in Brain Function. |

## Exercises

### Exercise 16-3 Meanings of Abbreviations

Provide the meaning for each of these abbreviations.

| Abbreviation | Definition |
|---|---|
| 1. ADHD | Attention Deficit Hyperactivity disorder. |
| 2. EEG | Electroencephalography |
| 3. IQ | Intelligent Quotient |
| 4. LP | Lumbar Puncture |
| 5. MA | Mental Age |
| 6. OBS | Organic Brain Syndrome |
| 7. OCD | Obsessive-Compulsive Disorder |
| 8. PERRLA | Pupils equal round + reactive to light + accomodation |
| 9. SAD | Seasonal affective disorder |
| 10. TENS | Transcutaneous electrical Nerve Stimulation |

## Exercises

### Exercise 16-4 Building Medical Terms

Build terms to satisfy the following definitions, and then analyze each term by identifying its word elements.

| Definition | Term | Analysis |
|---|---|---|
| 1. part of a neuron that conducts electrical impulses | AXON/ax | Axis /G/C |
| 2. one of the three parts of a neuron cell, the other two being the axon and dendrites | Cell body | two Common G/C words |
| 3. the gray matter surrounding the cerebrum | Cerebral Cortex | Brain / Bark |
| 4. neuron cell bodies grouped together in the PNS | Ganglion | Knot / GK |

| Definition | Term | Analysis |
|---|---|---|
| 5. the part of the brain that processes information from the sense of sight and other sensory and motor tasks | *occipital LOBE* | *Back of head / Lobes* |
| 6. loss of sensory input recognition | *Agnosia* | *without / knowledge Condition* |
| 7. a cerebral tumor occurring most frequently in adults | *Gliobastoma* | *Germ / GIC* |
| 8. disease of the CNS characterized by the formation of plaques in the brain and spinal cord | *Multiple Sclerosis* | *Hard Condition* |
| 9. a medical specialist who treats nervous system disorders | *Neurologist* | *Practitioner* |
| 10. radiograph of the spinal cord and nerve roots | *Myelography* | *Marrow / XRay* |

# Exercises

## Exercise 16-5 Multiple Choice

Circle the term in the Choices column that answers each of the following questions.

| Question | Choices |
|---|---|
| 1. What part of the brain controls functions that include heart rate, breathing, and body temperature? | basal nuclei; cerebrum; brain stem |
| 2. The axon is one of two processes that extend from a neuron cell body; what is the other? | effector; dendrite; neurotransmitter |
| 3. What is the term for the envelope of glial cells that provides protection and electrical insulation for neurons? | cell body; CNS; myelin sheath |
| 4. What part of the brain processes information from the sense of sight and other sensory and motor tasks? | frontal lobe; occipital lobe; parietal lobe |
| 5. What part of the brain stem passes information to the cerebellum and the thalamus to regulate subconscious somatic activities? | psychomotor; pons; receptor |
| 6. What is the term for a blood clot in the brain? | cerebrospinal; cerebellum; cerebral thrombosis |

| Question | Choices |
|---|---|
| 7. What is the clinical term for impaired speech? | dementia; dysphasia; delirium |
| 8. What is abnormal sensitivity to touch? | hydrocephalus; hyperesthesia; hypothalamus |
| 9. What is the word for inflamed gray matter of the spinal cord? | cerebral cortex; cerebrum; poliomyelitis |
| 10. What term means lack of muscular coordination? | ataxia; synapse; paraplegia |

# Exercises

## Exercise 16-6 Identifying the Major Areas of the Brain

Label the following parts in Figure 16-7.

* brain stem
* cerebellum
* cerebrum
* hypothalamus
* medulla oblongata
* pons
* thalamus

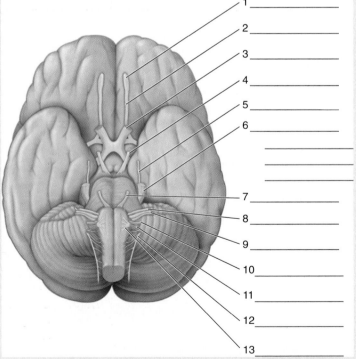

1 _____
2 _____
3 _____
4 _____
5 _____
6 _____
_____
_____
_____
7 _____
8 _____
9 _____
10 _____
11 _____
12 _____
13 _____

FIGURE **16-7** Identifying the major areas of the brain (Exercise 16-6). *From:* Cohen BJ, Taylor JJ, Memmler RL, eds. *Memmler's The Structure and Function of the Human Body.* 8th ed. Baltimore, MD: Lippincott Williams & Wilkins; 2005.

## Pre-Quiz Checklist

_____ Study the word roots given in Table 16-1.
_____ Using the study table, review the analyses and definitions.
_____ Review the exercises, and check your answers with the answers in the Appendix.
Consult the study table again to correct any errors before attempting the quiz.

## Chapter Quiz

Write the answers to the following items in the spaces provided.

1. What would be the destination of an electrical impulse traveling along a spinothalamic pathway?

    1. _to the Thalamus_ _____

2. What two body organs make up the central nervous system?

    2. _Brain + Spinal Cord_

3. What part of the nervous system is located outside the central nervous system?

    3. _Peripheral nervous System_

4. What abbreviations signify the central nervous system and the peripheral nervous system?

    4. _____

5. What two fundamental units make up the nervous system?

    5. _CNS + PNS_

6. What are the three principal parts of a neuron?

    6. _Cell bodies, dendrites, exon_

7. What are groups of neuron cell bodies in the CNS called?

    7. _Nucleus + Nuclei_

8. What are groups of neuron cell bodies in the PNS called?

    8. _Ganglion + Ganglia_

9. Between what two parts of the brain are the ventricles located?

    9. _Brain Stem + Cerebrum_

10. Briefly describe the essential differences between the autonomic and somatic subdivisions of the human nervous system.

    10. _Conscious + habitual actions are Somatic. Organs that work on their own are autoimmune_

11. Name the neurologic condition characterized by difficulty in controlling muscles.

    11. _Parkisons Disease_

12. Name the term for the brain disorder that involves a blood vessel.

    12. _Cerebral Vascular disease._

13. Multiple sclerosis is a disease of what system?

    13. _CNS_

## Chapter Quiz  (continued)

14. What is the name for a hereditary disorder of the CNS?

14. Huntingtons Disease

15. Briefly describe a craniotomy.

15. Incision into the Skull.

16. Inflamed gray matter in the spinal cord is referred to as what?

16. Cerebral Cortex

17. Define encephalitis.

17. Inflamation OF Brain

18. What word means loss of speech capability?

18. Aphasia

19. What is the common word for a CVA (cerebrovascular accident)?

19. Cerebral Vascular Accident ( Stroke )

20. A disturbance in the functioning of what part of the CNS causes a seizure?

20. Brain disturbance

# The Eye

CHAPTER CONTENTS

The eye works in conjunction with the nervous system, specifically the *visual cortex* of the brain. The process of vision begins when photoreceptors in the eye detect *photons*, which are basic units of visible light, and is completed by photon-generated impulses traveling along the *optic nerves* (one in each eye connecting to the brain) to the visual cortices of the cerebral hemispheres. The process depends on a highly complex series of physiologic events, but for ease of understanding it can be compared to the operation of a camera. For example, each eye has a *lens*, a mechanism for widening or narrowing the opening through which light is admitted, and ways of focusing on objects whether close by or far away.

This chapter will introduce you to the main parts of the eye and acquaint you with the terms that name them.

The eye is so complex that a terminology course, particularly a short one, can neither examine its deep inner workings nor broach the science of optics, which describes its basis. But you need not be concerned with this limitation, since learning the names of the main structures of the eye is by itself a big step in the direction of understanding.

## WORDS AND WORD ELEMENTS SPECIFIC TO THE EYE

The words and word elements shown in Table 17-1 are often found in terms related to the eye. You will recognize them in many of the terms you will learn in this chapter.

| TABLE 17-1 COMMON WORDS AND WORD ELEMENTS RELATED TO THE EYE | |
|---|---|
| Word or Root | Refers to |
| blephar/o | eyelid |
| conjunctiva (plural: conjunctivae) | mucous membrane covering the anterior surface of the eyeball |
| core/o | pupil of the eye |
| cornea (plural: corneas) | the outer wall of the eye; reflector of light |
| dacry/o | tears |
| dacryocyst/o | lacrimal sac |
| irid/o | iris (plural: irides) |
| ocul/o | eye |
| ophthalm/o | eye |
| opt/o | light |
| palpebra (plural: palpebrae) | eyelid |
| phak/o; phac/o | lens |
| retin/o | retina |
| scler/o | sclera |
| uve/o | middle layer of the eye containing muscles and blood vessels |
| -opia | suffix denoting vision; a condition of the eye |

## THE PRACTICE AND THE PRACTITIONERS

As noted in Table 17-1, the root *ophthalm/o* means "eye," and as you learned in Chapter 1, the suffix *-logy* means "study of." Coupling this root and suffix gives the term *ophthalmology,* which refers to the medical specialty dealing with the eye. Dropping the *y* from this term and adding the suffix *-ist* produces the term *ophthalmologist,* which refers to a physician who specializes in ophthalmology. An ophthalmologist (sometimes called an *oculist*) provides eye care ranging from prescribing corrective lenses to treating eye diseases or even performing ophthalmic surgery.

The term *optometry* refers to the practice of examining eyes for impaired vision and other disorders. It derives from the root *opt/o* ("light") and the suffix *-metry* ("act of measuring"). An *optometrist* "measures" a patient's ability to see and, like an ophthalmologist, can prescribe corrective lenses.

An *optician* is a specialist in the field of *optics,* which deals with the nature and characteristics of light. An optician uses the prescription for corrective lenses from an ophthalmologist or optometrist to make eyeglasses that improve a patient's vision.

## MAIN STRUCTURES OF THE EYE

The eyeball is a sphere filled with a jelly-like, transparent substance called the *vitreous body.* The outside of the eyeball has three distinctive outer layers or "coats": the *fibrous tunic,* the *vascular tunic,* and the *neural tunic (tunic* is the Latin word for "coat"). The fibrous tunic is the outermost layer, which connects with eye muscles. It consists of the *cornea* and the *sclera* (plural: sclerae). The vascular tunic, also called the *uvea,* is in the middle. It contains the *iris* (plural: irides), along with blood vessels and other tissues. The neural tunic, the innermost layer, is composed of the *retina,* where the nerves and light receptors (called rods and cones) are located.

The *photoreceptors* in the eye, which detect the presence of light, are of two kinds: cones and rods. The cones receive those photons that are traveling opposite to the direction one is looking, while the rods pick up those photons that strike the eye from the side. Most visual information comes through the cones, which enable us to see in full color. However, the rods are much more sensitive to light, which makes them more valuable than cones when we are in the dark. Unfortunately, the rods provide only black and white images that lack sharpness.

The visible parts of the eye include the *pupil* (the dark part in the very center of the eye), the iris (the colored part), and the sclera (the white part). The cornea, a transparent shield of tissue, covers the iris, and directly behind the iris is the *lens.* The sclera extends all the way around the eyeball to the *optic nerve,* which lies at the very back. The *retina* is a thin layer of tissue just inside the sclera (Figure 17-1). When light rays reflect off an object we are looking at, they travel through the

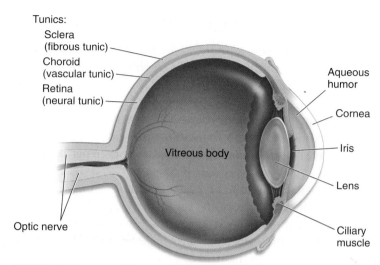

FIGURE **17-1** The layout of the eye. *Modified from:* Cohen BJ, Taylor JJ, Memmler RL, eds. *Memmler's The Structure and Function of the Human Body.* 8th ed. Baltimore, MD: Lippincott Williams & Wilkins; 2005.

cornea and lens, which focuses them onto photoreceptors in the retina. After receiving these light signals, the retina changes them into electrical impulses that travel through the optic nerve to the brain, where they are interpreted.

## ACCESSORY STRUCTURES OF THE EYE

Accessory structures of the eye comprise the eyelid and the *lacrimal apparatus,* which includes glands that produce tears, and the ducts and other cavities that contain tears. (*Lacrima* is the Latin word for "tears.") The *conjunctiva* (plural: conjunctivae) is the skin-like mucous membrane that covers the inside of the eyelid and the anterior part of eyeball. *Conjunctivitis* is a common childhood malady often referred to as "pinkeye."

Adjectives are used to designate the two different areas of the conjunctiva. *Palpebral conjunctiva* refers to conjunctiva covering the inside of the eyelid, because the Latin word for "eyelid" is *palbebra.* In contrast, *ocular conjunctiva* refers to conjunctiva covering the front of the eyeball, since the Latin word for "eye" is *oculus.*

## ABBREVIATION TABLE

### COMMON ABBREVIATIONS:
The Eye

| Abbreviation | Meaning |
|---|---|
| ECCE | extracapsular cataract extraction |
| EOC | extraocular movement |
| ERG | electroretinography |
| ICCE | intracapsular cataract extraction |
| IOP | intraocular pressure |
| OD | right eye |
| OS | left eye |
| OU | both eyes |
| PVD | posterior vitreous detachment (referring to the vitreous body) |

### DECIPHERING MEDICAL DOCUMENTS

**Read the following excerpt from a vision test and answer the questions that follow.**

*Slit lamp examination reveals normal lids, conjunctivae, and sclerae. Corneas are clear. Anterior chambers are clear and deep. Irides are within normal limits in the right eye. Evaluation of the lens reveals a 4+ posterior subcapsular plaquing with 3-4+ nuclear sclerosis. Intraocular pressures: OD, 18; OS, 17. Fundus examination in the right eye was severely hindered due to the dense cataract.*

1. What do the abbreviations OD and OS stand for?
2. What are the irides?
3. What are the singular forms of conjunctivae and sclerae?

## COMMON EYE DISORDERS AND PROCEDURES

Eye inflammation is a fairly common complaint. Conjunctivitis, commonly referred to as pinkeye, was mentioned earlier. *Uveitis* is inflammation of the uvea, and *iritis* is inflammation of the iris. Table 17-2 lists other common conditions and procedures associated with the eye.

| **TABLE 17-2** | COMMON CONDITIONS AND PROCEDURES ASSOCIATED WITH THE EYE |
|---|---|
| **Term** | **Definition** |
| aphakia | without a lens |
| astigmatism | fuzzy vision caused by the irregular shape of one or both eyeballs |
| blepharectomy | surgical removal of part or all of an eyelid |
| blepharitis | inflammation of the eyelid |
| blepharochalasis | relaxation of the eyelid |
| blepharoconjunctivitis | inflammation of the palpebral conjunctiva |
| blepharoplasty | surgery to correct a defective eyelid |
| blepharoplegia | paralysis of an eyelid |

| TABLE 17-2 | COMMON CONDITIONS AND PROCEDURES ASSOCIATED WITH THE EYE *(continued)* |
|---|---|
| Term | Definition |
| blepharoptosis | drooping eyelid(s) |
| blepharospasm | involuntary contraction of the eyelid |
| blepharotomy | surgical incision of an eyelid |
| conjunctivitis | inflammation of the conjunctiva |
| conjunctivoplasty | surgery on the conjunctiva |
| coreoplasty | surgical repair of the pupil |
| corepexy | surgical fixation of the iris |
| dacryocele | lacrimal sac filled with fluid; often called a *dacryocystocele*, because *dacryocyst* is a synonym for lacrimal sac |
| dacryocystalgia | pain in the lacrimal sac |
| dacryocystectomy | surgical removal of the lacrimal sac |
| dacryocystotomy | incision into the lacrimal sac |
| dacryolith | a "stone" in the lacrimal apparatus |
| dacryorrhea | excessive secretion of tears |
| emmetropia | normal vision |
| hyperopia | farsightedness |
| iridocele | hernia of the iris |
| iridomalacia | softening of the iris |
| iritis | inflammation of the iris |
| lacrimation | synonym for dacryorrhea |
| lacrimotomy | synonym for dacryocystotomy |
| myopia | nearsightedness |
| oculodynia | pain in the eyeball |
| oculopathy | generic term for eye disease; synonym for *ophthalmopathy* |
| ophthalmolith | synonym for *dacryolith* |
| ophthalmomalacia | softening of the eyeball |
| ophthalmoscope | device for examining the interior of the eyeball by looking through the pupil |
| ophthalmoscopy | examination of the eye with an ophthalmoscope |
| phacocele | hernia of the lens |
| phacolysis | operative removal of the lens in pieces |
| phacomalacia | softening of the lens |
| presbyopia | farsightedness resulting from loss of elasticity in the lens |
| retinectomy | surgical removal of part of the retina |
| retinitis | inflammation of the retina |
| retinopathy | disease of the retina |
| retinopexy | procedure to repair a detached retina |
| retinotomy | an incision through the retina |
| scleroiritis | inflammation of the sclera and iris |
| scleromalacia | softening of the sclera |
| uveitis | inflammation of the uvea |

By now, you have probably noticed that the names of anatomic structures and physiologic functions come from Latin words, while the abnormal conditions related to these same structures are derived from Greek. In connection with the eye, the Latin-derived word for "eyelid," *palpebral*, precedes *conjunctiva, veins, arteries*, etc., when those words are associated with the eyelid. But the Greek root *blephar/o* is combined with the suffix (again Greek) *-ptosis* to describe drooping eyelids (blepharoptosis). The Greek root *dacry/o*, which means tears, is preferred over the Latin word *lacrima* (which also means tear) when naming disorders associated with the lacrimal system. Thus, the term *dacryorrhea*, which refers to an excessive flow of tears, is more common than *lacrimation*.

## STUDY TABLE  THE EYE

| Term and Pronunciation | Analysis | Meaning |
|---|---|---|
| **STRUCTURE & FUNCTION** | | |
| aphakia (ah-FAY-kee-yah) | *a-* ("no," "without"); *phak/o* ("lens"); *-ia* ("condition") | without a lens |
| conjunctiva (kon-JUNK-tih-vuh); plural: conjunctivae (kon-JUNK-tih-vay) | from the Latin verb *conjungo* ("to join together") | the mucous membrane covering the anterior of the eyeball |
| cornea (KOR-nee-uh) | Latin word meaning "horn" | transparent shield of tissue forming the outer wall of the eyeball |
| corneal (KOR-nee-uhl) | Latin word meaning "horn"; *-al* (adjective suffix) | adjectival form of cornea |
| extraocular (EX-trah-AWK-yu-lahr) | *extra-* ("outside"); *ocul/o* ("eye"); *-ar* (adjective suffix) | situated outside the eye |
| fibrous tunic (FY-bruhs TOO-nik) | *fiber* (from the Latin word *fibra*, "filament"); *-ous* (adjective suffix); *tunic* (Latin for "coat") | the outermost layer of the eye, consisting of the cornea and sclera and connecting with eye muscles |
| iris (EYE-rihs); plural: irides (IHR-ih-deez) | Greek word for "rainbow" | the anterior part of the vascular tunic; it is the colored part of the eye |
| lacrimal apparatus (LAK-rih-mahl app-ah-RAT-uhs) | *lacrima* ("tear"); *-al* (adjective suffix); *apparatus* (common English word) | collectively: the lacrimal gland, lake, canaliculi (small canals), and sac, along with the nasolacrimal duct |
| lens (lenz) | Latin word for "lentil," a lens-shaped legume | the refractive structure of the eye, lying between the iris and the vitreous body |
| neural tunic (NUHR-ahl TOO-nik) | *neur/o* ("nerve"); *-ar* (adjective suffix); *tunic* (Latin for "coat") | the innermost layer, composed of the retina, where the nerves and light receptors (called rods and cones) are located |
| ocular (OK-yoo-lahr) | *ocul/o* ("eye"); *-ar* (adjective suffix) | adjective referring to the eye |
| optic nerve (OP-tik nuhrv) | *opt/o* ("light"); *-ic* (adjective suffix) | one of the cranial nerves (Chapter 16) |
| palbebra (pal-PEE-brah) | from the Latin word *palpebra* ("eyelid") | eyelid |

## STUDY TABLE THE EYE *(continued)*

| Term and Pronunciation | Analysis | Meaning |
|---|---|---|
| palpebral (PAL-peh-brahl) | from the Latin word *palpebra* ("eyelid") | adjectival form of palpebra; eyelid |
| photoreceptors (FOH-toh-ree-SEPP-tohrs) | *photo* (from the Greek word *phos*, "light"); *receptors* (from the Latin verb *recipio*, "to receive") | retinal cones and rods |
| pupil (PYOO-pihl) | from the French word *pupille* ("pupil of the eye") | the dark part in the center of the iris through which light enters the eye |
| retina (RETT-ih-nah) | from the Latin word *rete* ("net") | light-sensitive membrane forming the innermost layer of the eyeball |
| sclera (SKLER-ah); plural: sclerae (SKLER-ay) | from the Greek word *skleros* ("hard") | the outer surface of the eye; part of the fibrous tunic |
| uvea (YOO-vee-ah) | from the Latin word *uva* ("grape") | synonym for vascular tunic |
| vascular tunic (VASS-kyoo-lahr TOO-nik) | *vascul/o* ("vein"); *-ar* (adjective suffix); *tunic* (Latin for "coat") | middle layer of the eye; synonym for uvea, containing the iris, blood vessels, and other tissues |
| vitreous body (VIH-tree-uhs BOD-ee) | from the Latin word *vitreus* ("glassy"); *body* (common English word) | a transparent jelly-like substance filling the interior of the eyeball |
| **COMMON DISORDERS** | | |
| astigmatism (ah-STIG-mah-tizm) | *a-* ("not"); *stigmatism* (optical term meaning "focal point") | fuzzy vision caused by the irregular shape of one or both eyeballs |
| blepharitis (bleff-ah-RY-tiss) | *blephar/o* ("eyelid"); *-itis* ("inflammation") | inflammation of the eyelid |
| blepharochalasis (BLEFF-ahr-oh-cha-lay-sis) | *blephar/o* ("eyelid") *-chalasis* ("relaxation") | relaxation of the eyelid |
| blepharoconjunctivitis (BLEFF-ah-roh-kon-junk-tih-VY-tiss) | *blephar/o* ("eyelid"); *conjunctiva* (mucous membrane covering the anterior surface of the eyeball); *-itis* ("inflammation") | inflammation of the palpebral conjunctiva |
| blepharoplegia (BLEFF-ah-roh-pleej-ee-uh) | *blephar/o* ("eyelid"); *-plegia* ("paralysis") | paralysis of an eyelid |
| blepharoptosis (BLEFF-ahr-opp-TOH-sis) | *blephar/o* ("eyelid"); *-optosis* ("drooping") | drooping eyelid |
| blepharospasm (BLEFF-ahr-oh-SPAZ-um) | *blephar/o* ("eyelid"); *-spasm* ("contraction") | involuntary contraction of the eyelid |
| conjunctivitis (kon-junk-tih-VY-tiss) | from *conjungo* (Latin verb meaning "to join together"); *-itis* ("inflammation") | inflammation of the conjunctiva |
| dacryocele (DAKK-ree-oh-seel) | *dacry/o* ("lacrimal sac"); *-cele* ("hernia") | herniated lacrimal sac (filled with fluid); often called a *dacryocystocele*, because *dacryocyst* is a synonym for *lacrimal sac* |

## STUDY TABLE  THE EYE *(continued)*

| Term and Pronunciation | Analysis | Meaning |
|---|---|---|
| dacryocystalgia (dakk-ree-oh-sist-AL-jee-uh) | *dacryocyst/o* ("lacrimal sac"); *-algia* ("pain") | pain in a lacrimal sac |
| dacryolith (DAKK-ree-oh-lith) | *dacryo* ("lacrimal system"); *-lith* ("stone") | a "stone" in the lacrimal apparatus |
| dacryorrhea (DAK-ree-uh-REE-yuh) | *dacry/o* ("tear duct"); *rrhea* ("discharge") | excessive discharge of tears |
| hyperopia (hy-pur-OH-pee-ya) | *hyper-* ("above"); *-opia* ("condition of the eye") | farsightedness |
| iridocele (IHR-ih-doh-seel) | *irid/o* ("iris"); *-cele* ("hernia") | hernia of the iris |
| iridomalacia (IHR-ih-doh-muh-LAY-shee-uh | *irid/o* ("iris"); *-malacia* ("softening") | softening of the iris |
| iritis (eye-RY-tiss) | *irid/o* ("iris"); *-itis* ("inflammation") | inflammation of the iris |
| lacrimal (LAK-rih-muhl) | *lacrima* ("tear"); *-al* (adjective suffix) | teary |
| lacrimation (uncommon) | from the Latin word *lacrima* ("tear") | synonym for *dacryorrhea* |
| myopia (my-OHP-ee-ah) | *my/o* ("muscle"); *-opia* ("a condition of the eye") | nearsightedness |
| oculodynia (AWK-yu-loh-DIN-ee-ah) | *ocul/o* ("eye"); *-dynia* ("pain") | pain in the eyeball |
| oculopathy (AWK-yu-loh-path-ee) | *ocul/o* ("eye"); *-pathy* ("disease") | generic term for eye disease; synonym for *ophthalmopathy* |
| ophthalmolith (off-THAL-moh-lith) | *ophthalm/o* ("eye"); *-lith* ("stone") | synonym for *dacryolith* |
| ophthalmomalacia (off-THAL-moh-muh-LAY-shee-uh) | *ophthalm/o* ("eye"); *-malacia* ("softening") | softening of the eyeball |
| phacocele (FAK-oh-seel) | *phac/o* ("lens"); *-cele* ("hernia") | hernia of the lens |
| phacomalacia (FAY-koh-muh-LAY-she-uh) | *phac/o* ("lens"); *-malacia* ("softening") | softening of the lens |
| retinitis (rett-ih-NY-tiss) | *retin/o* ("retina"); *-itis* ("inflammation") | inflammation of the retina |
| retinopathy (rett-ihn-AWP-uh-thee) | *retin/o* ("retina"); *-pathy* ("disease") | disease of the retina |
| scleroiritis (skler-oh-RY-tiss) | *scler/o* ("sclera"); *-itis* ("inflammation") | inflammation of the sclera and iris |
| scleromalacia (SKLEHR-oh-muh-LAY-she-uh) | *sclero* ("sclera"); *-malacia* ("softening") | softening of the sclera |
| uveitis (YOU-vee-eye-tiss) | *uve/o* ("middle layer of the eyeball"); *-itis* ("inflammation") | inflammation of the uvea |
| **PRACTICE & PRACTITIONERS** | | |
| oculist (AWK-yu-list) | *ocul/o* ("eye"); *-ist* ("practitioner") | less common name for an ophthalmologist |
| ophthalmologist (off-thul-MAWL-uh-jist) | *ophthalm/o* ("eye"); *-logist* ("practitioner") | physician whose specialty is the eyes |
| ophthalmology (off-thul-MAWL-uh-jee) | *ophthalm/o* ("eye"); *-logy* ("study") | medical specialty dealing with the eye |
| optician (opp-TISH-ihn) | *opt/o* ("light"); *-ician* ("practitioner") | a maker of lenses |

## STUDY TABLE  THE EYE  (continued)

| Term and Pronunciation | Analysis | Meaning |
|---|---|---|
| **DIAGNOSIS & TREATMENT** | | |
| ophthalmoscope (off-THAL-moh-skope) | *ophthalm/o* ("eye"); *-scope* ("viewing") | device for examining the interior of the eyeball by looking through the pupil |
| ophthalmoscopy (OFF-thal-MAW-skuh-pee) | *ophthalm/o* ("eye"); *-scopy* ("viewing") | examination of the eye with an ophthalmoscope |
| optics (OPP-tiks) | from the Greek word *optikos* | science of the nature and characteristics of light |
| optometrist (opp-TOM-uh-trist) | *opt/o* ("light"); *-metrist* ("one who measures") | one trained in examining the eyes and prescribing corrective lenses |
| optometry (opp-TOM-uh-tree) | *opt/o* ("light"); *-metry* ("measurement") | science of examining eyes for impaired vision and other disorders |
| **SURGICAL PROCEDURES** | | |
| blepharectomy (bleff-ah-REK-tuh-mee) | *blephar/o* ("eyelid"); *-ectomy* ("removal") | surgical removal of part or all of an eyelid |
| blepharoplasty (BLEFF-ah-roh-plass-tee) | *blephar/o* ("eyelid"); *-plasty* ("repair") | surgery to correct a defective eyelid |
| blepharotomy (BLEFF-uh-rot-uh-mee) | *blephar/o* ("eyelid"); *-tomy* ("incision") | surgical incision of an eyelid |
| conjunctivoplasty (kon-JUNK-tih-voh-plass-tee) | from *conjungo* (Latin verb meaning "to join together"); *-plasty* ("repair") | surgery on the conjunctiva |
| coreoplasty (KOR-ee-oh-plass-tee) | *core/o* ("pupil"); *-plasty* ("repair") | surgery on the pupil |
| corepexy (KOR-ee-pexx-ee) | *core/o* ("pupil"); *-pexy* ("surgical fixation") | surgery on the iris to change the shape of the pupil |
| dacryocystectomy (dakk-ree-oh-sist-EKK-toh-mee) | *dacryocyst/o* ("lacrimal sac"); *-ectomy* ("removal") | surgical removal of the lacrimal sac |
| dacryocystotomy (dakk-ree-oh-sist-AW-toh-mee) | *dacryocyst/o* ("lacrimal sac"); *-tomy* ("incision") | incision into the lacrimal sac |
| lacrimotomy (lakk-rih-MAW-toh-mee) (uncommon) | from the Latin word *lacrima* ("tear"); *-tomy* ("incision") | rarely used synonym for *dacryocystotomy* |
| phacolysis (fah-KAWL-uh-sis) | *phac/o* ("lens"); *-lysis* ("disintegration") | operative removal of the lens in pieces |
| retinectomy (ret-ihn-EK-tuh-mee) | *retin/o* ("retina"); *-ectomy* ("removal") | surgical removal of part of the retina |
| retinopexy (RETT-ihn-oh-pexx-ee) | *retin/o* ("retina"); *-pexy* ("surgical fixation") | surgical fixation of a detached retina |
| retinotomy (rett-ihn-AW-tuh-mee) | *retin/o* ("retina"); *-tomy* ("incision") | incision through the retina |
| **ENHANCEMENT TERMS** | | |
| amblyopia (am-blee-OH-pee-ah) | from the Greek word *amblys* ("dull"); *-opia* ("a condition of the eye") | condition not caused by an ocular lesion and not fully correctable by an artificial lens |

## 📖 STUDY TABLE THE EYE (continued)

| Term and Pronunciation | Analysis | Meaning |
|---|---|---|
| cataract (KAT-ah-rakt) | from the Greek word *katarrhaktes* ("waterfall") | complete or partial opacity of the ocular lens |
| emmetropia (ehm-eh-TRO-pee-ah) | from the Greek word *emmetros* ("according to measure"); *-opia* ("a condition of the eye") | normal vision |
| extraocular (EX-trah-OK-yu-lahr) | *extra-* ("outside"); *ocul/o* ("eye"); *-ar* (adjective suffix") | adjective meaning "outside the eye"; used in referring to the eye muscles |
| glaucoma (glaw-KOH-mah) | from the Greek word *glaukos* ("bluish green") | disease of the eye characterized by increased intraocular pressure and atrophy of the optic nerve |
| presbyopia (prez-bee-OH-pee-ah) | from the Greek word *presbys* ("old man"); *-opia* ("a condition of the eye") | farsightedness resulting from loss of elasticity of the lens |
| refraction (re-FRAK-shun) | from the Latin verb *refringo* ("to break up") | deflection of a ray of light as it passes from one medium to another of different density |
| strabismus (stra-BIZ-muhs) | from the Greek word *strabismos* ("squinting") | lack of parallelism in the visual axes; crossed eyes |
| vitreous humor (VIH-tree-uhs HYU-mohr) | from the Latin words *vitreus* ("glassy") and *umor* ("liquid") | the fluid component of the vitreous body |

## 🖎 Exercises

### Exercise 17-1 Choosing the Correct Term
Fill in the blanks.

The visible parts of the eye are composed of a transparent shield of tissue called the 1) _Cornea_ ; the colored area, called the 2) _iris_ ; the white area, called the 3) _Schlera_ ; and the 4) _Pupil_ , which is the dark part in the center of the eye. The sclera extends all the way around the eyeball, to the 5) _optic Nerve_, which is responsible for carrying electrical impulses from the eye, to the 6) _Brain_ . When light is reflected off an object toward the eye, the rays travel through the 7) _Cornea_ and 8) _Lens_ , which focuses them onto 9) _Photo Receptor_, in the 10) _retina_ . The retina then changes them into 11) _Electrical impulses_ for the optic nerve to transport.

## Exercises

### Exercise 17-2 Converting Nouns to Adjectives

Convert each of the following nouns or roots to an adjective form using one of the following suffixes: *a, al, ic.*

| Noun | Adjective Form |
|------|----------------|
| 1. conjunctiva | Conjunctival |
| 2. cornea | Corneal |
| 3. retina | retinal |
| 4. sclera | Scleral |
| 5. ophthalmology | Ophtalmolog   Ophthalmic |
| 6. uvea | Uveal |
| 7. optics | Optic |
| 8. lacrima | Lacrimal |

## Exercises

### Exercise 17-3 Matching Terms with Definitions

Match the numbers in Column 1 with the letters in Column 2 according to the corresponding terms and definitions they designate.

| Term | Definition |
|------|------------|
| 1. __J__ ophthalmology | A. transparent shield of tissue covering the iris |
| 2. __G__ uvea | B. adjective associated with tears |
| 3. __E__ pupil | C. a thin layer of tissue, just inside the sclera, where light rays entering the eye converge |
| 4. __D__ iris | D. the "colored" part of the eye |
| 5. __H__ sclera | E. the dark part in the very center of the eye |
| 6. __A__ cornea | F. mucous membrane covering the anterior surface of the eyeball |
| 7. __F__ ocular conjunctiva | G. the vascular tunic in the middle of the eye |
| 8. __I__ ophthalmoscope | H. part of the outermost layer of the eye, which is white in color |
| 9. __C__ retina | I. a device for examining the interior of the eyeball by looking through the pupil |
| 10. __B__ lacrimal | J. name of the medical specialty dealing with the eye |

## Exercises

### Exercise 17-4 Identifying the Parts of the Eye

Label the following parts in Figure 17-1.

* cornea
* fibrous tunic
* iris
* lens
* pupil
* neural tunic
* optic nerve
* retina
* sclera
* vascular tunic
* vitreous body

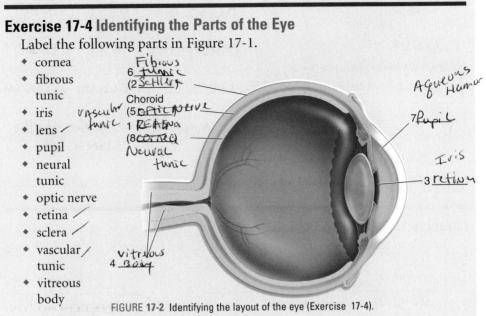

*Handwritten annotations:* Fibrous 6 tunic (2 Sclera) Choroid vascular tunic (5 OPTIC NERVE) 1 RETINA (8 CORNEA) Neural tunic vitreous 4 Body — Aqueous Humor 7 Pupil Iris 3 retina

FIGURE **17-2** Identifying the layout of the eye (Exercise 17-4).

## Exercises

### Exercise 17-5 Building Medical Terms

Build terms to satisfy the following definitions, and then analyze each term by identifying its word elements.

| Definition | Term | Analysis |
|---|---|---|
| 1. fuzzy vision caused by the irregular shape of one or both eyeballs | astigmatism | optical term/ Focal Point |
| 2. inflammation of the palpebral conjunctiva | Blepharoconjunctivitis | Conjunctive Mucos membrane (Line) eye |
| 3. involuntary contraction of the eyelid | Blepharospasm | Spasm of eyelid |
| 4. pain in a lacrimal sac | dacryocystalgia | Pain in lacrimal SAC |
| 5. farsightedness | Hyperopia | EYE condition/Abn |
| 6. teary | Lacrimal | Tearing of the EYE. |

| Definition | Term | Analysis |
|---|---|---|
| 7. nearsightedness | *Myopia* | *Condition of eye muscle* |
| 8. generic term for eye disease; synonym for ophthalmopathy | *Oculopathy* | *eye disease* |
| 9. inflammation of the retina | *retinitis* | *retina inflamation* |
| 10. disease of the retina | *retinopathy* | *disease of the retina* |

# Exercises

## Exercise 17-6 Multiple Choice

Circle the term in the Choices column that answers each of the following questions.

| Question | Choices |
|---|---|
| 1. What is the adjective form of cornea? | cataract; (corneal) corneous |
| 2. What is the name of the outermost layer of the eye, which consists of the cornea and sclera? | neural tunic; (fibrous tunic;) vascular tunic |
| 3. The colored part of the eye (the anterior part of the vascular tunic) is referred to as what? | (iris;) pupil; cornea |
| 4. What is the term for the innermost layer of the eye, composed of the retina, where the nerves and light receptors are located? | ocular tunic; vascular tunic; (neural tunic) |
| 5. What is the name for the middle layer of the eye which contains the iris, blood vessels, and other tissues? | ocular tunic; (vascular tunic;) fibrous tunic |
| 6. What is the name for the medical specialty dealing with the eye? | retinopathy; (ophthalmology;) optometry |
| 7. What is the term for an examination of the eye with an ophthalmoscope? | ophthalmology; blepharectomy; (ophthalmoscopy) |
| 8. What is the name for the science of the nature and characteristics of light? | (optics;) ocular; optometry |
| 9. What is the term for a condition not caused by an ocular lesion and not fully correctable by an artificial lens? | (amblyopia;) aphakia; astigmatism |
| 10. What term do we use to express the condition of farsightedness that results from loss of elasticity in the lens? | glaucoma; (presbyopia;) strabismus |

## Exercises

### Exercise 17-7 True, False, and Correction

Put an X in the True or False column next to each statement. Write the correct answer in the "Correction, if False" column for any you identify as false.

| Statement | True | False | Correction, if False |
|---|---|---|---|
| 1. When a disorder is classified as "corneal" it signifies that it's situated outside the eye. | | X | outside eye |
| 2. The abbreviations for the right eye and left eye are OD and OS, respectively. | X | | |
| 3. The abbreviation for both eyes is OSD. | | X | OU |
| 4. Photoreceptors are the retinal cones and rods. | X | | |
| 5. The dark part in the center of the iris through which light enters the eye is called the retina. | | X | Pupil |
| 6. The pupil is the light-sensitive membrane forming the innermost layer of the eyeball. | | X | Retina |
| 7. The sclera is the outer surface of the eye (part of the fibrous tunic). | X | | |
| 8. Glaucoma is a complete or partial opacity of the ocular lens. | | X | Cataract |
| 9. Cataracts are a disease of the eye characterized by increased intraocular pressure and atrophy of the optic nerve. | | X | Glaucoma |
| 10. Lack of parallelism in the visual axes (crossed eyes) is called a refraction. | | X | Strabismus |

### ✓ Pre-Quiz Checklist

_____ Study the words and word elements specific to the eye (Table 17-1).
_____ Using the study table, familiarize yourself with definitions and etymology.
_____ Since hearing and speaking the terms is a valuable memory aid, practice pronouncing the terms using the phonetic spellings in the study table or on the CD-ROM.
_____ Before attempting the quiz, review the exercises and compare your answers with those in the Appendix, correcting any errors you made.

## ✓ Chapter Quiz

Write the answers to the following items using the spaces provided.

1. What does an optometrist do?

   1. Measure Visability & Prescribe Corrective lens & detect disease

2. Name three distinctive outer layers of the eye.

   2. Fibrous Tunic, Vascular tunic, Neural tunic

3. What does the abbreviation OU stand for?

   3. Both Eyes

4. Where is the lens located in the eye, and what is its function?

   4. Behind the Iris, similar to a camera lens.

5. The word "iris" is derived from a Greek word meaning what?

   5. rainbow

6. What adjectives describe the two areas of the conjunctiva?

   6. Palpebral & Ocular

7. Describe how light rays reflected off an object travel through the eye.

   7. It travels through cornea & lens, which focus the onto photoreceptors in the retina.

8. What is the medical term for "pinkeye," and what is its definition?

   8. Conjunctivitis, eye inflamation

9. What is the collective name for retinal cones and rods?

   9. Photo receptors

10. What is dacryorrhea?

    10. Excessive discharge of tears.

# The Ear

CHAPTER CONTENTS

The brain cannot "hear" sound waves. Therefore, the job of the ears is to detect sound waves and then change them to electrical waves that the brain can use to interpret information (music, spoken words, etc.). The word that names the process of changing energy from one form to another is *transduction*. The verb is *tranduce*, and the devices that do the conversion (such as our ears) are *transducers*. Although these words are not medical terms, knowing their meanings will help you understand how the ear works.

## WORDS AND WORD ELEMENTS SPECIFIC TO THE EAR

The words and word elements shown in Table 18-1 are often found in terms related to the ear. You will recognize them in many of the terms you will learn in this chapter.

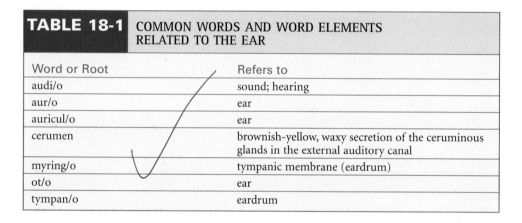

| **TABLE 18-1** | COMMON WORDS AND WORD ELEMENTS RELATED TO THE EAR |
|---|---|
| Word or Root | Refers to |
| audi/o | sound; hearing |
| aur/o | ear |
| auricul/o | ear |
| cerumen | brownish-yellow, waxy secretion of the ceruminous glands in the external auditory canal |
| myring/o | tympanic membrane (eardrum) |
| ot/o | ear |
| tympan/o | eardrum |

## THE PRACTICE AND THE PRACTITIONERS

Coupling the root *audi/o* with the suffix *-logy* yields the term *audiology*, which deals with hearing and hearing disorders. An *audiologist*, therefore, is a specialist who measures hearing efficiency and treats hearing impairment. An *otologist* is a specialist in *otology*, the branch of medical science concerned with the study, diagnosis, and treatment of diseases of the ear and its related structures.

## THE STRUCTURE OF THE EAR

The ear is divided into three parts: the external, middle, and inner ears (Figure 18-1).

### The External Ear

The external ear has two subparts. The outermost part, composed of flesh and cartilage, is called the *auricle* or *pinna* (both mean the same thing, but *auricle* is more commonly used). The other subpart, called the *external auditory canal,*

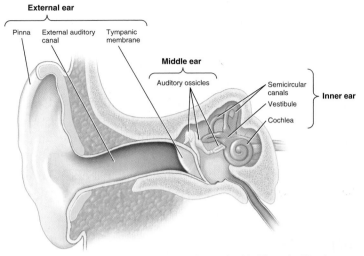

FIGURE **18-1** The ear. *Modified from:* Cohen BJ, Taylor JJ,  Memmler RL, eds.
*Memmler's The Structure and Function of the Human Body.* 8th ed.
Baltimore, MD: Lippincott Williams & Wilkins; 2005.

extends to the *tympanic membrane,* or eardrum. The tympanic membrane separates the external and middle ears. The external ear funnels sound waves into the
finer apparatus within the middle and inner ears. It also protects the ear from
injury and infection. The ear's chief infection fighter is *cerumen,* a wax-like substance
secreted by glands in the external auditory canal (Figure 18-2).

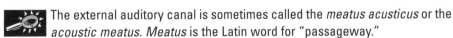 The external auditory canal is sometimes called the *meatus acusticus* or the
*acoustic meatus. Meatus* is the Latin word for "passageway."

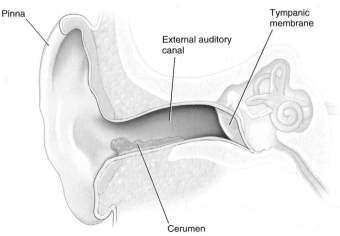

FIGURE **18-2** The external ear.

## The Middle Ear

The middle ear starts on the other side of the tympanic membrane and is called the *tympanic cavity*. The *eustachian tube*, or *auditory tube*, connects the middle ear to the nasal passages. The eustachian tube allows air on both sides of the tympanic membrane to stay at an equal pressure. When you have a bad cold, this tube sometimes gets blocked, which causes obstruction that adversely affects your hearing and makes your head feel heavy. Organisms in the nasal passages often travel through the eustachian tube, causing infection in the ears. The middle ear has three parts, which together are called the *auditory ossicles*. They consist of three bones: the *malleus* (hammer), the *incus* (anvil), and the *stapes* (stirrup) (Figure 18-3).

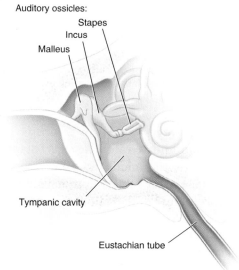

Auditory ossicles:
Stapes
Incus
Malleus
Tympanic cavity
Eustachian tube

FIGURE 18-3 The middle ear.

The auditory ossicles act as a kind of microphone, detecting and transmitting sound waves. In the mechanism of the ear, however, sound waves are not converted into electrical energy until after passing into the inner ear.

## The Inner Ear

The inner ear (Figure 18-4) picks up sound at the *oval window* (the opening to the inner ear) from the stapes and transfers it to the *vestibular duct*. Sound then travels through the *membranous labyrinth*, which is a collection of canals inside the *bony labyrinth*. Receptors in the *cochlea* then transduce the sound waves into electrical signals that our brains can interpret.

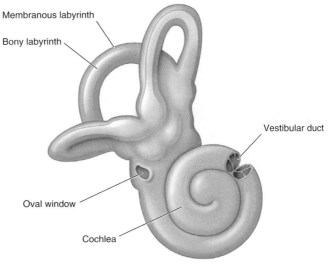

FIGURE **18-4** The inner ear.

## COMMON EAR DISORDERS AND PROCEDURES

Hearing impairment may be divided into three categories: *sensorineural, conductive,* and *presbyacusis.* Sensorineural hearing loss, as the name suggests, is caused by a neural condition—specifically, a disorder of the auditory nerve or some other part of the inner ear. Conductive hearing loss is caused by interference with sound transmission in the external auditory canal, middle ear, or ossicles. Presbyacusis is the hearing loss that occurs with aging.

Unlike electromagnetic waves, e.g., light and heat, sound does not travel through a vacuum. It does, however, travel through solids, liquids, and gases such as air. The density and compressibility of the medium through which it moves determines its speed. For example, sound moves through bone more than 12 times faster than it does through air, and the physics of sound travel can be used in detecting conductive hearing loss. Using a tuning fork, an audiologist can perform a Rinne test (Figure 18-5), which measures the differences between sound received through the ear from the air and that received through bone tissue.

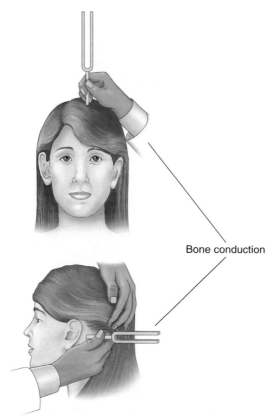

Bone conduction

FIGURE **18-5** Rinne test.

Table 18-2 lists common ear disorders and procedures to diagnose and treat them.

| **TABLE 18-2** | **COMMON DISORDERS AND PROCEDURES ASSOCIATED WITH THE EAR** |
|---|---|
| Term | Definition |
| audiogenic | caused by sound |
| audiogram | automatically recorded results of a hearing test with an audiometer (an electrical device for measuring hearing) |
| audiometer | electrical device for measuring hearing |
| audiometry | measuring hearing with an audiometer |
| cochlear implant | surgically implanted hearing aid in the cochlea |
| conductive hearing loss | hearing loss caused by interference with sound transmission in the external auditory canal, middle ear, or ossicles |

| TABLE 18-2 | COMMON DISORDERS AND PROCEDURES ASSOCIATED WITH THE EAR (continued) |
|---|---|
| **Term** | **Definition** |
| myringoplasty | surgical repair of the tympanic membrane (eardrum) |
| myringotomy | incision or surgical puncture of the eardrum |
| otalgia | pain in the ear |
| otitis | inflammation of the ear (otitis externa = the outer ear; otitis media = the middle ear; otitis interna = the inner ear) |
| otodynia | earache |
| otogenic | originating in the ear |
| otopathy | any disease of the ear |
| otoplasty | cosmetic surgery on the auricle |
| otorrhea | fluid discharge from the ear |
| otosclerosis | formation of spongy bone in the inner ear producing hearing loss |
| otoscope | device for looking into the ear |
| otoscopy | looking into the ear with an otoscope |
| presbyacusis | hearing loss that occurs with aging |
| sensorineural hearing loss | hearing loss caused by a neural condition; specifically, a disorder of the auditory nerve or some other part of the inner ear |
| tinnitus | sensation of noises (such as ringing) in the ears |
| tympanectomy | surgical removal of the eardrum |
| tympanocentesis | puncture of the tympanic membrane with a needle to aspirate middle ear fluid |
| tympanoplasty | surgery performed on the middle ear |
| tympanotomy; tympanostomy | synonyms for myringotomy |
| vertigo | sensation of spinning or whirling; can be caused by infection or other disorder in the inner ear |

 **DECIPHERING MEDICAL DOCUMENTS**

**Read the following excerpt from a patient history, and answer the questions that follow.**

The patient is a 4-year-old male with recurrent ear infections and ear congestion nonresponsive to antibiotic and decongestant therapy over the past 12 months. The patient also has a history of nasal obstruction and nasal speech. The patient is being admitted for myringotomy and examination of the nasopharynx and adenoidectomy.

1. What does nasal mean?
2. What word elements make up myringotomy?
3. What does myringotomy mean?
4. What does adenoidectomy mean?

## 📖 STUDY TABLE THE EAR

| Term and Pronunciation | Analysis | Meaning |
|---|---|---|
| **STRUCTURE & FUNCTION** | | |
| audiogenic (AW-dee-oh-JEN-ik) | *audio* ("hearing"); *-genic* ("origin") | caused by sound |
| auditory ossicles (AW-dih-tor-ee OSS-ih-kuhls) | from *audio* ("hearing") and the Latin word *os* ("bone") | three small bones in the inner ear: the malleus (hammer), the incus (anvil), and the stapes (stirrup) |
| auricle (AW-rik-uhl) | from *auris* (the Latin word for "ear") | one of the two parts of the external ear (the other part is the auditory canal) |
| bony labyrinth (LAB-ih-rinth) | from the Greek word *laburinthos* ("winding passageway") | collection of canals surrounding the membranous labyrinth of the inner ear |
| cerumen (seh-ROO-men) | from the Latin word *cera* ("wax") | wax-like secretion occurring in the external auditory canal |
| cochlea (KOK-lee-uh) | Latin word for "snail" | part of the bony labyrinth |
| eustachian tube (yu-STAY-shun) | after the 16th-century physician Bartolomeo Eustachio | the auditory tube, which connects the middle ear to the nasal passages |
| external auditory canal (ODD-ih tor-ee) | from *audio* ("hearing") and *canal* | one of the two parts of the external ear (the other part is the auricle) |
| incus (INK-uhs) | Latin word for "anvil" | one of the auditory ossicles (the anvil) |
| malleus (MAL-ee-uhs) | Latin word for "hammer" | one of the auditory ossicles (the hammer) |
| membranous labyrinth (MEM-brah-nuhs LAB-uh-rinth) | from the Latin word *membrana* ("skin or covering"); *-ous* (adjective suffix) | canals of the inner ear |
| otogenic (oh-toh-JENN-ik) | ot/o ("ear"); -genic ("origin") | originating in the ear |
| pinna (PIN-ah) | Latin word for "feather" | another term for *auricle* |
| stapes (STAY-peez) | Latin word for "stirrup" | one of the auditory ossicles (the stirrup) |
| tympanic cavity (tim-PAN-ik) | *tympan/o* ("eardrum"); *cavity* (common English word) | the middle ear |
| tympanic membrane (tim-PAN-ik MEM-brayn) | *tympan/o* ("eardrum"); *membrane* ("skin or covering") | the eardrum |
| **COMMON DISORDERS** | | |
| conductive hearing loss (kon-DUK-tihv) | adjectival form of the English verb *conduct* | hearing loss caused by interference with sound transmission in the external auditory canal, middle ear, or ossicles |
| otalgia (oh-TAHL-jee-ah) | ot/o ("ear"); -algia ("pain") | pain in the ear |
| otitis (oh-TY-tihs) | ot/o ("ear"); -itis ("inflammation") | inflammation of the ear (otitis externa = the outer ear; otitis media = the middle ear; otitis interna = the inner ear) |

## 📖 STUDY TABLE THE EAR *(continued)*

| Term and Pronunciation | Analysis | Meaning |
|---|---|---|
| otodynia (oh-toh-DIN-ee-uh) | *ot/o* ("ear"); *-dynia* ("pain") | earache |
| otopathy (oh-TOP-ahth-ee) | *ot/o* ("ear"); *-pathy* ("disease") | any disease of the ear |
| otorrhea (oh-toh-REE-uh) | *ot/o* ("ear"); *-rrhea* ("discharge") | fluid discharge from the ear |
| otosclerosis (OH-toh-skler-OH-sihs) | *ot/o* ("ear"); *-sclerosis* ("hardening") | formation of spongy bone in the inner ear producing hearing loss |
| presbyacusis (PREZ-be-ah-KOO-sihs) | from Greek words *presbys* ("old man") and *akousis* ("hearing") | hearing loss that occurs with aging |
| sensorineural hearing loss (SENTZ-oh-rih-NOO-rahl) | from the Latin verb *sentio* ("perceive"); *neur/o* ("nerve") | hearing loss caused by a neural condition |
| tinnitus (TIN-nih-nuhs) | Latin word for "ringing" | sensation of noises (such as ringing) in the ears |
| vertigo (VUR-tih-go) | Latin word for "dizziness" | sensation of spinning or whirling; can be caused by infection or other disorder in the inner ear |

### PRACTICE & PRACTITIONERS

| Term and Pronunciation | Analysis | Meaning |
|---|---|---|
| audiologist (awd-ee-AWL-oh-jist) | *audio* ("hearing"); *-logist* ("practitioner") | specialist who measures hearing efficiency and treats hearing impairment |
| audiology (awd-ee-AWL-oh-jee) | *audio* ("hearing"); *-logy* ("study") | specialty dealing with hearing and hearing disorders |
| otologist (oh-TOL-oh-jist) | *ot/o* ("ear"); *-logist* ("practitioner") | specialist in otology, the branch of medical science concerned with the study, diagnosis, and treatment of diseases of the ear and its related structures |
| otology (oh-TOL-oh-jee) | *ot/o* ("ear"); *-logy* ("study") | branch of medical science concerned with the study, diagnosis, and treatment of diseases of the ear and its related structures |

### DIAGNOSIS & TREATMENT

| Term and Pronunciation | Analysis | Meaning |
|---|---|---|
| audiogram (AW-dee-oh-gram) | *audio* ("hearing"); *-gram* ("written record") | automatically recorded results of a hearing test with an audiometer |
| audiometer (aw-dee-AWM-ih-tehr) | *audio* ("hearing"); *-meter* ("measure") | electrical device for measuring hearing |
| audiometry (aw-dee-AWM-ih-tree) | *audio* ("hearing"); *-meter* ("measure") | measuring hearing with an audiometer |
| cochlear implant (KOK-lee-ahr IM-plant) | *cochlea* (Latin word for "snail"); *-ar* (adjective suffix) | surgically implanted hearing aid in the cochlea |
| otoscope (OH-toh-skope) | *ot/o* ("ear"); *-scope* ("look") | device for looking into the ear |
| otoscopy (oh-TOSS-kuh-pee) | *ot/o* ("ear"); *-scopy* ("look") | looking into the ear with an otoscope |

📖 **STUDY TABLE** THE EAR *(continued)*

| Term and Pronunciation | Analysis | Meaning |
|---|---|---|
| Rinne test (rihn-eh) | an eponym | hearing test using a tuning fork; checks for differences in bone conduction and air conduction (Figure 18-5, A) |
| **SURGICAL PROCEDURES** | | |
| myringoplasty (mih-RIN-go-PLASS-tee) | *myring/o* ("tympanic membrane"); *-plasty* ("repair") | surgical repair of the tympanic membrane (eardrum) |
| myringotomy (mih-rin-GOT-uh-mee) | *myring/o* ("tympanic membrane"); *-tomy* ("incision") | incision or surgical puncture of the eardrum |
| otoplasty (OH-toh-plass-tee) | *ot/o* ("ear"); *-plasty* ("repair") | surgery on the auricle |
| tympanectomy (TIM-puh-NEK-tuh-mee) | *tympan/o* ("eardrum"); *-ectomy* ("removal") | surgical removal of the eardrum |
| tympanocentesis (TIM-puh-noh-senn-TEE-sihs) | *tympan/o* ("eardrum"); *-centesis* ("surgical puncture") | puncture of the tympanic membrane with a needle to aspirate middle ear fluid |
| tympanoplasty (TIM-puh-no-plass-tee) | *tympan/o* ("eardrum"); *-plasty* ("surgical repair") | surgery performed on the middle ear |
| tympanotomy (TIM-puh-NOT-oh-mee); tympanostomy (tim-puh-NOSS-toh-mee) | *tympan/o* ("eardrum"); *-tomy* ("incision"); *-ostomy* ("an artificial opening") | synonyms for *myringotomy* |
| **ENHANCEMENT TERMS** | | |
| adenoidectomy (AD-eh-noy-DEK-toh-mee) | *adenoid* ("pharyngeal tonsils"); *-ectomy* ("excision") | excision of adenoids |
| tuning fork (TOO-ning) | common English words | an instrument that vibrates when struck |
| Weber test (VAY-behr) | an eponym | hearing test using a tuning fork; distinguishes between conductive and sensorineural hearing loss (Figure 18-6) |

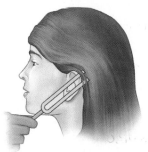

Air conduction

FIGURE **18-6** Webber test.

## ABBREVIATION TABLE

**COMMON ABBREVIATIONS:**
The Ear

| Abbreviation | Meaning |
|---|---|
| AD | right ear |
| AS | left ear |
| AU | both ears |
| BC | bone conduction |
| db or DB | decibel |
| TM | tympanic membrane (eardrum) |
| AC | air conduction |
| ENT | ear, nose, and throat |
| OM | otitis media |
| HL | hearing level |

## 🖎 Exercises

### Exercise 18-1 Choosing the Correct Term

Fill in the blanks.

The ear is divided into three parts, the 1) _External_, 2) _Middle_, and 3) _Inner_ ear. The external ear is made up of two subparts, called the 4) _Aurical_ or pinna, and the 5) _Auditory canal_. The middle ear begins on the other side of the 6) _Tympanic membrane_, also called the eardrum, and consists of three bones, which together are called the 7) _Auditory ossicles_. These three bones are referred to individually as the 8) _Malleus_ or hammer, the 9) _Incus_ or anvil, and the 10) _Stapes_ or stirrup.

## Exercises

### Exercise 18-2 Converting Nouns to Adjectives

Convert each of the following nouns to its adjective form using one of the following suffixes: -ic, -ar, -ous, -al.

| Noun | Adjective Form |
|---|---|
| 1. otoscopy | _Otoscopic_ |
| 2. cochlea | _Cochlear_ |
| 3. pinna | _Pinnal_ |
| 4. audiology | _Audiological_ |
| 5. membrane | _Membranous_ |

## Exercises

### Exercise 18-3 Matching Terms with Definitions

Match the numbers in Column 1 with the letters in Column 2 according to the corresponding terms and definitions they designate.

| Term | Definition |
|------|-----------|
| 1. C audiologist | A. the eardrum |
| 2. G cerumen | B. the process of changing energy from one form to another |
| 3. D otoscope | C. specialist treating abnormal hearing |
| 4. I tympanoplasty | D. device for looking in the ear |
| 5. B transduction | E. inflammation of the middle ear |
| 6. J auditory ossicles | F. part of the bony labyrinth (inner ear) |
| 7. E otitis media | G. wax-like secretion in the external auditory canal |
| 8. A tympanic membrane | H. auditory tube, which connects the middle ear to the nasal passages |
| 9. H Eustachian tube | I. surgery performed on the middle ear |
| 10. F cochlea | J. three small bones in the inner ear, the malleus, incus, and stapes |

## Exercises

### Exercise 18-4 Identifying the Parts of the Middle Ear

Label the following parts in Figure 18-7.

* auditory ossicles
* Eustachian tube (auditory tube)
* incus
* malleus
* stapes
* tympanic cavity

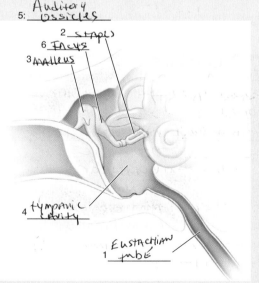

5: Auditory ossicles

2 stapes

6 incus

3 malleus

4 tympanic cavity

1 Eustachian tube

FIGURE 18-7 The middle ear (Exercise 18-4).

## Exercises

### Exercise 18-5 Identifying the Parts of the Inner Ear
Label the following parts in Figure 18-8.
* bony labyrinth
* cochlea
* membranous labyrinth
* oval window
* vestibular duct

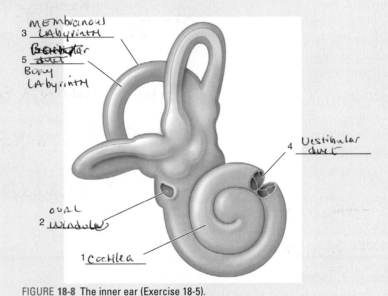

3 _MEMbranous LAbyrinth_

5 _Bestibular duct_

_Bony LAbyrinth_

4 _Vestibular duct_

2 _OVAL windows_

1 _CochleA_

FIGURE 18-8 The inner ear (Exercise 18-5).

## Exercises

### Exercise 18-6 Building Medical Terms
Build terms to satisfy the following definitions, and then analyze each term by identifying its word elements.

| Definition | Term | Analysis |
|---|---|---|
| 1. wax-like secretion occurring in the external auditory canal | Cerumen | wax |
| 2. canals of the inner ear | Membranous Labyrinth | Skin or covering |
| 3. hearing loss caused by interference with sound transmission in the | Conductive hearing loss | Conduct |

| Definition | Term | Analysis |
|---|---|---|
| external auditory canal, middle ear, or ossicles | | |
| 4. inflammation of the ear | *otitis* | *Ear inflamati* |
| 5. fluid discharge from the ear | *otorrhea* | *Ear discharge* |
| 6. sensation of noises (such as ringing) in the ears | *tinnitus* | *Ear Ringing* |
| 7. branch of medical science concerned with the study, diagnosis, and treatment of diseases of the ear and its related structures | *Otology* | *Ear Study of* |
| 8. surgically implanted hearing aid in the cochlea | *Cochlear implant* | *Looking in Ear* |
| 9. examination of the ear with an otoscope | *Otoscopy* | *Looking in Ear* |
| 10. excision of adenoids | *adenoidectomy* | *Excision of tonsils/adnods* |

# Exercises

## Exercise 18-7 Assembling and Defining Terms
Using the Term Analysis, write the term and a short definition.

| Term Analysis | Term | Analysis |
|---|---|---|
| 1. audio (hearing); -genic (origin) | *audiogenic* | *caused by Sound* |
| 2. alternate name for the auditory tube | *Eustachian tube* | *Connects middle Ear to Nasal Passage.* |
| 3. "anvil" of the ear mechanism | *Incus* | *1 of Auditory Ossicle* |
| 4. "hammer" of the ear | *Malleus* | *1 of Auditory Ossicle* |
| 5. ot/o (ear); -sclerosis (hardening) | *Otosclerosis* | *Hearing loss* |
| 6. from the Greek words *presbys* (old man) and *akousis* (hearing) | *Presbyacusis* | *Hearing loss w/ Aging.* |

| Term Analysis | Term | Analysis |
|---|---|---|
| 7. term taken directly from the Latin word for dizziness | *Vertigo* | *dizziness/Spinny Caused by inner ear.* |
| 8. audio (hearing); -gram (written record) | *audiometer* | *Measuring Hearig* |
| 9. tympan/o (eardrum); -ectomy (removal) | *tympanectomy* | *Surgical removal of ear drum* |
| 10. audio (hearing); -logist (practitioner) | *audiologist* | *Specializing in hearing & treatment.* |

# Exercises

## Exercise 18-8 True, False, and Correction

Put an X in the True or False column next to each statement. Write the correct answer in the "Correction, if False" column for any you identify as false.

| Statement | True | False | Correction, if False |
|---|---|---|---|
| 1. The auricle is one of the two parts of the external ear (the other is the auditory canal). | | ✓ | *auricle* |
| 2. The term for the middle ear is the tympanic membrane. | ✓ | ✓ | *tympanic cavity* |
| 3. Hearing loss caused by interference with sound transmission in the external auditory canal, middle ear, or ossicles is called conductive hearing loss. | ✓ | | |
| 4. The otologist checks ears by looking into them with an audiometer. | | ✓ | *Otoscope* |
| 5. To perform a surgical repair of the tympanic membrane, a doctor performs a myringoplasty. | ✓ | | |
| 6. The Rinne test is a hearing test that uses a tuning fork. | | ✓ | |
| 7. A tuning fork is an instrument that lights up when struck. | | ✓ | *vibrates when struck* |
| 8. The Weber test is a hearing test that uses a tuning fork. | ✓ | | |
| 9. The common abbreviation for the right ear is "AS." | | ✓ | *AD* |
| 10. The common abbreviation for both ears is ADAS. | | ✓ | *AU* |

## Pre-Quiz Checklist

_____ Study the word elements specific to the ear (Table 18-1).
_____ Using the study table, practice pronouncing the terms to help in memorizing them.
_____ Review the definitions and etymologies listed in the study table.
_____ Check your answers to exercises with the answers in Appendix, and consult the study table again to correct your errors before attempting the quiz.

## Chapter Quiz

Write the answers to the following items using the spaces provided.

1. To what does the word element myring/o refer?

2. What separates the external ear from the middle ear?

3. Describe the route that an infection often takes to travel to the ear.

4. Together, these three bones are called the auditory ossicles.

5. What two defenses does the external auditory canal have against infection?

6. Briefly describe the job of an audiologist.

7. Name three common types (locations) of ear infections.

8. Describe the function of the auditory ossicles.

9. What are the two subparts of the external ear?

10. Describe the job of the inner ear.

1. tympanic Membrane / eardrun
2. Eardrum
3. eustachian Auditory tube From Nasal Passage
4. Malleus, Incus & Stapes
5. Outer ear / Cerumen
6. To Treat abnormal hearing Conditions / Problems.
7. Outer Ear, Middle Ear Inner Ear,
8. To detect Soundwaves and make them louder.
9. Aurical & External Canal
10. To detect loud Sound and convert it to an electric Signal the brain can Process.

# Answers to Exercises and Quizzes

## CHAPTER 1: ANALYZING MEDICAL TERMS

### Exercise 1-1

1. psychopath — a mentally ill person
   psychology — the study of the mind and mental processes
2. pathology — the study of diseases and disorder (this term is also used informally as a synonym for "disease")
3. carditis — an inflamed heart muscle adjective form
   cardiology — the study of the heart, its functions, and diseases
4. hematology — the study of blood
5. dermatitis — inflamed skin
   dermatology — the study of the skin and its diseases
6. gerontology — the study of the aging process
7. neuralgia — pain in a nerve
   neurology — the study of the nervous system, its functions and diseases
8. osteology — the study of bone
   osteitis — inflammation of bone
   ostealgia — pain in a bone
   osteodynia — pain in a bone

## Exercise 1-2

1. F
2. G
3. A or B
4. D
5. H
6. A or B
7. E
8. C
9. K
10. J

### Answers to Chapter 1 Quiz

1. path and derm
2. knowledge of the aging process and the diseases of old age
3. the nervous system
4. -dynia
5. inflammation of the skin
6. the heart
7. psychology

## CHAPTER 2: COMMON SUFFIXES

### Exercise 2-1

| | | |
|---|---|---|
| 1. | cardiocele | a protrusion of the heart through the diaphragm or through a wound |
| | cardiodynia | pain in the heart |
| | cardiectasia | dilation of the heart |
| | carditis | inflammation of the heart |
| | cardiomalacia | softening of the heart |
| | cardioptosis | downward displacement of the heart |
| | cardioplegia | |
| | cardiorrhexis | |
| | cardiospasm | |
| 2. | dermatitis | inflamed skin |
| | dermatoma | tumor of the skin |
| | dermatomegaly | enlargement of the skin |
| | dermatosis | general term for abnormal skin condition |
| 3. | geroderma | thin, aged, or wrinkled skin |
| 4. | hematocele | blood cyst |
| | hematogenesis | formation of blood cells |
| | hematogenic | adjectival form of hematogenesis |
| | hematosis | abnormal blood condition |
| 5. | neuralgia | pain in a nerve |
| | neurectasis | stretched nerve |
| | neurectasia | synonym for neurectasis |
| | neuritis | inflamed nerve |
| | neuroma | nerve tumor |
| 6. | osteodynia | pain in a bone |
| | osteoectasia | stretched or bowed bones |

|                     |                                              |
|---------------------|----------------------------------------------|
| osteoma             | a benign bone tumor                          |
| osteomalacia        | softening of a bone                          |
| osteopenia          | decrease of bone density                     |
| osteosis            | abnormal bone condition                      |
| osteitis            | inflammation of bone                         |
| 7. pathosis         | diseased condition                           |
| 8. psychosis        | a mental illness                             |
| psychalgia          | distress caused by mental effort             |

## Exercise 2-2

|                       |                                                    |
|-----------------------|----------------------------------------------------|
| 1. cardiogenic        | originating in the heart                           |
| cardiogram            | graphic record of the heart                        |
| cardiograph           | the machine that produces a cardiogram             |
| cardiography          | process of electrically measuring heart function   |
| cardiopathy           | heart disease                                       |
| cardiorrhaphy         | suture of the wall of the heart                    |
| 2. dermatoplasty; also| loosening or atrophy of the skin;                  |
| dermoplasty           | surgical repair of skin                            |
| 3. hematogenesis      | originating with or in the blood                   |
| hematogenic           | adjectival form of *hematogenesis*                 |
| hematometry           | examination of blood                               |
| 4. neurectomy         | removal of a nerve or part of a nerve              |
| neurogenic            | adjectival form of *neurogenesis*                  |
| neurogenesis          | originating in the nervous system                  |
| 5. osteorrhaphy       | suturing broken bone together                      |
| osteoplasty           | surgical repair of bone                            |
| osteogenesis          | formation of bone                                  |
| ostectomy             | excision of bone                                   |
| osteotomy             | cutting of bone                                    |
| 6. pathogen           | a disease-causing agent                            |
| pathogenic            | adjectival form of *pathogen*                      |
| pathogenesis          | development of a disease                           |
| 7. psychogenic        | adjectival form of *psychogenesis*                 |
| psychogenesis         | mental development                                 |
| psychometry           | mental testing                                     |
| psychopath            | mentally ill person                               |

## Exercise 2-3

|                    |                                                                                        |
|--------------------|----------------------------------------------------------------------------------------|
| 1. cardiology      | the medical specialty dealing with heart disease                                       |
| cardiologist       | a heart specialist                                                                     |
| 2. dermatology     | the medical specialty dealing with the skin                                            |
| dematologist       | a skin specialist                                                                      |
| 3. geriatrics      | the medical specialty dealing with aging                                               |
| gerontology        | the study of the process and results of aging                                          |
| gerontologist      | a specialist in gerontology                                                            |
| 4. hematology      | the medical specialty dealing with the blood                                           |
| hematologist       | a blood specialist                                                                     |
| 5. neurology       | the medical specialty dealing with the nervous system                                  |
| neurologist        | a nervous system specialist                                                            |
| 6. oculist         | a medical specialist dealing with the eye; more often referred to as an *ophthalmologist* |

| | | |
|---|---|---|
| 7. | osteology* | the medical specialty dealing with the skeletal system |
| | osteologist* | a bone specialist* |
| 8. | pathology | study of disease; also the specialty practice in the study of disease |
| | pathologist | a practitioner of pathology |
| 9. | pediatrics | the medical specialty dealing with children |
| | pediatrician | a specialist in childhood development and diseases |
| 10. | psychology | the study of the mind |
| | psychiatry | the specialty of psychiatric medicine |
| | psychiatrist | a practitioner in psychiatry |
| | psychologist | an expert in psychology |
| | psychopath | mentally ill person |

*Orthopedics and orthopedist are also common terms for the study of the skeletal system and the specialist practitioners who deal with skeletal abnormalities.*

## Exercise 2-4

| | | |
|---|---|---|
| 1. | cardiac | both are adjectives referring to the heart |
| | cardial | |
| 2. | hematic | adjectives denoting blood |
| | hemic | |
| | hemoid | an adjective meaning "resembling blood" |
| 3. | dermal | adjectives denoting skin |
| | dermic | |
| | dermatic | |
| 4. | geriatric | adjectival form of the noun *geriatrics* |
| | gerontal | adjective meaning "old-age-related" |
| 5. | neural | adjective meaning "related to the nervous system" |
| | neurotic | adjectival form of *neurosis*; also acts as a noun to designate one with the condition |
| | neuroid | adjective meaning "resembling a nerve" |
| 6. | spinal | adjective referring to the spinal column |
| | spinous | adjective meaning "having spines" |
| 7. | osteal | adjective meaning "bone" |
| | osteoid | adjective meaning "resembling bone" |

## Exercise 2-5

1. G
2. J
3. T
4. Q
5. D
6. B
7. C
8. A
9. S
10. E
11. F
12. P
13. H
14. R
15. M
16. O

17.  K
18.  L
19.  N

### Answers to Chapter 2 Quiz
1.  -algia and -dynia
2.  angiectasia or angiectasis
3.  adjective
4.  suture of a blood vessel
5.  -graphy
6.  tumor of a blood vessel
7.  surgical procedure to repair or restore
8.  dermatologist
9.  old age
10.  Gerontology is the study of aging and diseases of the aged, and geriatrics is the medical specialty that deals with patients who fall into this category.

## CHAPTER 3: COMMON PREFIXES

## Exercise 3-1
1.  anteroom                     an outer room leading to a main room
2.  bradyseismic                 slow movements of the earth's crust
3.  neoclassic                   literally "new classic"; usually refers to creating new works of art in a classical style
4.  postglacial                  following the glacial period
5.  predominant                  important; prevailing
6.  tachymeter or, more          an instrument for measuring speed of rotation
    often, tachometer

## Exercise 3-2
1.  abnormal                     an adjective meaning "away from normal"; not normal
2.  adjoining                    an adjective meaning "next to"
3.  concentric                   having the same center
4.  contralateral                the other side
5.  diagram                      an illustration that gives an overall view or explanation; thus, something that permits one to "see through" the subject
6.  sympathetic                  sharing emotions with another person
7.  synthesis                    assembling parts, usually of a theory or idea, into a whole

## Exercise 3-3
1.  eccentric                    outside the center; unusual
2.  ectomorph                    slightly built person
3.  enslave                      to make a slave of
4.  endocardial                  adjective meaning "inside the heart"
5.  epidemic                     great number of occurrences of a particular disease in a particular community
6.  exchange                     give something in return for another
7.  exosphere                    the far reaches of the atmosphere
8.  extraterrestrial             beyond the earth
9.  hypersensitive               highly sensitive
10.  hypothesis                  a possible explanation underlying the facts

| | | |
|---|---|---|
| 11. | infrastructure | the internal framework of a system or organization |
| 12. | intercollegiate | participation involving at least two colleges |
| 13. | intramural | inside the walls; often applied to sports teams within a school |
| 14. | mesosphere | the middle part of the earth's atmosphere |
| 15. | metaphysics | beyond physics; the branch of philosophy that extends beyond simple measurement to an examination of first principles |
| 16. | panorama | a wide expansive view of everything |
| 17. | paralegal | a trained assistant to a lawyer |
| 18. | retrorocket | a rocket that provides thrust in the direction of motion to slow a vehicle |

## Exercise 3-4

| | | |
|---|---|---|
| 1. | biannual | occurring twice a year |
| 2. | hemisphere | half of a sphere |
| 3. | macrocosm | the universe |
| 4. | microscope | a device for viewing objects invisible to the human eye |
| 5. | monorail | a railway system on which the vehicle travels on one rail |
| 6. | oligarchy | rule by a small group of people |
| 7. | quadrilateral | having four sides |
| 8. | semiannual | twice a year |
| 9. | triangle | three-sided geometric shape |
| 10. | unicycle | a vehicle having one wheel |

### Answers to Chapter 3 Quiz
1. ad-
2. ante-
3. an abnormally slow heartbeat
4. beyond
5. hyper-
6. radar used to prevent collision
7. three
8. the size of the objects it was designed to make visible
9. Endocarditis is inflammation of the endocardium, i.e., the inner part of the heart.
10. Tachypnea is a rapid breathing rate. Dyspnea is difficulty in breathing.

# CHAPTER 4: THE BODY'S ORGANIZATION

## Exercise 4-1
1. abnormal enlargement of an organ
2. incision into the cranium
3. abnormal condition of any of the cranial bones

## Exercise 4-2
1. surgical repair by opening a clogged blood vessel by means of balloon dilation
2. x-ray of vessels
3. resembling blood vessels
4. muscle pain
5. protrusion of muscle tissue through surrounding tissue
6. protrusion of lung tissue through the chest wall
7. fixation of two layers of the lung

### Answers to Chapter 4 Quiz
1. Anatomy is the study of the structure of the body, and physiology is the study of body functions.
2. ventral and dorsal
3. ventral
4. lateral
5. the back of the body; after, in relation to time or space
6. proximal
7. forward
8. slowness of muscle response
9. abnormal enlargement of an organ
10. in a position toward the head

## CHAPTER 5: THE INTEGUMENTARY SYSTEM

### Answers to Deciphering Medical Documents
1. percutaneous (*per-* = through; *cutane* = skin; *ous* + *ly* = adverb)
2. after surgery; the prefix *post-* means after
3. B. the roots *hem/o* and *hemat/o* mean blood

## Exercise 5-1
1. epidermis
2. dermis
3. corium
4. sebaceous
5. sudoriferous
6. epithelial
7. keratin
8. stratus corneum

## Exercise 5-2
1. vascular
2. epidermal
3. sebaceous
4. cutaneous
5. cyanotic
6. follicular
7. keratinous

## Exercise 5-3
1. D
2. E
3. F
4. A
5. C
6. J
7. H
8. B
9. K
10. G

# Exercise 5-4
1. nerve endings
2. stratum germinativum
3. epidermis
4. subcutaneous tissue
5. dermis

# Exercise 5-5
1. False. Correction: a thin transparent layer of skin located at the nail root
2. False. Correction: the outermost sub-layer of the epidermis
3. False. Correction: hair-like in structure and appearance
4. True.
5. False. Correction: the inner layer of skin
6. False. Correction: an oil-producing gland
7. True.
8. False. Correction: an absence of veins
9. False. Correction: a tumor of the skin
10. False. Correction: the surgical repair of a nail
11. True.
12. False. Correction: softening of the nails

# Exercise 5-6
1. follicles
2. melanoma
3. lunula
4. keratin
5. epidermis
6. avascular
7. epidermal
8. skin
9. onychopathy
10. dermatology
11. melanin
12. epidermis

## Answers to Chapter 5 Quiz
1. the epidermis (outer layer) and the dermis (inner layer)
2. it protects the body from the environment
3. the dermis, because it contains blood vessels and nerves
4. subcutaneous tissue, and it is composed of connective tissue
5. keratin
6. hardened cells of the stratum corneum (outermost layer of the epidermis)
7. it colors the skin, and protects it from the sun's ultraviolet rays
8. the epidermis has five, and the dermis has two
9. sweat
10. the white, crescent-shaped area of a fingernail

## CHAPTER 6: THE SKELETAL SYSTEM

### Answers to Deciphering Medical Documents
1. CT is an abbreviation for computed tomography, a diagnostic procedure
2. Osteopenia means bone loss, which is part of the degenerative process.
3. the first and second lumbar vertebrae

## Exercise 6-1
The skeleton can be divided into two parts, the (axial) skeleton, and the (appendicular) skeleton. The bones covering the head are collectively called the (cranial) bones, of which there are six. The main facial bones are the (nasal ) bone, (zygomatic) bones, maxilla, and (mandible). The thoracic cage consists of the (sternum), the (ribs), and associated (cartilage). In the spinal cord, 24 vertebrae are numbered, and each one is also labeled with a prefix letter. The prefix "C", refers to the (cervix), the prefix "T" refers to the (thorax), and the "L" is for the (lumbar) vertebrae.

The main bones of the pectoral girdle are the (clavicle), or collarbone, and the (scapula), or the shoulder blade. The bones of the upper forearm include the (humerus), (ulna), and (radius). The wrist contains eight bones collectively called (carpals). Extending from the hip to the knee is the (femur), which joins the (tibia) and (fibula), which extend to the ankle. The tarsals and (metatarsals) of the ankle correspond with the carpal and (metacarpals) of the wrist and hand.

## Exercise 6-2
1. vertebral
2. thoracic
3. maxillary
4. mandibular
5. sternal
6. cervical
7. lumbar
8. sacral
9. appendicular
10. pectoral
11. ulnar
12. femoral
13. pelvic
14. tibial
15. clavicular
16. humeral
17. ischial
18. scapular

## Exercise 6-3
1. E
2. J
3. G
4. H
5. B
6. D
7. A
8. I
9. F

10. C
11. M
12. K
13. N
14. O
15. L

# Exercise 6-4

1. occipital
2. temporal
3. mandible
4. frontal
5. maxilla
6. sphenoid
7. nasal
8. zygomatic
9. parietal

# Exercise 6-5

1. lumbar vertebrae
2. sacrum
3. cervical
4. coccyx
5. thoracic
6. coccygeal vertebrae
7. sacral vertebrae

## Answers to Chapter 6 Quiz

1. 1) a framework for muscles and other tissues;
   2) protection for vital organs;
   3) producing and storing minerals to make blood cells
2. the cranial, facial and thoracic bones, and the spinal column
3. the frontal bone, the two parietal bones, two temporal bones, and the occipital bone
4. the sacrum and coccyx
5. the fourth cervical vertebra in the neck area
6. the maxilla and mandible
7. to protect the vital organs of the body
8. the joint where the humerus and radius meet
9. the knee and elbow; synovial indicates that they are highly moveable joints
10. There are 33 vertebrae in all, but only the first 24 are numbered.
11. the ilium, ischium, and pubis, located at the hip
12. carpal tunnel syndrome
13. the talus
14. the clavicle and scapula
15. The ulnar nerve causes a "pins and needles" sensation, when struck and is located where the humerus joins the elbow.
16. the fibula
17. the two hip bones (os coxae)

## CHAPTER 7: THE MUSCULAR SYSTEM

### Answers to Deciphering Medical Documents
1. serratus anterior and levator scapulae
2. in the shoulder
3. upward rotation

## Exercise 7-1
1. latissimus dorsi
2. flexor carpi ulnaris, extensor carpi ulnaris
3. flexor carpi radialis, extensor carpi radialis
4. quadriceps femoris
5. skeletal, striated
6. longus
7. toe
8. subclavius
9. styloglossus, genioglossus, hyoglossus, palatoglossus

## Exercise 7-2
1. muscular
2. digital
3. extensor
4. flexor
5. abductor
6. adductor
7. gluteal
8. erector
9. hyoglossal
10. digital

## Exercise 7-3
1. H
2. A
3. G
4. E
5. K
6. J
7. D
8. C
9. B
10. F

## Exercise 7-4
1. False. Correction: muscle around the eye
2. True.
3. False. Correction: the posterior thigh muscle
4. False. Correction: arm muscle that joins with the shoulder
5. False. Correction: an interior thigh muscle
6. True.
7. True.

8. False. Correction: formation of muscle cells
9. True.
10. False. Correction: are shoulder muscles that facilitate downward movement

## Exercise 7-5

1. tendonitis
2. tenalgia
3. myelitis
4. myocele
5. toes
6. fingers
7. tenontoplasty
8. tenotomy
9. digiti
10. kinesiology

## Exercise 7-6

1. biceps bra*chii*
2. correctly spelled
3. erec*tor* spinae
4. exten*sor* digitorum
5. exten*sor* hallucis long*us*
6. genioglos*sus*
7. correctly spelled
8. correctly spelled
9. orbicularis o*ris*
10. correctly spelled
11. correctly spelled
12. personatus ter*tius*
13. poll*icis*
14. correctly spelled
15. myomal*acia*
16. myo*cele*
17. *my*ology
18. correctly spelled
19. correctly spelled
20. tenorrh*aphy*

## Exercise 7-7

1. orbicular oculi
2. orbicularis oris
3. corrugator supercilii
4. genioglossus
5. hyoglossus
6. styloglossus
7. palatoglossus

## Exercise 7-8

1. triceps brachii
2. biceps brachii
3. flexor carpi ulnaris

4. extensor carpi ulnaris
5. flexor carpi radialis

### Answers to Chapter 7 Quiz

1. the genioglossus, hypoglossus, palatoglossus, and styloglossus; they effect movement of the tongue
2. the neck, body trunk, and shoulder girdle
3. the deltoid, biceps brachii, triceps brachii, and brachialis
4. the fingers
5. helps rotate the thigh
6. the vastus lateralis, vastus medialis, vastus intermedius, and rectus femoris, known collectively as the quadriceps femoris
7. the sartorius; it flexes and rotates the thigh, allowing for such movements as crossing the legs
8. the biceps femoris, semitendinosus, and semimembranosus; flex and extend the thigh
9. The voluntary muscles are striated or "grooved," and the involuntary muscles, except for the heart, are smooth.
10. the gluteus medius and the gluteus minimus

## CHAPTER 8: THE HEART

### Answers to Deciphering Medical Documents

1. ventricul/o (root) -graphy (suffix); a record of the ventricle
2. heart-related
3. obstruction

## Exercise 8-1

1. epicardium, pericardial sac, pericardium
2. right atrium, right ventricle, left atrium, left ventricle
3. right atrium; right ventricle
4. left atrium; left ventricle
5. arrest
6. electrical impulses
7. bradycardia; tachycardia
8. tachyarrhythmia and bradyarrhythmia; arrhythmia
9. myocardial infarction
10. MI

## Exercise 8-2

1. septal
2. ventricular
3. oxygenated
4. atrial
5. pericardial
6. aortic
7. valvular
8. serous
9. endocardial
10. epicardial
11. membranous
12. arrhythmic

13. tachycardic
14. bradycardic
15. stenotic

## Exercise 8-3

1. False. Correction: valvulitis is inflammation of a heart valve
2. True.
3. False. Correction: myocardial infarction (or) heart attack
4. True.
5. False. Correction: incision into the heart (or incision into the cardia of the stomach)
6. True.
7. False. Correction: a machine that electrically measures heart functions
8. False. Correction: a suturing of the wall of the heart
9. False. Correction: a cardiomyoplasty
10. True.

## Exercise 8-4

1. H
2. J
3. A
4. F
5. I
6. G
7. C
8. E
9. B
10. A
11. N
12. P
13. K
14. Q
15. T
16. L
17. S
18. O
19. M
20. R

## Exercise 8-5

1. atrium
2. epi
3. myo
4. pain
5. inflamed
6. endocardium
7. valvuloplasty
8. septa
9. atrioventricular
10. cardiogram

## Exercise 8-6
1. right atrium
2. right AV tricuspid valve
3. right ventricle
4. intraventricular septum
5. left ventricle
6. mitral valve
7. left atrium
8. aortic arch

### Answers to Chapter 8 Quiz
1. MI
2. the pulmonary semilunar valve
3. electrical impulses
4. the pericardial sac
5. an irregular heartbeat
6. the right atrium
7. ventricular
8. to allow fluid to flow in one direction only, eliminating backflow
9. no; it means that there is a narrowing of the coronary arteries and there is a potential for blockage or MI
10. the left ventricle, because it has to pump blood out to the entire body
11. valvulotomy or valvotomy
12. a "heart attack;" myocardial refers to the heart muscle, and this is the area affected
13. not necessarily; although the heart muscle will have been damaged, it may still be able to pump, and a cessation of heart function (cardiac arrest) may not necessarily have occurred
14. cardiology
15. a written tracing or record of the electrical activity of the heart
16. Bradycardia is a heart rate that is slower than normal, and tachycardia is one that is faster than normal.

## CHAPTER 9: THE BLOOD AND BLOOD VESSELS

### Answers to Deciphering Medical Documents
1. leuk/o (root), -cyte (suffix); white blood cell
2. hemoglobin
3. -emia; lack of or diminished number/amount

## Exercise 9-1
1. conducting arteries
2. arterioles
3. veins
4. superior vena cava; inferior vena cava
5. bad
6. bloodstream
7. liver
8. vasoconstriction
9. angioplasty
10. heart attack

## Exercise 9-2

1. artierial/arteriolar
2. venous
3. vascular
4. sclerotic
5. hemolytic
6. hemorrhagic
7. stenotic
8. vasospasmotic
9. vasculopathic
10. anginal

## Exercise 9-3

1. E
2. H
3. G
4. B
5. I
6. J
7. C
8. A
9. F
10. D
11. O
12. R
13. P
14. K
15. S
16. Q
17. T
18. N
19. L
20. M

## Exercise 9-4

1. False. Correction: azygos vein
2. True.
3. True.
4. False. Correction: Vasculopathy
5. True.
6. False. Correction: red blood cells
7. False. Correction: internal jugular vein
8. False. Correction: lower back
9. True.
10. False. Correction: fibrinogens, globulins and albumins

## Exercise 9-5

1. angiitis
2. arteriosclerosis
3. angina pectoris
4. hemolysis
5. hemophilia
6. hemopathy
7. angiotomy
8. angiography
9. angioplasty
10. angiogram

## Exercise 9-6

1. angi*ogen*ic
2. an*gi*oid
3. correctly spelled
4. capillar*ies*
5. erythroc*y*tes
6. g*l*obulins
7. correctly spelled
8. immunog*l*obulins
9. correctly spelled
10. plat*e*lets
11. correctly spelled
12. veno*us*
13. angiostenos*i*s
14. angi*i*tis
15. va*s*odilation
16. correctly spelled
17. angiotom*y*
18. angior*r*haphy
19. lipoprot*eins*
20. inferior *vena* cava

## Exercise 9-7

1. aortic trunk
2. brachiocephalic
3. left common carotid
4. pulmonary artery
5. right common carotid
6. left subclavian
7. right subclavian

### Answers to Chapter 9 Quiz

1. A bulge in an artery (or a heart chamber)
2. a narrowing of an artery's diameter by the constriction of arterial muscle tissue
3. it increases blood pressure because resistance to the blood flow is increased
4. the brachiocephalic trunk, the left common carotid artery, and the left subclavian artery
5. the great cerebral, internal jugular, brachiocephalic, vertebral, and azygos veins
6. erythrocytes (red blood cells), leukocytes (white blood cells), and platelets
7. albumins, globulins, and fibrinogens

8. Blood pressure lowers because widened arteries offer less resistance to blood flow.
9. the conducting arteries, medium-size or muscular arteries, and arterioles
10. the digital, tibial, femoral, lumbar, gonadal, and renal veins
11. myocardial infarction or MI
12. superior vena cava
13. hemoglobin
14. vasculitis and angiitis
15. hemophiliac
16. elevated body temperature, and discharging of blood
17. hemolytic
18. angina
19. hemopathy
20. vasculopathy

## CHAPTER 10: THE RESPIRATORY SYSTEM

### Answers to Deciphering Medical Documents
1. dys-; phag/o; -ia; difficulty in eating or swallowing
2. chronic obstructive pulmonary disease
3. acute lower respiratory infection

## Exercise 10-1
1. diaphragm
2. nose
3. nasal cavity
4. pharynx
5. larynx
6. trachea
7. bronchi
8. bronchioles
9. alveoli
10. capillaries
11. dyspnea
12. blood gas analysis
13. carbon dioxide
14. oxygen
15. blood
16. oxygen
17. bronchiostenosis
18. dyspnea

## Exercise 10-2
1. bronchial
2. laryngeal
3. pharyngeal
4. diaphragmatic
5. tracheal
6. nasal
7. basal
8. alveolar

9. apical
10. stenotic
11. apneic
12. dyspneic
13. asthmatic

## Exercise 10-3
1. E
2. D
3. I
4. F
5. A
6. H
7. B
8. J
9. C
10. G
11. R
12. N
13. T
14. S
15. M
16. Q
17. L
18. P
19. K
20. O

## Exercise 10-4

| Term | Analysis |
| --- | --- |
| 1. bronchiolitis | bronchiole (Latin for windpipe); -itis (inflammation) |
| 2. bronchorrhea | bronchi/o; -rrhea (flow) |
| 3. diaphragm | diaphragm (Greek, meaning partition) |
| 4. laryngectomy | laryng/o (larynx); -ectomy (excision) |
| 5. pharyngocele | pharyng/o (pharnyx); -cele (hernia) |
| 6. phrenalgia | phren/o (diaphragm); -algia (pain) |
| 7. phrenoplegia | phren/o (diaphragm); -plegia (paralysis) |
| 8. rhinitis | rhin/o (nose); -itis (inflammation) |
| 9. sinusotomy | sinus (cavity); -tomy (incision) |
| 10. tracheoplasty | trache/o (trachea); -plasty (surgical repair) |

## Exercise 10-5

| Term | Definition |
| --- | --- |
| 1. apnea | absence of breathing |
| 2. bronchiostenosis | narrowing of the bronchial tubes |
| 3. dyspnea | difficult breathing |
| 4. laryngospasm | involuntary contraction of the larynx |
| 5. pharyngoplegia | paralysis of the pharynx |
| 6. pneumolith | calculus in a lung |
| 7. rhinalgia | pain in the nose |
| 8. rhinorrhea | discharge from the nose |
| 9. rhinostenosis | narrowing or obstruction occurring in the nasal passages |
| 10. tracheomegaly | abnormal dilation of the trachea |

## Exercise 10-6

1. lungs
2. bronchi
3. nose
4. pharynx
5. lower respiratory tract
6. trachea
7. nasal cavity
8. diaphragm
9. larynx
10. upper respiratory tract
11. epiglottis

## Answers to Chapter 10 Quiz

1. hemoglobin
2. the nose, the nasal cavity, and the pharynx
3. the larynx
4. the larynx and the epiglottis
5. narrowing of the bronchial tube; it would likely cause shortness of breath
6. the larynx, trachea, bronchi, bronchioles, and lungs (including alveoli)
7. at the base of the thoracic cavity beneath both lung bases
8. inflammation of the larynx
9. the left lung must accommodate the heart, which is located in the left side of the chest
10. the body's cells cannot store oxygen
11. the lungs
12. laryngostenosis, pharyngostenosis, and tracheostenosis
13. laryngitis is inflammation of the larynx or "voice box"
14. emphysema
15. bronchiostenosis is defined as narrowing of bronchial tubes, and bronchostenosis is a chronic narrowing of a bronchus
16. pneumonitis
17. bronchoplasty, laryngoplasty, pharyngoplasty, rhinoplasty, and tracheoplasty
18. to restore air flow to the lungs
19. bronchopneumonia
20. apnea is the absence of breathing, and dyspnea is difficulty in breathing

## CHAPTER 11: THE DIGESTIVE SYSTEM

### Answers to Deciphering Medical Documents
1. the stomach
2. the section of the small intestine that connects with the stomach
3. scope
4. a visual inspection

## Exercise 11-1
1. esophagus
2. stomach
3. small intestine
4. large intestine
5. peristalsis
6. chyme
7. small intestine
8. large intestine
9. colon
10. colitis
11. enterorrhagia
12. enterospasm
13. enterologist
14. colonoscope
15. colostomy
16. colectomy

## Exercise 11-2
1. jejunal
2. pancreatic
3. esophageal
4. digestive
5. enzymatic
6. biliary
7. antral
8. intestinal
9. duodenal
10. salivary
11. intestinal
12. diabetic
13. cholecystic
14. colonic
15. pancreatic

## Exercise 11-3
1. F
2. G
3. E
4. J
5. D
6. H
7. C

8. A
9. B
10. I
11. M
12. S
13. R
14. Q
15. L
16. N
17. P
18. T
19. K
20. O

## Exercise 11-4
1. cardia
2. esophagus
3. diabetes mellitus
4. enterostenosis
5. enterorrhagia
6. enteropathy
7. gastrocele
8. gastrocolitis
9. gastritis
10. gastroenteritis

## Exercise 11-5
1. False. Correction: the antrum.
2. True.
3. True.
4. False. Correction: the ileum.
5. False. Correction: the stomach.
6. False. Correction: colorraghia.
7. False. Correction: inflammation.
8. True.
9. False. Correction: enterectomy.
10. True.

## Exercise 11-6
1. stomach
2. small intestine
3. esophagus
4. large intestine

### Answers to Chapter 11 Quiz
1. the fundus, cardia, body, and antrum
2. endocrine function: producing insulin and delivering it to the bloodstream; exocrine function: producing enzymes and secreting them into the small intestine to aid digestion
3. parotid, sublingual, and submandibular
4. keeping the body's metabolism balanced by extracting and storing nutrients and fat-soluble vitamins from the GI tract, and releasing them when needed; the liver also produces and recycles bile, which emulsifies fat

5. the duodenum, jejunum, and ileum
6. Saliva is more than 99% water and contains antibiotics that kill bacteria and essential enzymes that break down complex carbohydrates.
7. storing, condensing, and delivering bile, produced by the liver, to the small intestine
8. the ascending, transverse, descending, and sigmoid colon
9. the jejunum
10. The stomach temporarily stores food, secretes enzymes and acid to reduce food particle size, and liquefies and chemically changes food to produce protein, fat, and carbohydrate molecules to fuel the body's cells.
11. diagnoses and treatment of ailments of the digestive tract
12. cancer originating in the liver
13. jejunoplasty
14. Diabetes is a disease caused by failure of the pancreas to produce insulin in the required amounts, causing a rise in blood sugar.
15. bleeding in the intestinal tract
16. colectomy
17. gallbladder
18. incision of the duodenum
19. gastrocele
20. gastric; duodenal

# CHAPTER 12: THE ENDOCRINE SYSTEM

## Answers to Deciphering Medical Documents
1. hyper- (high or excessive); cholesterol; -emia (blood)
2. the type that is not caused by an insufficient production of insulin
3. oste/o (bone); arthritis; (arthr/o (joint); -itis (inflammation)
4. high blood pressure

## Exercise 12-1
1. seasonal affective disorder
2. hypophysis
3. anterior
4. adenohypophysis
5. neurohypophysis
6. suprarenal
7. kidney
8. epinephrine
9. norepinephrine
10. inflammation
11. gland
12. adenohypophysitis
13. adrenalitis
14. hypophysitis
15. thyroiditis

## Exercise 12-2
1. adrenal
2. hypothalamic
3. hormonal

4. steroidal
5. diuretic
6. glandular

## Exercise 12-3

1. D
2. H
3. G
4. I
5. A
6. E
7. F
8. C
9. J
10. B
11. Q
12. N
13. O
14. S
15. T
16. M
17. K
18. L
19. R
20. P

## Exercise 12-4

1. pineal
2. thyroid
3. adrenal
4. pituitary

## Exercise 12-5

1. GH
2. TSH
3. ACTH
4. FSH
5. ICSH
6. LH
7. PRL
8. MSH

## Exercise 12-6

| Term | Analysis |
| --- | --- |
| 1. adenohypophysis | aden/o (gland); hypophysis from the Greek word for undergrowth (because of its location below the hypothalamus) |
| 2. adenohypophysitis | aden/o (gland); hypophysis from the Greek word for undergrowth (it's located below the hypothalamus); -itis (inflammation) |

| | |
|---|---|
| 3. endocrinology | endo- (inside); crin/o from the Greek word *krino* (to separate); -logy (study) |
| 4. antidiuretic hormone | anti- (against); di- (through); -uret (from *uresis* (urination); -ic (adjective suffix) |
| 5. epinephrine | epi- (around); nephr/o (kidney); -ine (suffix often used in the names of chemical substances) |
| 6. hyperpituitarism | hyper- (greater or above); pituitary, from the Latin word *pituita* (phlegm); -ism (condition) |
| 7. adrenalectomy | adrenal/o (adrenal gland); -ectomy (excision) |
| 8. thyroparathyroidectomy | thyr/o (thyroid gland); parathyroid/o (parathyroid gland); -ectomy (excision) |
| 9. oxytocin (OT) | from the Greek word *oxytokos*, meaning swift birth |
| 10. thyroaplasia | thyr/o (thyroid gland); -aplasia (deficiency) |

## Exercise 12-7

| Term | Definition |
|---|---|
| 1. adrenal gland | glands located at the top of each kidney |
| 2. corticosteroids | steroid produced by the cortices of the adrenal glands |
| 3. gonadotropin (LH) | stimulates ovulation |
| 4. adrenomegaly | enlargement of the adrenal glands |
| 5. hypopituitarism | condition of diminished hormone secretion from the anterior pituitary gland |
| 6. endocrinologist | medical specialist in endocrinology |
| 7. triiodothyronine | another secretion of the thyroid gland, which is often synthesized from thyroxine ($T_4$) by bodily organs |
| 8. adenectomy | excision of a gland |
| 9. thyromegaly | enlargement of the thyroid gland |
| 10. thyrotomy | surgery performed on the thyroid gland |

### Answers to Chapter 12 Quiz

1. the endocrine system and the nervous system
2. exocrine glands: secretions are directed onto the skin or other epithelial surface; endocrine glands: secretions are deposited into extracellular fluid
3. amino acid derivatives, peptide hormones, and lipid derivatives
4. the pineal gland, pituitary gland, thyroid glands, and adrenal glands
5. somatotropin, thyrotropin, corticotropin, gonadotropin (FSH), gonadotropin (ICSH), prolactin, and melanocyte-stimulating hormone
6. thyroxine ($T_4$) and triiodothyronine ($T_3$) regulate metabolism, and calcitonin (CT) helps keep bones strong by preventing excessive absorption of calcium
7. aldosterone; it helps the body retain the correct amount of sodium ions
8. they are located at the top of each kidney
9. antidiuretic hormone (ADH) regulates the amount of electrolytes in extracellular fluid by preventing the kidneys from expelling too much water, and oxytocin (OT) helps the muscles used in childbirth and assists in the production of mother's milk
10. seasonal affective disorder (SAD)
11. a) adenectomy; b) adrenalectomy; c) hypophysectomy; d) parathyroidectomy; e) thyroidectomy; f) thyroparathyroidectomy
12. chronic enlargement of the thyroid gland; the anterior neck (throat) area
13. adenogenous
14. endocrinologist

15. a congenital condition characterized by insufficient thyroid secretion
16. enlarged adrenal glands
17. hyperpituitarism
18. a common form of hyperthyroidism resulting from overproduction of thyroxine; caused by a false immune system response
19. thyrotomy
20. an insufficient amount of iodine in the diet

# CHAPTER 13: THE IMMUNE SYSTEM

### Answers to Deciphering Medical Documents
1. Type I reactions
2. IgE
3. hem/o (blood); lysis (destruction); -ic (adjective suffix); destructive of blood cells)
4. cyt/o (cell); -toxin (poison); -ic (adjective suffix); poisonous to (destructive of) cells

## Exercise 13-1
1. white blood cell
2. lymphatic
3. lymphocytes
4. natural killer
5. perforins
6. thymus
7. antigen
8. lymph tissue
9. T cells
10. immune

## Exercise 13-2
1. pharyngeal
2. lymphatic
3. lymphocytic
4. phagocytic
5. leukocytic
6. lymphoid
7. sternal
8. palatine
9. tonsillar
10. pathogenic
11. splenic
12. cellular
13. thoracic
14. inflammatory
15. allergenic

## Exercise 13-3

1. D
2. H
3. G
4. A
5. J
6. C
7. E
8. B
9. I
10. F
11. M
12. T
13. S
14. Q
15. L
16. K
17. O
18. N
19. R
20. P

## Exercise 13-4

1. lingual
2. pharyngeal (adenoids)
3. palatine

## Exercise 13-5

| Term | Analysis |
|------|----------|
| 1. antibody | anti- (against); body (a foreign substance, and antigen) |
| 2. leukocyte | leuk/o (white); -cyte (cell) |
| 3. lymphocyte | lymphat/o (lymphatic system); -cyte (cell) |
| 4. immunodeficiency | immun/o (immune system) |
| 5. splenitis | splen/o (spleen); -itis (inflammation) |
| 6. splenomalacia | splen/o (spleen); -malacia (softening) |
| 7. splenopathy | splen/o (spleen); -pathy (disease) |
| 8. thymitis | thym/o (thymus); -itis (inflammation) |
| 9. immunologist | from the Latin word *immunis* (free from service) or from the common English word (immune); -logist (practitioner) |
| 10. tonsillotomy | tonsil/o (tonsil); -tomy (incision) |

## Exercise 13-6

1. antigen
2. autoimmunity
3. immunology
4. spleen
5. lymphadentitis
6. lymphangitis
7. lymphangiography
8. lymphangiectomy

9. lymphangioplasty
10. splenotomy

**Answers to Chapter 13 Quiz**
1. mostly water
2. NK cells, T cells, and B cells
3. first on the scene of injury and prevent infection by cleaning away pathogens and debris; the two types are microphages and macrophages
4. thoracic duct and right lymphatic duct
5. gets rid of damaged red blood cells; recycles and stores reclaimed iron; works with the thymus
6. secretes hormones called thymosin, which helps T cells develop
7. structures of variable size within the lymph vessels; contain macrophages that filter out pathogenic antigens and debris as lymph flows through
8. swelling is produced by large numbers of phagocytes and lymphocytes in the node
9. the palatine, pharyngeal, and lingual tonsils
10. in the chest area, behind the sternum
11. lymphadenitis is inflammation of a lymph node or nodes, and lymphangitis is inflammation of lymph vessels
12. a) lymphadenectomy, b) lymphangiectomy, c) splenectomy, d) tonsillectomy, e) thymectomy
13. the thymus and the spleen
14. blood-type antigens
15. they are named according to the antigen contained in the red blood cells of the person
16. the antigens in the transfused blood would signal the recipient's immune system to attack
17. lymphadenopathy
18. *lympha* means water; lymph is mostly water
19. the palatine tonsils
20. immunodeficiency

# CHAPTER 14: THE URINARY SYSTEM

**Answers to Deciphering Medical Documents**
1. radiography of the urinary bladder
2. frontal radiograph of the abdomen
3. ureter/o (ureter); -al (adjective suffix)

## Exercise 14-1
1. kidneys
2. ureters
3. urinary bladder
4. peristalsis
5. urine
6. urethra
7. internal sphincter
8. micturition
9. external urethral sphincter
10. urethra
11. renal calculus
12. ureteralgia

13. ureteritis
14. urologist
15. ureterography
16. ureterolithotomy
17. urethralgia
18. urethritis

## Exercise 14-2

1. G
2. D
3. I
4. A
5. B
6. J
7. H
8. F
9. E
10. C
11. P
12. R
13. N
14. T
15. L
16. S
17. K
18. M
19. Q
20. O

## Exercise 14-3

1. left ureter
2. urinary bladder
3. right kidney
4. left kidney
5. right ureter
6. urethra

## Exercise 14-4

| Term | Analysis |
| --- | --- |
| 1. electrolyte | electr/o (electricity); -lyte from the Greek word *lytos* (soluble) |
| 2. hilum | Latin word for trifle |
| 3. cystalgia | cyst/o (bladder); -algia (pain) |
| 4. ureteralgia | ureter/o (ureter); -algia (pain) |
| 5. urinalysis | urin/o (urine); analysis (common English word) |
| 6. urology | from the Greek word *ouron* (urine); -logy (study) |
| 7. cystopexy | cyst/o (bladder); -pexy (surgical fixation) |
| 8. nephrotomy | nephr/o (kidney); -tomy (incision) |
| 9. renal capsule | ren/o (kidney); -al (adjective suffix) |
| 10. urethrectomy | excision of all or part of the urethra |

## Exercise 14-5

| Term | Definition |
| --- | --- |
| 1. oliguria | diminished urine production |
| 2. polyuria | excessive urine production |
| 3. micturition reflex | reflex that signals the external sphincter to open |
| 4. renal fascia | protective outer covering of the kidney |
| 5. renal calculus | kidney stone |
| 6. renal hypoplasia | underdeveloped kidney |
| 7. renomegaly | enlargement of one or both kidneys; nephromegaly |
| 8. ureterography | radiography of the ureter |
| 9. nephrology | medical specialty dealing with the kidneys |
| 10. renopathy | any disease of the kidney; the preferred term is *nephropathy* |

## Exercise 14-6

1. uremia
2. glomerulus
3. kidneys
4. nephrons
5. nephromegaly
6. nephropathy
7. urethra
8. urethralgia
9. ureterectomy
10. ureterorrhaphy

## Exercise 14-7

1. True.
2. False. Correction: perirenal fat
3. False. Correction: ureters
4. False. Correction: uric acid
5. True.
6. True.
7. False. Correction: practitioner
8. False. Correction: nephrolithotomy
9. True.
10. False. Correction: urethritis

### Answers to Chapter 14 Quiz

1. the indented, narrowest part of the kidney, where blood vessels and nerves enter
2. renal capsule, perirenal fat, and renal fascia
3. urea and uric acid
4. the micturition reflex
5. the internal sphincter muscle
6. glomerulus; it assists in filtration
7. two tubes connecting the kidneys to either side of the urinary bladder; their job is to move urine from the kidneys to the bladder
8. by peristalsis
9. tube connected to the bottom of the bladder; carries urine from the bladder to be expelled from the body

10. nephrology
11. cystectomy
12. renal hypoplasia
13. cystalgia, nephralgia, ureteralgia, and urethralgia
14. urinalysis and urinometry
15. removal of the gallbladder; removal of a cyst.
16. surgical removal of a kidney
17. a kidney, a ureter, and part of the urinary bladder
18. renomegaly
19. renopathy
20. nephropathy

## CHAPTER 15: THE REPRODUCTIVE SYSTEM

### Answers to Deciphering Medical Documents
1. second pregnancy, one child previously delivered
2. extraction and diagnostic examination of amniotic fluid from the amniotic sac
3. inside the uterus

## Exercise 15-1
1. testes
2. androgens
3. testosterone
4. spermatogenesis
5. epididymis
6. testes
7. ductus deferens
8. urethra
9. prostatic fluid
10. semen
11. hormonal
12. uterine
13. menstrual
14. progestins
15. progesterone
16. oocytes
17. gametes
18. uterine
19. fallopian

## Exercise 15-2
1. testicular
2. chromosomal
3. androgenous
4. epididymal
5. prostatic
6. urethral
7. spermatogenetic
8. oogenetic
9. uterine

10. ovulatory
11. cervical
12. ovarian
13. gestational
14. fetal
15. embryonic

## Exercise 15-3

1. D
2. F
3. E
4. I
5. B
6. H
7. A
8. J
9. G
10. C
11. O
12. Q
13. R
14. M
15. T
16. L
17. K
18. S
19. P
20. N

## Exercise 15-4

1. testis
2. ductus deferens
3. epididymis
4. urethra

## Exercise 15-5

1. uterus
2. oviduct (fallopian tube)
3. ovary
4. cervix

## Exercise 15-6

| Term | Analysis |
| --- | --- |
| 1. androgens | from the Greek *andros* (man); -gen (origin) |
| 2. epididymus | epi (on); didymus from the Greek word *didumos* (testes) |
| 3. gonad | from the Greek word *goneos* (generation) |
| 4. oocytes | oo (egg); -cyte (cell) |
| 5. prostatic fluid | -ic (adjective suffix added to prostate); fluid (common English word) |
| 6. uterus | Latin word for womb |

7. cervicoplasty                    cervic/o (cervix); -plasty (repair)
8. oophorotomy                      oophor/o (ovary); -tomy (incision)
9. testosterone                     from the Latin word *testiculus* (testes) and sterol (class of
                                    complex alcohols)
10. amenorrhea                      a- (not); men/o (menses); -rrhea (flow)

## Exercise 15-7

1. False. Correction: gestation
2. True.
3. False. Correction: fertilization
4. False. Correction: mitosis
5. False. Correction: ovulation
6. True.
7. True.
8. False. Correction: obstetrics
9. False. Correction: dysmenorrheal
10. False. Correction: Pap test

### Answers to Chapter 15 Quiz

1. sperm and spermatozoon
2. meiosis is cell division that produces cells with only one set of chromosomes, those of the potential father or potential mother; mitosis is a process of cell division, by which one cell becomes two, both of which contain a full complement of chromosomes, paternal and maternal
3. collective name for any male or female organ that produces a gamete
4. a combination of gametes, their associated glandular secretions, and prostatic fluid
5. ovum
6. the secretion of androgens, and most significantly, testosterone
7. the single cell formed at fertilization, containing a full complement of chromosomes and DNA
8. a haploid cell contains only one set of chromosomes, those of the potential mother or potential father; a diploid cell contains both maternal and paternal chromosomes
9. it acts as a male reproductive duct, secreting semen, and also as a urinary system duct, secreting urine
10. the ductwork leading from the epididymus to the outside of the body, which would include the vas (ductus) deferens and the urethra
11. secretory phase: secretion of hormones; proliferative phase: proliferation of ovum; menses: the end of one cycle and the beginning of another
12. proliferative phase
13. the fallopian (uterine) tubes
14. as soon as it divides the first time
15. from about the eighth week of gestation until birth
16. during the proliferative phase, at the time of ovulation
17. at the lower end of the uterus
18. oogenesis
19. the secretion of hormones called progestins, the principal one of which is progesterone
20. gametes for fertilization

# CHAPTER 16: THE NERVOUS SYSTEM

## Answers to Deciphering Medical Documents
1. lack of muscular coordination
2. pupils equal, round, and reactive to light and accommodation
3. organic brain syndrome

## Exercise 16-1
1. cerebrum
2. cerebral cortex
3. cerebellum
4. thalamus
5. hypothalamus
6. diencephalon
7. mesencephalon
8. pons
9. medulla oblongata
10. spinal cord
11. meninges
12. dura mater

## Exercise 16-2
1. loss of sensory input recognition
2. dilated blood vessel
3. brain disorder involving a blood vessel
4. excision of part of the skull
5. impaired consciousness
6. impaired speech
7. inflammation of the brain
8. tumor of glial tissue
9. partial paralysis of one side of the body
10. benign tumor of meninges
11. disease of the CNS characterized by the formation of plaques in the brain and spinal cord
12. pain in a nerve
13. a neurologic condition characterized by difficulty in controlling muscles
14. inflamed gray matter in the spinal cord
15. sudden disturbance in brain function sometimes producing a convulsion

## Exercise 16-3
1. attention deficit hyperactivity disorder
2. electroencephalography
3. intelligence quotient
4. lumbar puncture
5. mental age
6. organic brain syndrome
7. obsessive-compulsive disorder
8. pupils equal, round, and reactive to light and accommodation
9. seasonal affective disorder
10. transcutaneous electrical nerve stimulation

## Exercise 16-4

| Term | Analysis |
|------|----------|
| 1. axon | Greek for axis |
| 2. cell body | two common English words |
| 3. cerebral cortex | cerebr/o (brain); -al (adjective suffix); *cortex* (Latin for bark as on a tree and rind as on a lemon) |
| 4. ganglion | *ganglion* (Greek word for knot) |
| 5. occipital lobe | adjective form of *occiput* (back of the head); *lobos* (Greek word for lobe) |
| 6. agnosia | a- (without); -gnosis (knowledge); -ia (condition) |
| 7. glioblastoma | gli/o (glue); *blastos* (Greek word for germ); -oma (tumor) |
| 8. multiple sclerosis | multiple (common English word); *scleros* (Greek word for hard); -osis (condition) |
| 9. neurologist | neur/o (nerve); -logist (practitioner) |
| 10. myelography | myel/o (marrow); -graphy (x-ray) |

## Exercise 16-5

1. brain stem
2. dendrite
3. myelin sheath
4. occipital lobe
5. pons
6. cerebral thrombosis
7. dysphasia
8. hyperesthesia
9. poliomyelitis
10. ataxia

## Exercise 16-6

1. cerebellum
2. thalamus
3. pons
4. cerebrum
5. hypothalamus
6. medulla oblongata
7. brain stem

### Answers to Chapter 16 Quiz

1. the thalamus
2. the brain and spinal cord
3. the peripheral nervous system
4. CNS and PNS
5. neurons and neuroglia
6. cell bodies, dendrites, axons
7. nucleus (singular); nucleii (plural)
8. ganglion (singular); ganglia (plural)
9. the brain stem and cerebrum
10. conscious and habitual actions are somatic; the performance of organs that work on their own are autonomic
11. Parkinson disease (also sometimes called Parkinson's disease)

12. cerebrovascular disease
13. CNS
14. Huntington disease (also sometimes called Huntington's disease)
15. an incision into the skull
16. poliomyelitis
17. inflammation of the brain
18. aphasia
19. a stroke
20. a sudden disturbance in brain function, sometimes producing a seizure

# CHAPTER 17: THE EYE

### Answers to Deciphering Medical Documents
1. right eye and left eye, respectively
2. irides is the plural form of iris
3. conjunctiva and sclera

## Exercise 17-1
1. cornea
2. iris
3. sclera
4. pupil
5. optic nerve
6. brain
7. cornea
8. lens
9. photoreceptors
10. retina
11. electrical impulses

## Exercise 17-2
1. conjunctival
2. corneal
3. retinal
4. scleral
5. ophthalmic
6. uveal
7. optic
8. lacrimal

## Exercise 17-3
1. J
2. G
3. E
4. D
5. H
6. A
7. F
8. I
9. C
10. B

## Exercise 17-4

1. lens
2. sclera
3. retina
4. vitreous body
5. optic nerve
6. fibrous tunic
7. pupil
8. cornea
9. neural tunic
10. iris
11. vascular tunic

## Exercise 17-5

| Term | Analysis |
|------|----------|
| 1. astigmatism | a- (not); stigmatism (optical term meaning focal point) |
| 2. blepharoconjunctivitis | blephar/o (eyelid); conjunctiva (mucous membrane covering the anterior surface of the eyeball); -itis (inflammation) |
| 3. blepharospasm | blephar/o (eyelid); -spasm (contraction) |
| 4. dacryocystalgia | dacryocyst/o (lacrimal sac); -algia (pain) |
| 5. hyperopia | hyper- (above); -opia (condition of the eye) |
| 6. lacrimal | lacrima (tear); -al (adjective suffix) |
| 7. myopia | my/o (muscle); -opia (a condition of the eye) |
| 8. oculopathy | ocul/o (eye); -pathy (disease) |
| 9. retinitis | retin/o (retina); -itis (inflammation) |
| 10. retinopathy | retin/o (retina); -pathy (disease) |

## Exercise 17-6

1. corneal
2. fibrous tunic
3. iris
4. neural tunic
5. vascular tunic
6. ophthalmology
7. ophthalmoscopy
8. optics
9. amblyopia
10. presbyopia

## Exercise 17-7

1. False. Correction: extraocular – outside the eye
2. True.
3. False. Correction: OU
4. True.
5. False. Correction: pupil
6. False. Correction: retina
7. True.
8. False. Correction: cataract
9. False. Correction: glaucoma
10. False. Correction: strabismus

**Answers to Chapter Quiz**
1. measures a patient's ability to see and, like an ophthalmologist, can prescribe corrective lenses
2. the fibrous tunic, the vascular tunic, and the neural tunic
3. both eyes
4. directly behind the iris; it works much the same way as a camera lens does
5. rainbow
6. palpebral and ocular
7. Light rays travel through the cornea and lens, which focuses them onto photoreceptors in the retina. The retina changes them into electrical impulses that travel through the optic nerve to the brain.

# CHAPTER 18: THE EAR

**Answers to Deciphering Medical Documents**
1. adjective for nose
2. myring/o (eardrum); -tomy (incision)
3. incision or surgical puncture of the ear drum
4. excision of adenoids (pharyngeal tonsils)

# Exercise 18-1
1. external
2. middle
3. inner
4. auricle
5. auditory canal
6. tympanic membrane
7. auditory ossicles
8. malleus
9. incus
10. stapes

# Exercise 18-2
1. otoscopic
2. cochlear
3. pinnal
4. audiological
5. membranous

# Exercise 18-3
1. C
2. G
3. D
4. I
5. B
6. J
7. E
8. A
9. H
10. F

## Exercise 18-4

1. Eustachian tube
2. stapes
3. malleus
4. tympanic cavity
5. auditory ossicles
6. incus

## Exercise 18-5

1. cochlea
2. oval window
3. membranous labyrinth
4. vestibular duct
5. bony labyrinth

## Exercise 18-6

1. cerumen — from the Latin word *cera* meaning wax
2. membranous labyrinth — from the Latin word *membrana* (skin or covering); -ous (adjective suffix)
3. conductive hearing loss — adjectival form of the English verb *conduct*
4. otitis — ot/o (ear); -itis (inflammation)
5. otorrhea — ot/o (ear); -rrhea (discharge)
6. tinnitus — Latin for ringing
7. otology — ot/o (ear); -logy (study)
8. cochlear implant — cochlea (Latin word for snail); -ar (adjective suffix)
9. otoscopy — ot/o (ear); -scopy (look)
10. adenoidectomy — adenoids (pharyngeal tonsils); -ectomy (excision)

## Exercise 18-7

1. audiogenic — caused by sound
2. eustachian tube — connects the middle ear to the nasal passages
3. incus — one of the auditory ossicles
4. malleus — one of the auditory ossicles
5. otosclerosis — formation of spongy bone in the inner ear producing hearing loss
6. presbyacusis — hearing loss that occurs with aging
7. vertigo — sensation of spinning or whirling; can be caused by infection or other disorder in the inner ear
8. audiometer — electrical device for measuring hearing
9. tympanectomy — surgical removal of the ear drum
10. audiologist — specialist who measures hearing efficiency and treats hearing impairment

## Exercise 18-8

1. False. Correction: the auricle
2. False. Correction: the tympanic cavity
3. True.
4. False. Correction: an otoscope
5. True.
6. True.
7. False. Correction: vibrates when struck

8. True.
9. False. Correction: AD
10. False. Correction: AU

## Answers to Chapter Quiz

1. tympanic membrane; eardrum
2. the tympanic membrane (eardrum)
3. through the eustachian (auditory) tube from the nasal passages
4. the malleus (hammer), incus (anvil), and stapes (stirrup)
5. the outer ear and cerumen
6. treats abnormal hearing conditions
7. otitis externa (outer ear), otitis media (middle ear), otitis interna (inner ear)
8. the malleus (hammer) and incus (anvil) detect sound waves, and the stapes (stirrup) amplifies them
9. the auricle (pinna) and the external auditory canal
10. detects amplified sound and converts it to an electrical signal that the brain can process

# Appendix B

# Commonly Prescribed Drugs

The following alphabetical list of commonly prescribed drugs (trade and generic) is based on listings of prescriptions dispensed in the United States in 2003. The classification and major therapeutic uses for each are also provided. Trade-name drugs begin with a capital letter; their generic names accompany them in parentheses. All generic names are set in lowercase.

| Name | Classification | Major Therapeutic Uses |
|---|---|---|
| Accupril (quinapril hydrochloride) | angiotensin-converting enzyme (ACE) inhibitor | hypertension, congestive heart failure (CHF) |
| Accutane (isotretinoin) | retinoid | acne |
| acetaminophen and codeine | analgesic/antipyretic and opiate (narcotic) combination | moderate to severe pain, fever |
| AcipHex (rabeprazole) | proton pump inhibitor (PPI) (gastric acid secretion inhibitor) | peptic ulcer disease (PUD), gastroesophageal reflux disease (GERD) |
| Actonel (risedronate) | bisphosphonate (bone resorption inhibitor) | osteoporosis, Paget disease |
| Actos (pioglitazone) | oral antidiabetic | type 2 diabetes mellitus |
| Adderall XR (amphetamine mixed salts) | amphetamine | attention deficit hyperactivity disorder (ADHD) |
| Advair Diskus (salmeterol/ fluticasone) | adrenergic agonist (bronchodilator) and glucocorticoid (anti-inflammatory) | asthma |
| albuterol | adrenergic agonist (bronchodilator) | asthma, bronchitis |
| Allegra (fexofenadine) | antihistamine | allergy |
| Allegra D (fexofenadine/ pseudoephedrine) | antihistamine and decongestant combination | allergy with nasal congestion |
| allopurinol | xanthine oxidase inhibitor | gout |
| Alphagan P (brimonidine) ophthalmic solution | $\alpha_2$-adrenergic agonist (antihypertensive) | glaucoma |
| alprazolam | benzodiazepine (anxiolytic, sedative, hypnotic) | anxiety |
| Altace (ramipril) | angiotensin-converting enzyme (ACE) inhibitor | hypertension, congestive heart failure (CHF) |
| Amaryl (glimepiride) | oral antidiabetic | type 2 diabetes mellitus |
| Ambien (zolpidem) | hypnotic | insomnia |
| amitriptyline | antidepressant | depression |
| amoxicillin | penicillin (antibiotic) | bacterial infections |
| amoxicillin/clavulanate | penicillin (antibiotic) and $\beta$-lactamase inhibitor combination | bacterial infections |
| Apri (desogestrel/ethinyl estradiol) | oral contraceptive | birth control |
| Aricept (donepezil) | acetylcholinesterase inhibitor | Alzheimer disease |
| Atacand (candesartan) | angiotensin receptor blocker (antihypertensive) | hypertension |
| atenolol | cardioselective $\beta$ blocker/ $\beta_1$-adrenergic antagonist (antihypertensive, antiarrhythmic, antianginal) | hypertension, angina pectoris, cardiac arrhythmias |
| Atrovent (ipratropium) | anticholinergic (bronchodilator) | chronic obstructive pulmonary disease (COPD) |
| Augmentin (amoxicillin/clavulanate) | penicillin (antibiotic) and $\beta$-lactamase inhibitor combination | bacterial infections |

| | | |
|---|---|---|
| Avalide (irbesartan/hydrochlorothiazide) | angiotensin receptor blocker (antihypertensive) and diuretic combination | hypertension |
| Avandia (rosiglitazone) | oral antidiabetic | type 2 diabetes mellitus |
| Avapro (irbesartan) | angiotensin receptor blocker (antihypertensive) | hypertension |
| Avelox (moxifloxacin) | fluoroquinolone (antibiotic) | bacterial infections |
| Aviane (levonorgestrel/ethinyl estradiol) | oral contraceptive | birth control |
| Bactrim (trimethoprim/ sulfamethoxazole) | antibacterial and sulfonamide (antibiotic) combination | bacterial infections |
| Bactroban (mupirocin) | topical antibiotic | bacterial skin infections |
| Bextra (valdecoxib) | cox-2 inhibitor (nonsteroidal anti-inflammatory drug [NSAID]) | pain, inflammation, fever, arthritis |
| Biaxin (clarithromycin) | macrolide (antibiotic) | bacterial infections |
| carisoprodol | skeletal muscle relaxant | skeletal muscle spasms and spasticity |
| Cartia XT (diltiazem) | calcium channel blocker | hypertension, angina pectoris, cardiac arrhythmias |
| Cefzil (cefprozil) | cephalosporin (antibiotic) | bacterial infections |
| Celebrex (celecoxib) | cox-2 inhibitor (nonsteroidal anti-inflammatory drug [NSAID]) | pain, inflammation, fever, arthritis |
| Celexa (citalopram) | selective serotonin reuptake inhibitor (SSRI) (antidepressant) | depression |
| cephalexin | cephalosporin (antibiotic) | bacterial infections |
| Cipro (ciprofloxacin) | fluoroquinolone (antibiotic) | bacterial infections |
| ciprofloxacin | fluoroquinolone (antibiotic) | bacterial infections |
| clonazepam | benzodiazepine (sedative/hypnotic, anticonvulsant, anxiolytic) | epilepsy, seizures, anxiety (panic disorder) |
| clonidine | $\alpha_2$-adrenergic agonist (antihypertensive) | hypertension |
| clotrimazole and betamethasone | topical antifungal and anti-inflammatory combination | fungal infections, some parasites |
| Combivent (ipratropium/ albuterol) inhalation aerosol | anticholinergic and adrenergic agonist combination (bronchodilators) | asthma, chronic bronchitis, emphysema |
| Concerta (methylphenidate) extended release | central nervous system stimulant | attention deficit hyperactivity disorder (ADHD) |
| Coreg (carvedilol) | cardioselective $\beta$ blocker/$\beta_1$-adrenergic antagonist (antihypertensive, antiarrhythmic, antianginal) | hypertension, congestive heart failure (CHF) |
| Coumadin (warfarin sodium) | anticoagulant | thromboembolic disorders |
| Cozaar (losartan) | angiotensin receptor blocker (antihypertensive) | hypertension |
| cyclobenzaprine | skeletal muscle relaxant | skeletal muscle spasms and spasticity |

| Depakote (divalproex) | anticonvulsant | epilepsy, migraine prophylaxis, bipolar mania |
| --- | --- | --- |
| Detrol LA (tolterodine) | anticholinergic | overactive bladder |
| diazepam | benzodiazepine (sedative/hypnotic, anticonvulsant, anxiolytic) | anxiety, skeletal muscle spasms, epilepsy, seizures |
| Diflucan (fluconazole) | antifungal | fungal infections |
| Digitek (digoxin) | cardiac glycoside | congestive heart failure (CHF), cardiac tachyarrhythmias |
| Dilantin (phenytoin) | hydantoin (anticonvulsant) | epilepsy, seizures |
| diltiazem hydrochloride | calcium channel blocker | hypertension, angina pectoris, cardiac arrhythmias |
| Diovan (valsartan) | angiotensin receptor blocker (antihypertensive) | hypertension |
| Diovan HCT (valsartan/ hydrochlorothiazide) | angiotensin receptor blocker and diuretic combination (antihypertensive) | hypertension |
| Ditropan XL (oxybutynin) | anticholinergic (urinary antispasmodic) | overactive bladder |
| doxycycline | tetracycline (antibiotic) | bacterial, rickettsial, and chlamydial infections |
| Duragesic (fentanyl) | analgesic, opiate (narcotic) | pain, sedation |
| Effexor XR (venlafaxine) | antidepressant | depression |
| Elidel (pimecrolimus) topical cream | immunosuppressant agent | atopic dermatitis |
| enalapril | angiotensin-converting enzyme (ACE) inhibitor | hypertension, congestive heart failure (CHF) |
| Endocet (oxycodone/acetaminophen) | opiate (narcotic) and nonsteroidal anti-inflammatory (NSAID) (analgesic/antipyretic) combination | moderate to severe pain |
| Evista (raloxifene) | selective estrogen receptor modulator (SERM) | prevention and treatment of osteoporosis |
| Flomax (tamsulosin) | $\alpha_1$-adrenergic antagonist (antihypertensive, vasodilator) | benign prostatic hypertrophy (BPH) |
| Flonase (fluticasone) nasal spray | glucocorticoid (anti-inflammatory, immunosuppressant) | allergic rhinitis |
| Flovent (fluticasone) oral inhalation | glucocorticoid (anti-inflammatory, immunosuppressant) | asthma control |
| fluoxetine | selective serotonin reuptake inhibitor (SSRI) (antidepressant) | depression |
| folic acid | vitamin | nutritional supplement |
| Fosamax (alendronate) | bisphosphonate (bone resorption inhibitor) | osteoporosis, Paget disease |
| furosemide | diuretic | hypertension, edema associated with congestive heart failure (CHF) or renal disease |
| gemfibrozil | antihyperlipidemic | hypertriglyceridemia, hyperlipidemia |
| Glucophage XR (metformin) | oral antidiabetic | type 2 diabetes mellitus |

| Glucotrol XL (glipizide) | oral antidiabetic | type 2 diabetes mellitus |
|---|---|---|
| Glucovance (glyburide/metformin) | oral antidiabetic (combination product) | type 2 diabetes mellitus |
| glyburide | oral antidiabetic | type 2 diabetes mellitus |
| Humalog (insulin lispro) | insulin, antidiabetic | types 1 and 2 diabetes mellitus |
| Humulin (insulin preparation) | insulin, antidiabetic | types 1 and 2 diabetes mellitus |
| hydrochlorothiazide | diuretic | hypertension, edema associated with congestive heart failure (CHF) or renal disease |
| hydrocodone and acetaminophen | opiate (narcotic) and nonsteroidal anti-inflammatory drug (NSAID) (analgesic/antipyretic) combination | moderate to severe pain |
| Hyzaar (losartan/hydrochlorothiazide) | angiotensin receptor blocker and diuretic combination (antihypertensive) | hypertension |
| ibuprofen | analgesic, nonsteroidal anti-inflammatory drug (NSAID) | pain, inflammation, fever |
| Imitrex (sumatriptan succinate) | triptan (antimigraine agent) | migraine headache |
| Inderal LA (propranolol) | β blocker (antihypertensive, antiarrhythmic, antianginal) | hypertension, angina pectoris, cardiac arrhythmias, migraine headache prophylaxis |
| isosorbide mononitrate | coronary vasodilator (antianginal) | angina pectoris |
| Kariva (desogestrel/ethinyl estradiol) | oral contraceptive | birth control |
| Klor-Con (potassium chloride) | potassium salt, electrolyte supplement | potassium deficiency |
| Lanoxin (digoxin) | cardiac glycoside | congestive heart failure (CHF), cardiac tachyarrhythmias |
| Lantus (insulin glargine) | insulin, antidiabetic | type 1 and 2 diabetes mellitus |
| Lescol XL (fluvastatin) | HMG-CoA reductase inhibitor (statin) | hyperlipidemia, hypercholesterolemia |
| Levaquin (levofloxacin) | fluoroquinolone (antibiotic) | bacterial infections |
| Levothroid (levothyroxine) | thyroid hormone | hypothyroidism |
| Levoxyl (levothyroxine sodium) | thyroid hormone | hypothyroidism |
| Lexapro (escitalopram) | selective serotonin reuptake inhibitor (SSRI) (antidepressant) | depression |
| Lipitor (atorvastatin) | HMG-CoA reductase inhibitor (statin) | hyperlipidemia, hypercholesterolemia |
| lisinopril | angiotensin-converting enzyme (ACE) inhibitor | hypertension |
| lorazepam | benzodiazepine (sedative/hypnotic, anticonvulsant, anxiolytic) | anxiety, preoperative sedation, epilepsy, seizures |
| Lotensin (benazepril) | angiotensin-converting enzyme (ACE) inhibitor | hypertension |
| Lotrel (amlodipine/benazepril) | calcium channel blocker and angiotensin-converting enzyme (ACE) inhibitor combination | hypertension |

| Low-Ogestrel (norgestrel/ethinyl estradiol) | oral contraceptive | birth control |
|---|---|---|
| Macrobid (nitrofurantoin) | antibiotic | bacterial infections of urinary tract |
| meclizine | anticholinergic | motion sickness, vertigo |
| metformin | oral antidiabetic | type 2 diabetes mellitus |
| methylprednisolone | glucocorticoid (anti-inflammatory, immunosuppressant) | inflammation, immunological disorders, allergies |
| metoprolol | cardioselective β blocker (β$_1$-adrenergic antagonist) | hypertension, angina pectoris |
| Miacalcin (calcitonin) | hormone | osteoporosis, Paget disease |
| Microgestin Fe (norethindrone ethinyl estradiol) | oral contraceptive | birth control |
| MiraLax (polyethylene glycol) | laxative | constipation |
| Mobic (meloxicam) | nonsteroidal anti-inflammatory drug (NSAID) | osteoarthritis |
| Monopril (fosinopril) | angiotensin-converting enzyme (ACE) inhibitor | hypertension |
| naproxen | analgesic, nonsteroidal anti-inflammatory drug (NSAID) | pain, fever, arthritis |
| Nasacort (triamcinolone) AQ topical nasal spray | glucocorticoid (anti-inflammatory, immunosuppressant) | allergic rhinitis |
| Nasonex (mometasone) topical nasal spray | glucocorticoid (anti-inflammatory, immunosuppressant) | allergic rhinitis |
| Necon (ethinyl estradiol/norethindrone) | oral contraceptive | birth control |
| Neurontin (gabapentin) | anticonvulsant | postherpetic neuralgia, epilepsy (partial seizures) |
| Nexium (esomeprazole) | proton pump inhibitor (PPI) (gastric acid secretion inhibitor) | peptic ulcer disease (PUD), gastroesophageal reflux disease (GERD) |
| Niaspan (niacin) | vitamin | dyslipidemia |
| nifedipine | calcium channel blocker | hypertension, angina pectoris |
| NitroQuick (nitroglycerin) | antianginal | coronary vasodilator |
| Norvasc (amlodipine) | calcium channel blocker | hypertension, angina pectoris |
| omeprazole | proton pump inhibitor (PPI) (gastric acid secretion inhibitor) | peptic ulcer disease (PUD), gastroesophageal reflux disease (GERD) |
| Omnicef (cefdinir) | cephalosporin (antibiotic) | bacterial infections |
| Ortho Evra (norelgestromin/ethinyl estradiol) | contraceptive patch | birth control |
| Ortho Novum (norethindrone/ethyl estradiol) | oral contraceptive | birth control |
| Ortho Tri-Cyclen (norgestimate/ethyl estradiol) | oral contraceptive | birth control |
| oxycodone and acetaminophen | opiate (narcotic) and nonsteroidal anti-inflammatory drug (NSAID) (analgesic/antipyretic) combination | moderate to severe pain |

| | | |
|---|---|---|
| OxyContin (oxycodone) | opiate (narcotic) analgesic | moderate to severe pain |
| Patanol (olopatadine) | ophthalmic antihistamine | allergic conjunctivitis |
| Paxil (paroxetine) | selective serotonin reuptake inhibitor (SSRI) (antidepressant) | depression |
| Penicillin VK (penicillin V potassium) | penicillin (antibiotic) | bacterial infections |
| Percocet (oxycodone and acetaminophen) | opiate (narcotic) and nonsteroidal anti-inflammatory drug (NSAID) (analgesic/antipyretic) combination | moderate to severe pain |
| phenobarbital | barbiturate (sedative/hypnotic, anticonvulsant, anxiolytic) | insomnia, epilepsy, seizures, anxiety |
| phenytoin | hydantoin (anticonvulsant) | epilepsy, seizures |
| Plavix (clopidogrel) | antiplatelet agent | reduction in stroke or myocardial infarction risk by excessive clot prevention |
| Plendil (felodipine) | calcium channel blocker | hypertension, angina pectoris |
| potassium chloride | potassium salt, electrolyte supplement | potassium deficiency |
| Pravachol (pravastatin) | HMG-CoA reductase inhibitor (statin) | hyperlipidemia, hypercholesterolemia |
| prednisone | glucocorticoid (anti-inflammatory, immunosuppressant) | inflammation, immunologic disorders, allergy |
| Premarin (conjugated estrogens) | estrogen derivative | hormone replacement |
| Prempro (estrogen/medroxyprogesterone) | estrogen/progestin | hormone replacement |
| Prevacid (lansoprazole) | proton pump inhibitor (PPI) (gastric acid secretion inhibitor) | peptic ulcer disease (PUD), gastroesophageal reflux disease (GERD) |
| Prilosec (omeprazole) | proton pump inhibitor (PPI) (gastric acid secretion inhibitor) | peptic ulcer disease (PUD), gastroesophageal reflux disease (GERD) |
| promethazine | antihistamine, sedative, antiemetic | allergy, motion sickness, nausea |
| promethazine and codeine | antihistamine and opiate (narcotic) antitussive combination | cold and cough |
| propoxyphene and acetaminophen | opiate (narcotic) analgesic and nonsteroidal anti-inflammatory drug (NSAID) (analgesic/antipyretic) combination | mild to moderate pain |
| propranolol | β blocker (antihypertensive, antiarrhythmic, antianginal) | hypertension, angina pectoris, cardiac arrhythmias, migraine headache prophylaxis |
| Proscar (finasteride) | 5α-reductase inhibitor | benign prostatic hyperplasia (BPH) |
| Protonix (pantoprazole) | proton pump inhibitor (PPI) (gastric acid secretion inhibitor) | peptic ulcer disease (PUD), gastroesophageal reflux disease (GERD) |

| Pulmicort (budesonide) inhalant | glucocorticoid (anti-inflammatory, immunosuppressant) | asthma |
| --- | --- | --- |
| ranitidine hydrochloride | H2 receptor antagonist | peptic ulcer disease (PUD), gastroesophageal reflux disease (GERD) |
| Remeron (mirtazapine) | atypical antidepressant | depression |
| Rhinocort Aqua (budesonide) nasal spray | glucocorticoid (anti-inflammatory, immunosuppressant) | allergic rhinitis |
| Risperdal (risperidone) | atypical antipsychotic (neuroleptic) | psychoses (e.g., schizophrenia) |
| Roxicet (oxycodone and acetaminophen) | opiate (narcotic) and nonsteroidal anti-inflammatory drug (NSAID) (analgesic/antipyretic) combination | moderate to severe pain |
| Seroquel (quetiapine) | atypical antipsychotic (neuroleptic) | psychoses (e.g., schizophrenia) |
| Singulair (montelukast) | leukotriene receptor antagonist | asthma |
| Skelaxin (metaxalone) | skeletal muscle relaxant | skeletal muscle spasms and spasticity |
| spironolactone | potassium-sparing diuretic | hypertension, edema |
| Strattera (atomoxetine) | selective norepinephrine reuptake inhibitor (SNRI) | attention-deficit hyperactivity disorder (ADHD) |
| Synthroid (levothyroxine) | thyroid product | hypothyroidism |
| temazepam | benzodiazepine (hypnotic) | insomnia |
| terazosin | $\alpha_1$-adrenergic antagonist (antihypertensive, vasodilator) | hypertension, benign prostatic hypertrophy (BHD) |
| timolol | $\beta$ blocker (antihypertensive, antiarrhythmic, antianginal) | hypertension, angina pectoris, cardiac arrhythmias, glaucoma (ophthalmic solution) |
| TobraDex (tobramycin and dexamethasone) ophthalmic solution | antibiotic and corticosteroid combination | external ocular bacterial infections |
| Topamax (topiramate) | anticonvulsant | epilepsy (partial seizures) |
| Toprol-XL (metoprolol) | cardioselective $\beta$ blocker ($\beta_1$-adrenergic antagonist) | hypertension, angina pectoris, congestive heart failure (CHF) |
| trazodone | atypical antidepressant | depression |
| triamcinolone | glucocorticoid (anti-inflammatory, immunosuppressant) | inflammation, immunologic disorders, allergy |
| triamterene and hydrochlorothiazide (HCTZ) | diuretic combination | hypertension, edema in congestive heart failure (CHF) |
| Tricor (fenofibrate) | fibric acid derivative | hyperlipidemia, hypertriglyceridemia, hypercholesterolemia |
| trimethoprim/sulfamethoxazole (TMP-SMX or co-trimoxazole) | antibacterial and sulfonamide (antibiotic) combination | bacterial infections |
| Trimox (amoxicillin) | penicillin (antibiotic) | bacterial infections |
| Trivora-28 (levonorgestrel/ethinyl estradiol) | oral contraceptive | birth control |
| Tussionex (hydrocodone and chlorpheniramine) | narcotic antitussive and antihistamine combination | cough and cold |

| Ultracet (tramadol/acetaminophen) | opioid analgesic and nonsteroidal anti-inflammatory drug (NSAID) (analgesic/antipyretic) combination | pain |
|---|---|---|
| Valtrex (valacyclovir) | antiviral | herpes viruses |
| verapamil | calcium channel blocker | hypertension, cardiac arrhythmias, angina pectoris |
| Viagra (sildenafil) | phosphodiesterase (type 5) enzyme inhibitor | erectile dysfunction (ED) |
| Vioxx (rofecoxib) | cox-2 inhibitor (nonsteroidal anti-inflammatory drug [NSAID]) | pain, inflammation, fever, arthritis |
| warfarin | anticoagulant | thromboembolic disorders |
| Wellbutrin SR (bupropion) | atypical antidepressant | depression |
| Xalatan (latanoprost) ophthalmic solution | prostaglandin | glaucoma |
| Yasmin 28 (drospirenone/ethinyl estradiol) | oral contraceptive | birth control |
| Zetia (ezetimibe) | cholesterol absorption inhibitor | hypercholesterolemia |
| Zithromax (azithromycin dihydrate) | macrolide (antibiotic) | bacterial infections |
| Zocor (simvastatin) | HMG-CoA reductase inhibitor (statin) | hyperlipidemia, hypercholesterolemia |
| Zoloft (sertraline) | selective serotonin reuptake inhibitor (SSRI) (antidepressant) | depression |
| Zyprexa (olanzapine) | atypical antipsychotic (neuroleptic) | psychoses (e.g., schizophrenia) |
| Zyrtec (cetirizine) | antihistamine | allergy |

## REFERENCES

Appendix: Commonly prescribed drugs and their applications. In: Stedman TL. *Stedman's Medical Dictionary for the Health Professions and Nursing.* 5th ed. Lippincott Williams & Wilkins; 2005.

*Quick Look Drug Book.* Hudson, OH: Lexi-Comp; Baltimore, MD: Lippincott Williams & Wilkins; 2004.

The top 200 prescriptions for 2003 by number of US prescriptions dispensed. RxList: The internet drug index. Available at: www.rxlist.com/top200.htm

# Index